Acclaim for

"Rebecca Fett's stellar constellation of perspective, experience, knowledge, and scientific background may well revolutionize our current global conversation, understanding, and practices related to fertility... It is hard to overestimate the impact that this book may have on the lives of many."

— DR. CLAUDIA WELCH, AUTHOR OF *BALANCE YOUR HORMONES, BALANCE YOUR LIFE*

"With detailed, up-to-date research, Rebecca Fett provides a clear, cool-headed guide to both the science that determines IVF success and the practical changes that patients can make to drastically increase their chances of IVF success."

— DR. LINDSAY WU, LABORATORY FOR AGEING RESEARCH, UNIVERSITY OF NEW SOUTH WALES MEDICAL CENTER, AUSTRALIA

"This is a very useful resource: well-researched, accessibly written, and with easy-to-follow take-home messages and action plans. I would recommend this to any woman who is trying to conceive."

— DR. CLAIRE DEAKIN, UNIVERSITY COLLEGE LONDON, INSTITUTE OF CHILD HEALTH

"A thoroughly researched and eye-opening account of how small, simple lifestyle changes can have powerful, positive effects on your health and fertility. A must-read for women wanting the best chance of conceiving a healthy baby."

— BETH GREER, BESTSELLING AUTHOR OF *SUPER NATURAL HOME*

"*It Starts with the Egg* presents a reasoned and balanced review of the latest science linking environmental chemicals to reduced fertility and other health problems. Readers will find sound advice for how to avoid chemicals of concern, providing a useful guide for couples that want to improve their chances of a healthy pregnancy."

— DR. LAURA VANDENBERG, UNIVERSITY OF MASSACHUSETTS AMHERST SCHOOL OF PUBLIC HEALTH

"This timely synthesis of scientific literature is essential reading for both women and men wanting practical, evidence-based recommendations to enhance their fertility."

— DR. LORETTA MCKINNON, EPIDEMIOLOGIST,
PRINCESS ALEXANDRA HOSPITAL

"With *It Starts with the Egg*, Rebecca Fett delivers a much-needed overview on the available scientific evidence regarding the influence of nutrition on fertility and fertility treatment, providing a valuable resource for couples trying to conceive."

— DR. JOHN TWIGT, DEPARTMENT OF OBSTETRICS AND GYNECOLOGY,
ERASMUS MEDICAL CENTER, NETHERLANDS

"Rebecca has done a great service for all women, children, and future generations by starting at the beginning of a human life and examining which toxic chemicals cause harm to the egg... This book is a wonderful addition to the growing library of information on toxic exposures."

— DEBRA LYNN DADD, AUTHOR OF *TOXIC FREE: HOW TO PROTECT
YOUR HEALTH AND HOME FROM THE CHEMICALS THAT ARE MAKING
YOU SICK*

"Rebecca Fett did a stellar job of researching and summarizing the current understanding of the impact of egg quality on IVF pregnancy chances."

— DR. NORBERT GLEICHER, REPRODUCTIVE ENDOCRINOLOGIST,
THE CENTER FOR HUMAN REPRODUCTION, NEW YORK

"Rebecca Fett's *It Starts with the Egg* is a complete guide to everything a woman can do to improve her egg quality before trying to conceive... *It Starts with the Egg* also breaks information down in easy-to-digest bullet points that show exactly what to do to get to where you want to be: the parent of a happy, healthy, gorgeous baby."

— CHERYL ALKON, AUTHOR OF *BALANCING PREGNANCY WITH
PRE-EXISTING DIABETES: HEALTHY MOM, HEALTHY BABY*

The Science of **Egg Quality** for
Fertility, Miscarriage, and **IVF**

Third Edition

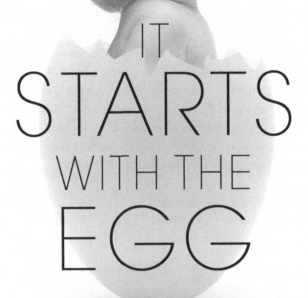

IT
STARTS
WITH THE
EGG

REBECCA FETT

FRANKLIN
FOX

FRANKLIN FOX PUBLISHING

First edition: © 2014 by Rebecca Fett
Second edition: © 2019 by Rebecca Fett
Third edition: © 2023 by Rebecca Fett

Published in the United States by Franklin Fox Publishing LLC, New York
Interior/cover design: Steven Plummer / SPDesign

ISBN-13 (print): 979-8-9886751-0-5
ISBN-13 (ebook): 979-8-9886751-1-2

www.itstartswiththeegg.com

Contents

Introduction

WHETHER YOU ARE just starting to think about having a baby, find yourself on the long road of fertility treatments and failed IVF cycles, or have suffered multiple miscarriages, it is critically important to provide your eggs with the specific nutrients needed to support embryo development and avoid the toxins that cause the most harm. This book will explain the simple things you can do to have the best possible chance of getting pregnant and bringing home a healthy baby. And it starts with the egg.

The conventional thinking is that women are born with all the eggs they will ever have and that the quality of those eggs declines drastically with age. But this is not the whole story. Most of our lives, our eggs are in a state of suspended animation as immature cells, but in the three to four months before ovulation, an egg must undergo a major transformation. It grows dramatically in size and starts producing much more energy. The egg must then execute a precise process of separating and ejecting copies of chromosomes. If this process goes wrong, and it often does, the egg will have chromosomal abnormalities. These chromosomal abnormalities are the single most important cause of early miscarriages and failed IVF cycles, as well as the reason it takes older women so much longer to conceive.

Many women are told there is little they can do to improve egg quality, but the latest research defies that old assumption. The four-month growth phase before ovulation is a critical time during which many things can happen that affect the quality of the egg, both positively and negatively. These include harmful effects from exposure to toxins such as BPA and phthalates, as well as protective effects from antioxidants, hormones, and other nutrients. As a result, there is a brief window of opportunity in which you can make a difference in your egg quality.

This book will be your guide to specific strategies that are supported by strong scientific research. Importantly, the advice in this book is not based on isolated animal studies that provide enticing hints as to the causes of and solutions for poor egg quality. Individual studies, and particularly animal or test-tube studies, provide only limited evidence and must be taken with a grain of salt. Instead, this book is based on a comprehensive analysis of a large body of medical research involving studies that have been confirmed by multiple groups and that involve real patients.

If you are currently being treated by a fertility specialist, you may have already received advice about supplements that can improve egg quality. The advice of some doctors will be more up-to-date and supported by scientific research than that of others. My goal in writing this book is to provide a tool for thoroughly understanding what helps and why, so you can make your own informed decisions and tailor your supplement plan to your own unique situation.

But first, the story of how I became obsessed with the science of egg quality.

My Story

My mission started with the same fears and anxieties faced by many women struggling with infertility. I was about to begin an IVF cycle and could not help worrying that the massive financial and physical toll could all be for nothing.

In any IVF cycle, there are so many opportunities for things to go wrong and so much at stake. In our IVF cycle, there was also another person counting on me to produce enough eggs: our gestational surrogate. If this cycle failed, not only would I have to repeat all the injections and doctors' appointments, but so would she.

I had started the process with so much confidence, thinking that because I was under 30, conceiving through IVF would be easy. But then the unexpected happened. I was diagnosed with diminished ovarian reserve and told by our fertility specialist that the most aggressive drug protocol would be required to help us conceive. If they were able to retrieve only a few eggs, our chance of having an embryo to transfer was not good. I asked our fertility specialist if there was anything I could do to improve our chances, but there were no clear answers. So, I put my training in molecular biology and biochemistry to work. I embarked on a mission to find out for myself what the scientific research showed.

In the process of earning my molecular biology degree, I had studied mechanisms of DNA damage and repair, the detailed process of energy production inside cells, and how both processes relate to antioxidants. I had also studied the complex system in which chromosomes in an egg are recombined and then mechanically separated before and after fertilization. As I delved deeper into the scientific papers addressing egg quality, all the pieces I had learned about years earlier started to fit together with groundbreaking recent studies to form a picture of the various causes of chromosomal abnormalities in eggs and the influence of external factors. In short, the research revealed a quiet revolution in the way we think about egg quality.

I started putting into practice everything I had learned. I improved my diet by cutting out refined carbohydrates (to lower insulin, which is shown to impact egg quality), started taking a small handful of daily supplements, and took extra steps to limit my exposure to household toxins, such as replacing plastic with glass and buying fragrance-free cleaning products.

I also decided to take the hormone DHEA, which, as I will explain later in this book, has now been shown in numerous clinical trials to improve the chance of success for those with diminished ovarian reserve and specific hormone deficiencies. Many years later, I learned that this was likely one of the most important decisions I made because it later became clear that autoimmune disease was compromising my hormone production and ovarian function; DHEA is helpful on both fronts.

During those months, I started thinking of myself as

"pre-pregnant" and protected my eggs the way I would protect a growing baby if I was pregnant. I found it reassuring that even if this particular IVF cycle failed, I could at least take comfort in the knowledge that I had done absolutely everything I could to make healthy embryos.

That said, I was not expecting any miracles. I still suspected that with a diminished reserve of eggs, I had an uphill battle. I had seen the statistics showing IVF success rates in relation to ovarian reserve, and they were not grounds for optimism.

A couple of months after beginning my quest for egg quality, I went back to the fertility clinic for a routine check of my ovaries before starting stimulation medication for IVF. I was shocked to witness how much had changed. Instead of a couple of follicles in each ovary, the ultrasound showed that I probably had about 20 eggs maturing. This number was perfectly normal, and our odds had suddenly become a lot better.

Nevertheless, I remained nervous. The weeks passed, and each day became a routine of injections, pills, ultrasounds, and blood tests. The tests gave us every reason to expect a good outcome, but as our doctor explained, there are never any guarantees in an IVF cycle because so much can go wrong. Every morning and evening when I took out my boxes of syringes, needles, and vials of expensive fertility drugs, preparing to give myself several injections, I felt the anxiety that is so familiar to anyone going through IVF.

The next stages went better than anyone could have expected. On the day of the egg retrieval, I woke up after the procedure to discover that 22 eggs had been retrieved, and all were mature. Even through the haze of the anesthetic, this news brought huge relief. I tried not to get too excited, knowing there were still quite a few hurdles to go, but suddenly we were faced with the very real prospect that this cycle could actually work.

Five days later, we received more good news. Of the 19 eggs that had fertilized, every single one had survived to become a good-quality blastocyst. This result was simply unheard of.

We transferred a single embryo and two weeks later were elated to find out that our surrogate was pregnant. It is impossible to know if the same result would have happened without my mission to improve my egg quality and ovarian function, but the scientific research shows that egg quality is the single most important factor in determining whether an egg will fertilize and survive to the blastocyst stage. It also determines whether an embryo is capable of implanting and leading to a viable pregnancy.

I knew the scientific research I had uncovered could benefit thousands of other women facing similar struggles. I found myself wanting to delve even deeper into this research in order to develop a comprehensive plan others could follow. It is one thing to make a determination for myself on whether the research shows that a particular supplement is safe and worthwhile, but if I was going to share my knowledge with other women who were trying to get pregnant or who had suffered multiple miscarriages, I had a much greater responsibility to investigate the issue from every angle. And so I began an even more exhaustive search and analysis of the latest research relating to egg quality.

I carefully analyzed hundreds of scientific papers investigating specific effects of toxins and nutrients on biological processes, identifying influences on fertility and miscarriage rates in large, population-based studies, and uncovering the factors that influence success rates in IVF. (You can find these scientific papers listed in the references section, along with information on how to access them online.) This comprehensive research was an undertaking most fertility specialists are simply too busy to do, and, unsurprisingly, many doctors are not up-to-date on recent findings.

I quickly learned that the standard advice of IVF clinics and fertility books was not keeping pace with research. At that time, in 2013, no one was talking about the new research showing that BPA has a significant negative effect on fertility. Even CoQ10 was considered controversial, and clinics were simply not telling their patients about it.

Even now, these and other issues are often overlooked, and many doctors simply do not have time to keep up with every relevant area of research. As just one example, numerous studies have now reported that for the purpose of preventing miscarriage and pregnancy complications, the optimal vitamin D level is much higher than previously thought. Yet many doctors still follow old guidelines for vitamin D levels that are woefully inadequate.

This is not to suggest that all fertility doctors are neglecting the issue of egg quality. Many have started recommending the supplements I outline in this book, but they may only share these recommendations with patients a month or two before treatment begins, which misses the key early stages of egg development. And clinics generally do not explain the fascinating story of how each supplement is thought to work, or refine their recommendations on the basis of individual factors or the latest scientific studies.

Many women are aware that they may not be getting the most up-to-date advice about which supplements can improve their chances, and so they turn to the internet for information. This path often leads them to supplements that are not supported by any scientific research or that may actually be harmful for egg quality or pregnancy. This book not only discusses the measures that may help but also debunks myths about some supplements that may do more harm than good, and explains how to determine which supplements are right for your situation.

The supplement DHEA provides an example of why personalization is so important. This supplement is only likely to help if lab testing shows your level is low, but whether or not you will be advised to take DHEA depends more on whether you are preparing for IVF and which clinic you happen to be attending than on any logical basis. Many clinics also leave the decision of whether to take DHEA up to the individual patient, without performing any testing or providing any detailed information about the strength of the clinical evidence. We deserve better and have a right to make truly informed decisions.

Seeing the immense gap between the research and conventional fertility advice, I felt compelled to help by distilling the clinical research into concrete, comprehensible information. As I became more convinced of the impact of external factors on egg quality and the importance of egg quality to the chance of conceiving, whether naturally or through IVF, I felt an urgent need to help educate other women struggling with infertility. And so this book was born.

Over the past ten years, I have continued to follow the science of egg quality and fertility, always asking what the evidence shows and what else can make a difference, to ensure that this book is a complete and up-to-date guide.

Seeing our growing baby on the 12-week ultrasound and hearing his heartbeat for the first time were moments of such pure joy that I desperately want the same for everyone going through the process of fertility treatment or planning to have a baby.

In the world of infertility there is always uncertainty, with many variables and unique challenges. My results are unusual and likely due in part to my age, since I was in my twenties. Not everyone will end up with a large number of eggs or all of their eggs becoming good-quality embryos, but that is not the outcome that matters. What matters is shifting the odds—doing what you can to optimize the quality of the eggs you have and giving every egg the best possible chance of leading to a healthy pregnancy.

How to Use This Book

This book is structured as a path for you to follow, with detours and additional areas to explore based on the unique challenges you may be facing. The first few steps along the path are similar for everyone, with the chapters that make up part 1.

Part 1 begins with understanding exactly what egg quality means and why it is so critical. In chapter 2, you will learn how common toxins can impact fertility and the practical steps that make the most difference. Chapter 3 will introduce you to preliminary lab testing that can help you uncover potential obstacles to fertility and a healthy pregnancy, and chapter 4 explains the hormone lab tests that will later help you identify which supplements will be most helpful. From there, you will be ready to start building your supplement plan.

Navigating the supplement chapters

If you are just starting out

If you have just begun trying to get pregnant and have no reason to expect fertility challenges, you are unlikely to need an extensive supplements regime. By following the supplement recommendations in the *basic plan* (covered in chapters 5 and 6, and summarized in chapter 11), you may be able to increase the proportion of healthy eggs, which can help you get pregnant faster and reduce the risk of miscarriage.

If you are freezing your eggs

Even if you have no fertility issues, you will likely get a better result from egg retrieval if you prepare with a supplement regime to support egg quality. The *intermediate plan* for egg freezing includes the core supplements in chapters 5 and 6, along with one or more antioxidants, as discussed in chapter 7. See chapter 11 for a summary of the egg-freezing supplement recommendations.

If you are having difficulty conceiving

Poor egg quality is the common factor that unites many different infertility diagnoses, including age-related infertility, PCOS, endometriosis, and unexplained infertility. We need to address egg quality in different ways in these different situations, but they share the common feature that fertility can be significantly improved by addressing energy production and oxidative damage in developing eggs. For that reason, we start with the core supplements in chapters 5 and 6, and then add specific antioxidants discussed in chapter 7. From there, the path depends on your lab tests and specific concerns.

If you have a pattern of hormonal imbalance reminiscent of PCOS, such as high testosterone, high AMH, insulin resistance, or long or irregular cycles, you will continue with chapter 8 on myo-inositol and likely follow the *intermediate plan* for PCOS.

On the other hand, if you have low AMH, chapter 9 on DHEA may be more relevant to you. Chapter 10 then explains some supplements to avoid, and complete supplement plans are summarized in chapter 11.

If you are over 40 or trying to conceive through IVF

If you have been battling infertility for a substantial length of time, are in your late thirties or early forties, or you are trying to conceive through IVF, you have the most to gain from a systematic plan for improving egg quality.

As the next chapter explains, poor egg quality is often the culprit in women with unexplained and age-related infertility, and also in those who have had unsuccessful IVF cycles. Research shows that only good-quality eggs are likely to become good-quality embryos that can survive the critical first week and successfully implant to result in a pregnancy. It is therefore critical to maximize the number of good-quality eggs that have the potential to become a healthy baby.

This requires a comprehensive approach that includes minimizing toxin exposure and adopting the eating habits shown to boost IVF success rates, along with taking the supplements listed in the *advanced plan*. These supplements are intended to help those with age-related infertility, endometriosis, diminished ovarian reserve, or the catch-all diagnosis of unexplained infertility. The precise supplements most helpful for each situation are discussed in chapters 6 through 10, with chapter 11 providing examples of overall supplement plans. The lab testing discussed in chapter 4 will also help guide you as to which supplements may be most useful for you.

If lab tests show you have a pattern of hormonal imbalance reminiscent of PCOS, such as high testosterone, high AMH, insulin resistance, long or irregular cycles, or many immature eggs in IVF, myo-inositol is likely to be helpful, as discussed in chapter 8. If you have low AMH, age-related infertility, short cycles, or very few eggs retrieved in IVF, it is important to read chapter 9, which covers DHEA. Chapter 10 then explains some supplements to avoid or use with caution, and chapter 14 will help you prepare for a frozen embryo transfer.

If you have extremely low ovarian reserve and want to explore additional supplements and advanced treatments, you will find an explanation of these options in chapter 16.

If you are facing recurrent miscarriage

There are many potential causes of early miscarriage, but egg quality is a major factor. That is because an embryo with DNA damage or an incorrect number of chromosomes may implant and lead to a pregnancy, but with very little chance of surviving beyond the first trimester. Chromosomal abnormalities are thought to account for up to 40–50% of early miscarriages.[1] As the next chapter explains, these chromosomal abnormalities often originate in the egg and become even more frequent with maternal age.[2]

In this book, you will learn how chromosomal abnormalities often occur during the last phase of egg maturation before ovulation and what you can do to reduce the likelihood of your next pregnancy being affected. Research has also established that sperm quality can be a major contributor to miscarriage, likely by raising the risk of chromosomal abnormalities.

If you have had two or more miscarriages and your doctor cannot find a medical cause, or you know that chromosomal abnormalities affected a previous pregnancy, consider following the *advanced plan* for at least three months before trying to conceive again. This starts with the common supplements in chapters 5 through 7.

From there, the supplements differ depending on your hormone levels. If you have insulin resistance or many immature eggs in IVF, myo-inositol is likely to be helpful, as discussed in chapter 8. If you have low AMH or age-related infertility, chapter 9 on DHEA may be helpful. See chapter 10 for a discussion of supplements to avoid and chapter 11 for a summary of the supplement recommendations for this plan.

For everyone: the path beyond supplements

Once you have your supplement plan in place, the different pathways rejoin and you will be back on the common track applicable to everyone. The next step on this path is learning how to rebalance hormones and support egg quality through nutrition, with a particular focus on balancing blood sugar and insulin, increasing nutrient density, and reducing inflammation. That is the focus of chapter 12.

From there we move on to sperm quality in chapter 13. Although this chapter is especially important if testing shows any abnormality in male fertility, or if you are preparing for IVF, it is something all couples should pay attention to for the best possible chance of getting pregnant and reducing the risk of miscarriage. It is just as important for men to take preconception supplements, eat well, and avoid toxins as it is for women—a topic that has long been neglected.

At this point, you will have completed the key steps necessary to optimize egg quality, hormone balance, and sperm quality. For many, that will be enough, and by the end of chapter 14 on male fertility you will be able to set the book down and focus on implementing what you have learned. But for others, more help is needed. The remaining chapters of the book, new in the third edition, explain some of the more advanced testing and treatment strategies that go beyond egg and sperm quality to address other potential factors that can contribute to infertility and pregnancy loss.

Immune & implantation factors

Even with good egg and sperm quality, some couples continue to struggle with unexplained infertility, failed embryo transfers, or recurrent miscarriage. When the cause is not chromosomal errors or embryo quality, what remains is a collection of potential factors relating to the immune system, hormones, blood clotting, and the uterus. This includes endometriosis, silent infections, autoimmunity, and scar tissue in the uterine lining.

If you have unexplained infertility, failed embryo transfers, recurrent miscarriage, a history of autoimmune disease or infections, or an extremely limited number of embryos available and want to ensure that all your bases are covered, you will find information on advanced testing and treatment options for immune and implantation factors in chapter 15.

Possible ovarian reserve boosters

Chapter 16 covers some additional strategies to consider for those with very low ovarian reserve or age-related infertility. These are somewhat experimental and controversial treatments, such as the ketogenic diet, platelet-rich plasma, red light therapy, and additional supplements. Some of these strategies are not yet supported by clear evidence, but they are discussed so you are aware of the options available and can make informed decisions.

Getting started

By the end of this book, you will have a clear strategy in place to optimize hormone balance, egg quality, sperm quality, and embryo implantation. You will be armed with the knowledge to advocate for yourself and take back some control in this difficult process, and you will be in the best possible position to improve your egg quality and have a healthy pregnancy.

The first step is understanding what egg quality means and how chromosomal abnormalities occur, so you can appreciate why all the strategies you will put into action are so important. That is the focus of chapter 1.

PART 1

PUTTING THE SCIENCE INTO ACTION

Chapter 1

Understanding Egg Quality

"When you know better you do better."
— MAYA ANGELOU

THE DECLINE IN fertility as we age is almost entirely due to a decline in egg quality. We know this because older women who use donor eggs have pregnancy rates similar to younger women. But what does egg quality mean? Broadly, it describes the potential of an egg to become a viable pregnancy after fertilization. And this is no trivial matter—the vast majority of eggs simply do not have what it takes.

Egg Quality Is Essential to Fertility

For any embryo, the first few weeks after fertilization represent a major hurdle, and many embryos stop developing at some point during this time. In fact, most naturally conceived embryos are lost before a woman even knows she is pregnant.[1] Only about a third of fertilized embryos survive to become a baby.[2] The odds may be even worse in the IVF context, where many fertilized eggs are unable to progress to the day-5 embryo stage (known as the blastocyst stage). Even many embryos that do make it this far and are transferred to the uterus often do not successfully implant, resulting in a failed IVF cycle.

The fact that most fertilized eggs never become a successful pregnancy is an issue that receives very little attention because of the common misconception that getting an egg fertilized is the real challenge in conceiving. Most natural fertility advice therefore focuses on ovulation and timing to achieve fertilization. This approach misses the mark because the potential of a fertilized egg to continue developing is often a much bigger issue. In reality, egg quality plays a critical role in how long it takes to become pregnant, whether naturally or through IVF, and the secret is in the egg's DNA.

Although an embryo's potential to develop into a pregnancy depends on many factors, by far the most important is having the correct number of copies of each chromosome. Chromosomal abnormalities in eggs have a profound impact on fertility because at every stage of development from fertilization onward, an embryo formed from a chromosomally abnormal egg has much less potential to continue developing.[3] This may manifest as an inability to get pregnant or as early miscarriage. For many women, chromosomal abnormalities in eggs become the greatest obstacle to conceiving and carrying to term.

It comes as no surprise that poor egg quality is significantly more common in women who have had a difficult time conceiving. High rates of chromosomal abnormalities are seen in eggs of women who have a history of multiple miscarriages, women who have had repeated IVF cycles in which embryos were transferred but no pregnancy occurred (so-called "repeated implantation failure"), and women with polycystic ovary syndrome. For example, the proportion of abnormal embryos in women with a history of repeated implantation failures in IVF cycles can be up to 70%.[4]

Chromosomal errors in eggs not only impact the ability to get pregnant but are also a major cause of miscarriage. Miscarriages are unfortunately very common, occurring in about 10–15 % of recognized pregnancies.[5] However, most pregnancy losses are not even noticed because they happen so early—before the woman knows she is pregnant. When such pregnancies are taken into account, up to 70% end in miscarriage.[6] Part of the reason for this incredibly high rate is that from the moment of conception, a continuous process of selection against chromosomally abnormal embryos is taking place.

In fact, *chromosomal abnormalities cause more miscarriages than every other known cause of miscarriage combined.* In one study in women with a history of two or more miscarriages, researchers found that 41% of miscarriages were caused by a chromosomal abnormality, whereas all the other known causes of miscarriage together accounted for less than 30% of cases.[7] Other studies have found that more than half of all first-trimester miscarriages are caused by chromosomal abnormalities.[8]

It is also important to note that these studies were investigating miscarriages from *recognized* pregnancies. When we include all the losses that occur in the short time after fertilization, the rate of chromosomal abnormalities is likely to be much higher.[9]

A common reaction to this information is to assume that chromosomal errors in eggs are beyond our control, but recent scientific research shows that is not true. The proportion of eggs with chromosomal abnormalities can be influenced by nutrients, hormones, and lifestyle factors you can control, as you'll learn throughout this book.

The best-known example of a chromosomal abnormality originating in the egg is Down syndrome, which becomes much more common as women age and egg quality declines. Down syndrome is almost always caused by the egg providing an extra copy of chromosome 21, which results in the fetus having three copies instead of the usual two.[10]

Down syndrome is just one example of a chromosomal abnormality, but it is perhaps the best known because it is one of the few compatible with life. Some babies with an extra copy of chromosome 13 or 18 can also survive to term, but with serious medical problems. An extra or missing copy of other chromosomes will prevent the embryo developing past the first few days or weeks, or will cause an early miscarriage.[11] This is why we rarely hear about chromosomal errors involving extra copies of these other chromosomes, even though they are very common.

These types of genetic errors explain much of the drop in fertility and increase in miscarriage rates that occurs with age. In women in their early thirties, about 10–25% of eggs are genetically abnormal. This percentage starts increasing exponentially in the mid- to late thirties, and by the time a woman is in her early forties, 50–80% of her eggs may be chromosomally abnormal.[12]

The main lesson from the data is that these errors are incredibly common. Even if you are young and have no specific fertility issues, you will still have many months with little potential to conceive. If the egg that you ovulate in a given month is chromosomally abnormal and unable to support a pregnancy, using ovulation prediction kits and charts to achieve fertilization with perfect timing will not make any difference; you will not be able to conceive a viable pregnancy until the next cycle in which you ovulate a good egg.

In other words, regardless of your age, fertility issues, or whether you are trying to conceive naturally or by IVF, your chance of becoming pregnant and carrying to term is very much determined by your egg quality, and specifically by the proportion of your eggs that are chromosomally normal. Luckily, this is not entirely out of your hands. It is something you have the power to influence.

There is, in fact, an enormous variation in chromosomal abnormality rates between different women of the same age.[13] One study found that some women may have very few chromosomally normal eggs over a given time frame, whereas another woman's eggs may all be normal.[14] The number of normal eggs can also vary widely over time for the same person, with big differences in the proportion of normal eggs between two consecutive IVF cycles. Researchers have described the variation over time and between different women as random and unpredictable, but we know that is not really true.

The fascinating research discussed in the remainder of this

book establishes that this variability is not purely random; on the contrary, a wide range of external factors impact egg quality and the rate of chromosomal abnormalities.

Countless clinical studies have shown that avoiding certain toxins, correcting hormonal imbalances, and adding specific supplements can increase the percentage of eggs that can develop into a good-quality embryo, increase the odds of an embryo implanting, and reduce the risk of early-pregnancy loss. There is strong scientific evidence that these improvements are due in part to a reduction in the proportion of eggs with chromosomal abnormalities. In short, egg quality is something we have the power to change.

How Do Eggs Become "Chromosomally Abnormal"?

The process of egg production is very long and error-prone. By the time an egg is ovulated, it is decades old. Eggs are formed before a woman is even born—stored in a state of suspended animation throughout a woman's life until it is each egg's turn to begin the development process. From the time an egg leaves the stage of being completely dormant until it is ready to be ovulated, it takes almost a year, with most of the development activity taking place in the final four months.

In these last few months, a group of dozens of immature eggs start developing, but most die off naturally. Each cycle, only one lead egg is selected from the pool to finish maturing.[15] The fully grown egg completes ovulation by bursting from its follicle and traveling down the fallopian tube, ready to be fertilized.

During the decades-long interval between when an egg is first formed and ovulation, eggs have many opportunities to accumulate damage as a part of normal aging. The traditional belief is that by the time a woman is 40, her eggs have already accumulated chromosomal abnormalities, and nothing can be done to reverse that damage. But that is not scientifically correct, because most chromosomal errors actually occur shortly before ovulation, in later stages of the development process.

An egg ends up with the incorrect number of chromosomes when meiosis goes awry. Meiosis involves carefully aligning chromosome copies along the middle of the egg, then pulling one set to each end of the egg with a network of microscopic tubules. One set of chromosomes is then pushed out of the egg in what is called a "polar body." A developing egg actually does this twice; it starts out with four copies of each chromosome and, if the process goes correctly, ends up with just one copy of each chromosome.

If this process fails at any stage, the end result is an extra or missing copy of a chromosome. Although the first round of meiosis begins before a girl is born, most of the chromosomal processing activity happens in the months immediately before an egg is ovulated.

The critical point to note—and a point that many doctors are not aware of—is that most of the chromosomal abnormalities in eggs do not accumulate gradually over 30 or 40 years as an egg ages, but instead happen in the couple of months before an egg is ovulated. In other words, aging does not directly cause chromosomal abnormalities; rather, it creates conditions that predispose eggs to mature incorrectly shortly before ovulation.[16]

This means that by changing those conditions before ovulation, you can increase the odds of an egg maturing with the correct number of chromosomes. In short, you may be able to influence the quality of eggs that you ovulate a couple of months from now because chromosomal errors in those eggs have probably not occurred yet.

This leads us to the fundamental issue: How can an egg be predisposed to mature with an incorrect number of chromosomes, and what can you do about it? Every chapter in this book addresses different aspects of that question, but a common theme is the egg's energy supply.

Energy production in the egg

It takes an enormous amount of energy for the egg to process chromosomes correctly. It turns out that the energy-producing structures inside eggs can become damaged with age and in response to certain cellular conditions.[17] These structures, called mitochondria, are found in nearly every cell in the body. They act as miniature power plants to transform various fuel sources into energy that the cell can use in the form of ATP.

ATP is quite literally the energy of life. It moves muscles, makes enzymes work, and powers nerve impulses. Just about every other biological process depends on it. And it is the primary form of energy used by eggs. A growing egg needs a lot of ATP and has a lot of mitochondria. In fact, each egg has more than fifteen thousand mitochondria—over ten times more than any other cell in the body.[18] The follicle cells surrounding the egg also contain many mitochondria and supply the egg with additional ATP.[19] But these mitochondria must be in good condition to make enough energy.

Over time, and in response to oxidative stress (explained in chapter 6), mitochondria become damaged and less able to produce energy.[20] Without sufficient energy, egg and embryo development may go awry or stop altogether.[21] As explained by Dr. Robert Casper, a leading fertility specialist in Toronto, "the aging female reproductive system is like a forgotten flashlight on the top shelf of a closet. When you stumble across it a few years later and try to switch it on, it won't work, not because there's anything wrong with the flashlight but because the batteries inside it have died."[22]

A growing body of evidence suggests that the ability of an egg to produce energy when needed is critically important to being able to mature with the correct number of chromosomes. It is also vital to an embryo's potential to survive the first week and successfully implant.

Poorly functioning mitochondria may be one of the most important reasons some women's eggs are more likely to end up with chromosomal abnormalities or otherwise lack the potential to become a viable embryo. What you can do to help "recharge" your mitochondria and thereby boost your eggs' energy supply is the subject of several chapters later in this book, but first we turn to another contributor to chromosomal errors in developing eggs: environmental toxins.

Chapter 2

Protecting Eggs from Toxins

"Big, sweeping life changes really boil down to small, everyday decisions."

— ALI VINCENT

I F YOU WANT the best possible chance of getting pregnant and having a healthy baby, one of the first steps you should take is reducing your exposure to certain toxins that can harm fertility. There is a lot of confusion and misinformation on this subject, but it is incredibly important to learn about if you are trying to conceive.

The two types of chemicals to pay most attention to are bisphenols and phthalates. Avoiding an unusually high level of exposure to these chemicals can help protect developing eggs and sperm, reduce the risk of miscarriage, and protect your future baby's health.

Ten years after I first shed light on this topic in the first edition of this book, there is now much more awareness of the importance of avoiding these chemicals when trying to conceive. However, many people still find it difficult to know where to start or how careful they need to be. It is common to fall into one of two extremes: either not paying attention to this issue at all because it seems too difficult, or not feeling comfortable that you've done enough and becoming worried about every source of plastic and fragrance.

In this chapter, I want to provide you with the facts so you can take a reasonable middle ground—understanding not only why it is worth making a few changes to avoid very high levels of exposure, but also why we don't have to worry about every single source.

The reality is that BPA and phthalates are all around us, found in foods, plastics, and the whole array of fragranced products, from perfumes to fabric softener to cleaning products. The sheer range of products that can contain bisphenols and phthalates is daunting, but there is no need to replace every product in your home.

The most recent studies suggest that these chemicals may only impact fertility in couples with unusually high levels of exposure. The goal, then, is not a complete lifestyle overhaul, but rather making a few changes that have the most impact. This will not only help protect egg quality and get your body ready for a healthy pregnancy, but will have the added bonus of creating a healthy and nontoxic home for your future baby.

Bisphenols and Fertility

The story of bisphenols and fertility begins with a chance discovery so unexpected that researchers spent years verifying their results before going public. In 1998, Dr. Patricia Hunt and her research group were using mice to study egg development and saw something very unusual: a sudden increase in the number of chromosomally abnormal eggs. In mice, typically only 1–2% of eggs are unable to properly align the chromosomes in the middle of the egg. However, in Dr. Hunt's laboratory, this specific problem abruptly increased and affected 40% of the eggs, along with other severe chromosomal aberrations. When the eggs matured, they were much more likely to have an incorrect number of chromosomes. As Dr. Hunt observed, "I was really horrified because we saw this night and day change."[1]

The researchers began a thorough investigation and eventually found the culprit. BPA, which stands for Bisphenol A, had started leaching out of the mice's plastic cages and water bottles after they were washed with harsh detergent. When all of these damaged plastic cages and bottles were replaced, the percentage of eggs with chromosomal errors began to return to normal. Dr. Hunt's group did not publish this finding for several years because the implications for human fertility were so troubling that they wanted to do further investigation to make sure they were right.[2]

To confirm that BPA was the specific cause of the egg abnormalities, the researchers gave controlled doses of BPA to the mice—and the same thing happened. Through a series of investigations over several years, the group determined that exposure to BPA during the final stages of egg development is enough to cause chromosomal abnormalities. The researchers noted that this had obvious relevance for human fertility because of the extraordinary similarity in chromosome processing between the two species.[3]

Other researchers were inspired to investigate further, and their work revealed further evidence that BPA is not only toxic to developing eggs but can also interfere with the hormones that carefully coordinate the reproductive system.[4]

In the years following Dr. Hunt's accidental experiment showing the effect of BPA on eggs from laboratory mice, subsequent studies indicated a clear impact of BPA on human fertility. In the IVF context, numerous studies from 2008 to 2012 reported that women with higher BPA levels before IVF ended up with fewer eggs retrieved, fewer embryos, and a lower pregnancy rate.[5] At that time, most women trying to conceive were not told about this important research, a problem I felt strongly about correcting when I was writing the first edition of this book in 2013.

The situation has improved dramatically since then. Most people now have a general awareness that BPA is something to avoid, particularly when trying to conceive. In response to consumer demand, many companies have also started phasing out its use. The net effect is that there has been a significant reduction in BPA exposure in recent years, particularly in women trying to conceive through IVF.[6] At the current typical levels of exposure, BPA may not be negatively impacting IVF success rates. It is only unusually high levels of exposure that seem to pose a concern.[7]

Another positive development in the research is that diet and supplements may make a difference in the link between

BPA and fertility. Researchers at the Harvard School of Public Health and the CDC reported that a higher intake of natural folate from food sources appeared to cancel out much of the effect of BPA on IVF outcomes.[8]

Interestingly, the researchers noted that folate from supplements did not have the same protective effect. It could be that supplements were ineffective because most brands at that time contained synthetic folic acid, which may be inferior to natural forms of folate, or there could be some other compound in folate-rich foods that is responsible for the protective effect. Either way, the research provides reason to eat more folate-rich foods, particularly berries, oranges, broccoli, cauliflower, kale, asparagus, avocado, and lentils.

BPA and miscarriage

Even if there is reason to be optimistic that BPA is having less impact on fertility than in the past, some caution is still warranted because researchers are continuing to find a link between BPA exposure and miscarriage.[9] Again, it is only unusually high levels of BPA that raise concern, but researchers have found that women with the highest levels may be almost twice as likely to miscarry.[10]

Part of the explanation for the link is an increase in chromosomal abnormalities, which fits with what we know about how BPA interferes with chromosome processing in developing eggs.[11] That is only part of the issue, however, because research has shown that women with higher BPA levels are also more likely to miscarry even when the fetus is chromosomally normal. This could be the result of BPA interfering with progesterone signaling, which plays a key role in preparing the uterine lining for early pregnancy.[12] BPA may also impact development of the placenta.[13]

To counteract this risk factor, all that is necessary is bringing your BPA level down to average levels. Studies have consistently found that the increase in miscarriage rate is only significant in the quarter of women with the highest BPA level. To both improve the odds of conceiving and prevent miscarriage, the goal is simply to avoid having higher than normal exposure to BPA.

Before getting into the specifics of how to do that, it is useful to learn about phthalates, another group of chemicals that can impact fertility. The same practical steps you will take to minimize BPA have the double benefit of helping reduce your exposure to phthalates.

Phthalates and Fertility

Phthalates (pronounced THAL-lates) are a group of chemicals known as plasticizers. They help make plastic strong and flexible, provide structure for products such as hairsprays and nail polish, and help fragrances last longer. Given all those roles, it is not surprising that phthalates are widely used in plastic and fragranced products.[14] Just like BPA, these chemicals can disrupt the careful balance of hormones needed for optimal fertility.[15]

By avoiding a small number of the "worst offenders" that contribute most to daily phthalate exposure, you can quickly reduce the level of these chemicals in your body and create a safer environment for your developing eggs and your future pregnancy.

The backstory

In the 1990s, evidence began to emerge that a high level of exposure to phthalates during pregnancy could impact the development of baby boys, causing specific physical changes to their reproductive system. Following a public outcry, governments around the world responded by banning certain phthalates, starting with children's toys. As the European Commission said in 1999, the ban was intended "to protect the youngest and most vulnerable amongst us. We received scientific advice that phthalates pose a serious risk to human health."[16]

But banning phthalates in toys does not go far enough to protect the most vulnerable, because it does little to protect babies from phthalate exposure before birth, when these chemicals can have an even greater impact. Studies have found that exposure to phthalates during pregnancy may compromise infant brain development and increase the risk of preterm birth.[17]

Fortunately, governments have become more and more proactive on this issue in recent years, prohibiting the use of many phthalates in food-contact materials and personal care products.

These restrictions may not go far enough, because companies are still allowed to use alternate phthalates in place of the old ones, but it is clear that progress is being made. We know this because the data shows that at a broad population level, total exposure to phthalates is declining. At an individual level, we can do even more. We have the opportunity to go even further in protecting our fertility and the health of our future children by making informed decisions about the products we buy and use on a daily basis.

Phthalates and antioxidants

The latest research on the extent to which phthalates impact fertility is perplexing. Some studies have found that phthalates clearly compromise sperm quality, and that couples with higher phthalate levels before IVF have a lower chance of pregnancy.[18] Yet other studies on phthalates and fertility have reported a limited impact. [19]

These inconsistent results likely flow from the key issue being the overall balance between pro-oxidants and antioxidants. Phthalates are most likely to compromise egg and sperm quality by weakening our natural antioxidant defense systems.[20] How much impact phthalates have on fertility for a given individual may therefore depend on other factors that are either compromising or supporting cellular antioxidants in that particular individual.

In couples with conditions contributing to oxidative stress, such as age-related infertility, endometriosis, PCOS, or male fertility challenges such as varicocele, phthalates may have more negative impact. In all these situations, antioxidant defenses are not only much more important but also are already under stress. On the other hand, phthalates may have less impact in couples with no complicating medical issues and a higher intake of antioxidants from food and supplements.

This is backed up by studies finding that zinc and selenium, which are found in prenatal supplements and are necessary cofactors for antioxidant enzymes, can counteract some of the negative effects of phthalates on fertility.[21] So too can supplementing with antioxidants such as NAC and vitamins C and E.[22]

Phthalates and miscarriage

Even with a good intake of antioxidants and no predisposing conditions, it is worth being mindful of phthalates when trying to conceive because phthalate exposure may also impact the risk of miscarriage.

Numerous studies have now reported that women with unusually high levels of phthalates in their system before they conceive are more likely to miscarry.[23] This is particularly true for very early losses occurring before six weeks. One explanation for the link is that phthalates may reduce progesterone levels, which could compromise implantation and development of the placenta.[24]

The potential link between phthalates and miscarriage is troubling, but it provides one more opportunity to improve the odds by making some simple changes.

Reducing Exposure

Bisphenols and phthalates are found in a variety of different places—from cosmetics to cleaning products to kitchenware to processed food. But the latest studies provide guidance on the sources of exposure that matter most. As a result, we can avoid unusually high levels of BPA and phthalates with just a few changes to the food we eat, the plastic we use in the kitchen, and the cosmetics and cleaning products we buy.

Research also shows that by tackling the worst offenders in each category, the amount of bisphenols and phthalates in your system will decrease rapidly.[25] It is up to you whether to do this mini-overhaul all at once to get ready for pregnancy or whether to replace products gradually as needed. Either way, it makes sense to start with the most important category: food.

Category 1: food

The general rule: healthy food matters more than packaging

As companies have started phasing out bisphenols and phthalates in products marketed directly to consumers, the problem has shifted to a surprising source. The single greatest contributor to BPA and phthalate exposure is now food—specifically fast food and highly processed food. [26] The reason for this is likely the use of plastic during processing.

The more processing a food undergoes, the more time it will spend in contact with plastic equipment and storage containers. In factories and fast-food chains, these plastics are often sterilized regularly with hot water and harsh cleaners, turning you into the mouse exposed to BPA after the water bottle was washed with a harsh cleaning agent.

As a result, one of the most effective ways to reduce your exposure to bisphenols and phthalates is to emphasize minimally processed food made from natural ingredients.[27] That does not mean completely avoiding processed foods; it just means shifting the balance toward more whole, natural foods when you can. This shift will have the added payoff of greater nutrient density and better blood sugar control, both of which can help support hormone balance and fertility.

To ease a common concern that often arises, it appears that we generally do not have to worry about plastic food packaging. Researchers have found that packaging of fresh fruit, vegetables, meats, and dry goods does not seem to transfer chemicals to the food in significant amounts. By limiting highly processed foods, you can dramatically lower your level of BPA exposure, even if you are still eating foods that are packaged in plastic.[28] One study on this issue concluded that "processing—and not packaging—was the most important contamination source."[29] But the research does suggest a few items for which it is worth paying attention to packaging.

Where it pays to avoid plastic

Specifically, we should be mindful of plastic bottles for oils, vinegars, sauces, and condiments. That is because liquids that are high in fat or acid can act as highways for BPA and phthalates to leach more easily from plastic containers. It is therefore worth buying oil, salad dressings, and sauces in glass bottles and jars. Shelf life also matters. Items that are packaged in plastic for many months or even years are more of an issue than fresh items such as milk and yogurt.

Heat is another factor that can cause chemicals to leach rapidly from plastics, so it is worth limiting how often you eat hot takeout items in plastic containers. Better options include salads, sushi, or ordering from restaurants that use cardboard containers.

Drinking hot coffee from disposable paper cups is a gray area. It is not clear how often the plastic lining of these cups contains BPA or phthalates, but researchers have seen that the plastic lining can break down quickly in hot liquid, releasing microplastics into the coffee. We do not yet know if this is a problem, but to be extra cautious, you may decide to order iced coffee more often or bring your own stainless steel travel cup when you can.

Canned food and drinks

The final category in which packaging matters is food and drinks packaged in cans. Even though many canned foods are now labeled BPA-free, researchers have found that cans are still a major source of BPA and related bisphenols, such as bisphenol S and bisphenol F. If you regularly eat canned foods such as beans, tuna, or chopped tomatoes, it is worth swapping these items for alternatives that are either fresh, frozen, or packaged in glass jars, cardboard cartons, or foil pouches. This is particularly worthwhile for acidic items such as tomatoes, because high acid encourages leaching of chemicals from the can lining.[30] Canned beans are less problematic, but it is still preferable to use frozen or pressure-cooked dried beans when you have time.

Are cans or plastic bottles better?

Studies have produced conflicting results on whether canned beverages are a concern, but glass bottles are the safest option. If you have a choice between a beverage in a can or plastic bottle, the research points toward choosing plastic.[31] Single-use plastic water bottles are not too problematic. They are unlikely to contain BPA, but they can release a small amount of phthalates into the water if stored for a long period of time. For that reason, it is better to buy bottled water from stores with a high turnover so the bottles haven't been stored as long.[32]

With drinks, as with food, the ingredients and degree of processing matter more than packaging. It is far better to drink water from a plastic bottle than soda or another highly processed drink from a glass bottle. When you are at home, the best option is filtered tap water, particularly if your filter can remove chemicals found in many public water supplies. There is little concern over plastic parts in water filters because most companies use safer plastics, no heat is involved, and the water is not in contact with the plastic for a long period of time.

BPA in receipts

One other potential source of BPA at the supermarket is paper receipts, but this is likely only an issue for those who handle receipts or tickets throughout their workday.[33] The most recent studies indicate that occasionally handling receipts while shopping does not make a significant difference to your overall exposure to BPA. (If you do work in retail or handle tickets printed on thermal paper, the best solution is to use rubber fingertip protectors on your thumb and index finger. Also known as thimblettes, they are designed for gripping banknotes and preventing paper cuts, so they should not look too out of place.)

Category 2: kitchenware

To figure out which plastic items in your kitchen are worth replacing, the key question to ask is whether an item will come in contact with hot food or drinks for any substantial length of time. Typically, these are the top items to replace:

- Coffee machines with internal plastic parts
- Travel coffee mugs
- Reusable food storage containers
- Bowls used in the microwave

- Plastic tea kettles
- Colanders
- Blender containers used with hot soups or sauces

For these items, glass and stainless steel are the best choice. To make coffee without plastic, stainless steel options include a French press, pour-over, or classic percolator. See **itstartswiththeegg.com/resources** for recommended products.

Sometimes plastic kitchenware is simply the more practical option, and for these times it is useful to know which types are safest. For cutting boards or containers for storing dry goods or cold foods, the best plastics are polypropylene ("PP" or number 5) or high-density polyethylene (HDPE or number 2). Silicone cooking utensils are also safer than other plastics, although silicone baking mats are not recommended because they can leach chemicals when heated for a substantial length of time. Name-brand Ziploc bags and Glad plastic wrap are claimed to be BPA-free and phthalate-free, although it may be best to allow food to cool before contact with these plastics. A glass plate cover can be helpful for microwaving.

Category 3: cosmetics & personal care

Phthalates used to be a key ingredient in a vast number of cosmetics and personal care products, used in everything from nail polish to hair-styling products. Thankfully, times have changed, and manufacturers have reformulated many products to remove these chemicals. Testing by the FDA has confirmed that the use of phthalates in cosmetics has decreased considerably in recent years.[34]

The improvement has not happened across the board, however. Although more and more products are testing as phthalate-free or with very low levels, most perfumes and colognes are still extremely high in phthalates. This is likely because phthalates act as good solvents for fragrances and help scents linger. A labeling loophole also allows companies to add phthalates to perfumes and simply list "fragrance" as an ingredient. Even in Europe, where most phthalates have been banned in personal care products for several years, perfumes continue to contain high levels of banned phthalates.[35]

The end result is that wearing perfume or cologne regularly can drastically raise phthalate levels. A 2020 study found that men who wore cologne had eight times higher exposure to a particular phthalate than men who never wore cologne, and this was associated with much lower sperm concentration.[36]

The good news is that you can have a significant impact on your exposure to phthalates and potentially improve your fertility just by retiring your perfume. If you would like to go further, the next step is to replace other skin-care and hair-care products with fragrance-free versions. Body lotion is a higher priority than other products because it is applied over a large surface area, which provides more opportunity for chemicals to be absorbed.

Other potential culprits for phthalate exposure include lipsticks and eyelash glue, where phthalates can be added to help the product stick to the skin.[37] In theory, a product containing phthalates should include one of the following on the label:

- Fragrance
- Diethyl phthalate (DEP)
- Dibutyl phthalate (DBP)
- Dimethyl phthalate (DMP)
- Di(2-ethylhexyl) phthalate (DEHP)

Most major brands of nail polish now claim to be phthalate-free, but nail polish remains a source of many other questionable chemicals, so it is better to choose a brand that relies on nontoxic ingredients. Alternatively, a Japanese nail buffer can give the look of clear polish without the chemicals.

When choosing safer skin-care products, another ingredient to watch out for is the preservative propylparaben, which has been linked to diminished ovarian reserve.[38] Numerous studies over the past ten years have reported that women with higher levels of propylparaben tend to have a lower follicle count and higher FSH.[39] Fortunately, many companies have now stopped using parabens and opted for safer preservatives, but it is worth checking labels for propylparaben in products you use often.

Category 4: cleaning & laundry products

Changing your cleaning and laundry products is a lower priority than upgrading the products you apply to your skin, but two small changes can have a significant impact. The first is to stop using room fragrances, including fragranced plug-ins, candles, and air-freshener sprays, which can have a high concentration of phthalates. The second is to stop using fabric softeners and dryer sheets.

Fabric softeners not only contain high concentrations of phthalates but also chemicals known as quaternary ammonium compounds, which have been found in animal studies to compromise both male and female fertility.[40] A better alternative is to use natural wool dryer balls or half a cup of vinegar diluted in an equal amount of water (full-strength vinegar may damage washing machines).

Quaternary ammonium compounds are also the active ingredient in disinfectants such as Lysol (listed on the ingredients as benzalkonium chloride, benzyl ammonium chloride, or alkyl C14 C12 C16). The safest disinfectants are alcohol, hydrogen peroxide, and vinegar.

How much further you choose to go in replacing your laundry and cleaning products is up to you. I typically use cleaning products from Seventh Generation or Better Life but use conventional brands of fragrance-free laundry detergent.

When shifting toward fragrance-free products, it is natural to start wondering about sources of fragrance around you, whether that may be someone else's perfume or the air freshener in your workplace. Occasional exposures will not have a significant impact, and this is not usually worth worrying about. If you are exposed to a lot of fragrance on a daily basis from a particular source and you are in a position to ask a favor, one option is to gently communicate that you are sensitive to fragrances. The chemicals in synthetic fragrances often trigger headaches, allergies, and asthma, so it is not necessary to go into details about potential impacts on fertility.

BPA and phthalates during pregnancy

Creating a nontoxic home while trying to conceive will have added benefits during pregnancy by protecting the health of your future baby. As explained by Dr. Shanna Swan, a leading researcher on phthalates and fertility, "I think we have now have a lot of data that environmental chemicals can and do lower sperm count, impact time to conception, increase fetal loss in early pregnancy, and affect pregnancy outcomes. Do we need more studies? Of course we do. But do we have enough information to act on these studies that we have? I say that we do."[41]

Reducing BPA and phthalates during pregnancy seems to be particularly beneficial for infant brain development, with studies linking lower levels of these chemicals during pregnancy to fewer behavioral disorders and better language development in young children.[42] Minimizing exposure to phthalates during pregnancy may also help prevent premature birth and reduce the risk of rare reproductive abnormalities in baby boys.[43]

Action Steps

Reducing exposure to BPA and phthalates can help protect fertility and improve pregnancy outcomes. We can make the most impact by

- preparing more meals at home, using whole, natural ingredients.
- minimizing canned and highly processed foods.
- replacing plastic kitchenware used with hot food or drinks with glass or stainless steel.
- avoiding perfume, air freshener, certain disinfectants, and fabric softener.
- replacing fragranced products with fragrance-free.

For up-to-date product recommendations, visit **itstartswiththeegg.com/resources**

Chapter 3

Unexpected Obstacles to Fertility

*"Discovery consists of seeing what everybody has
seen and thinking what nobody has thought."*
— ALBERT SZENT-GYORGYI

I F YOU ARE having trouble conceiving or have had one or
more miscarriages, it is worth asking your doctor to test you
for several easily treated conditions that are often missed:
vitamin B12 deficiency, vitamin D deficiency, and underactive thyroid. Each condition has a surprisingly strong link
to infertility and miscarriage, and the standard benchmarks
for levels considered normal may be quite different from the
optimal levels for fertility. Any one of these factors could be
the missing link in your treatment plan that, once corrected,
will greatly improve your chances of a healthy pregnancy.

Surprising Factor 1: Vitamin B12

Vitamin B12 is essential to fertility and preventing miscarriage, but it is unfortunately very common to be severely deficient and never find out, or find out only after a miscarriage that could have been prevented.

There are several reasons why B12 deficiency is so often overlooked. First, many people assume that with a balanced diet and a prenatal multivitamin providing more than 100% of the recommended daily intake of B12, a deficiency is unlikely. That is wrong for reasons that will be discussed in this chapter.

Second, performing a standard test for B12 in the bloodstream and looking to the standard reference range of what is considered normal will often miss a *functional* deficiency, which refers to the ability of cells to access and utilize enough B12 for cellular functions.

Part of the problem is that the level of B12 in the blood considered normal is far too low. Doctors typically only diagnose a deficiency when total B12 is below 200 pg/ml. But studies have found that many people with levels between 200 and 350 pg/ml are in fact deficient when assessed by other measures.[1] In a study of IVF patients at the prestigious Massachusetts General Hospital, women had the highest chance of live birth when their serum B12 was over 700 pg/mL.[2]

Perhaps more importantly, this conventional test for B12 in the blood cannot accurately measure the amount of B12 available to cells. It is possible to have normal or even higher than normal levels of B12 in the blood but still have a functional deficiency because the B12 may be bound to proteins and biologically inactive, or there may be some other problem with transportation or processing.

For this reason, it is more useful to assess whether the body has enough B12 to perform necessary detoxification functions. This can be done by measuring the level of a toxin produced by normal metabolism and normally broken down with the help of B12. This toxin is called methylmalonic acid (MMA). If MMA is higher than normal, that indicates a functional deficiency of B12. Another similar marker is homocysteine, but high homocysteine can reflect low B12, low folate, or other issues, so it is a less specific test than measuring MMA.

Optimal lab values for vitamin B12

Most useful test:
Serum methylmalonic acid (MMA): less than 270 nmol/L

Additional tests:
Total B12: over 350 pg/mL
Active B12 (Holo-Tc): over 60 pmol/L
Homocysteine: less than 9 μmol/L

Identifying and addressing a B12 deficiency can be extremely helpful because the metabolic toxins that build up in the absence of B12 can harm egg quality, increase the risk of miscarriage, and cause problems during pregnancy. Deficiencies are also very common, even when supplementing with a multivitamin containing a significant amount of B12.

B12 deficiencies are so common because absorption and conversion of B12 into its active forms requires numerous steps and can be compromised by a whole array of factors, including

- genetic variations, especially MTHFR and B12 transport proteins
- low stomach acid
- medications for acid reflux (PPIs)
- Metformin
- autoimmune conditions
- celiac or Crohn's disease
- intestinal problems such as bacterial overgrowth (SIBO)

The amount of B12 in a prenatal multivitamin may appear very high compared to the recommended daily intake, but it is typically not enough to correct a deficiency if you have any of these issues or if you follow a largely plant-based diet.

It is particularly important to test for a B12 deficiency if you have any of the common symptoms or complications, which include

- weakness, fatigue, or lightheadedness
- heart palpitations
- shortness of breath
- mouth sores
- numbness or tingling
- depression or memory loss
- migraine
- unexplained infertility
- recurrent pregnancy loss
- a pregnancy impacted by a neural tube defect

If you are deficient in B12, correcting that deficiency could help you get pregnant sooner and reduce the risk of a range of pregnancy complications. A recent study found that women taking B12 supplements before IVF had a significantly higher chance of success.[3] Addressing high homocysteine levels caused by B12 deficiency is also likely to reduce the risk of early pregnancy loss, neural tube defects, and low birth weight.[4]

Addressing a B12 deficiency is especially critical if you have a variant in the MTHFR gene associated with poor processing of folate, such as A1298C or C677T. The biological functions of folate and B12 are intricately linked, and problems with the MTHFR gene appear to reduce the availability of B12. Studies have found that B12 deficiencies are four times more common in people who are homozygous for the C677T variant, for example.[5] In addition, having an MTHFR variation can magnify the consequences of a slight B12 deficiency by causing an even higher level of homocysteine.

Correcting B12 deficiency

There is a long-standing controversy over the best way to correct B12 deficiency, with many arguing that oral tablets are not effective and that either injections or lozenges are needed. This makes some intuitive sense, given that one of the major causes of B12 deficiency is poor absorption through the digestive system. But the data shows that oral tablets are in fact effective. When the dose of B12 in a supplement is high enough, it appears to compensate for poor absorption.[6]

Most studies that have compared oral tablets with injections and lozenges have found that all three methods are similarly effective at addressing B12 deficiency in most people as long as an active form of B12 is used and the dose is at least 1,000–2,000 mcg per day.[7]

The standard form of B12 found in supplements is called cyanocobalamin. This form is not recommended because it is not biologically active, and some people may have difficulty processing it into the natural bioactive forms.

There are three natural forms of B12 used in the body: hydroxocobalamin, adenosylcobalamin, and methylcobalamin. These forms have different activites, with methylcobalamin participating in detoxification and adenosylcobalamin participating in energy production within mitochondria. But the body can convert between these forms as needed. All forms are broken down into the same core compound, which then enters cells and is converted into adenosyl and methyl cobalamin in the proportion needed by that particular cell.[8] For this reason, any of these three natural supplement forms will be effective.[9]

Some people may tolerate one form better than another, however. Supplementing with high-dose methylcobalamin sometimes causes anxiety, itching, rapid heartbeat, or headache. Given that, starting with either hydroxocobalamin or a combination of hydroxocobalamin and adenosylcobalamin may be a better option.

The supplement dose needed to address a deficiency is vastly higher than the recommended daily intake, since only 1–2% will be absorbed even without any specific factors impairing absorption.[10] As mentioned above, studies have found that 1,000–2,000 mcg per day is often required to correct a deficiency.[11] Some doctors advise starting with 4,000–5,000 mcg per day for one month to quickly replenish B12 stores in the liver, followed by a maintenance dose of 1,000 mcg per day long-term.[12]

If you are unable to access proper testing and have symptoms or risk factors for a B12 deficiency, it is better to err on the side of supplementing rather than waiting for answers, because a B12 deficiency is so problematic when trying to conceive. If you take more B12 than needed, most will be excreted and the rest used to replenish long-term stores of B12 in the liver.

Ideally, you will be able to build up your B12 stores while trying to conceive and then reduce your dose when pregnant. Initial reports have flagged a possible link between either very low or very high levels of B12 in the bloodstream during pregnancy and a slightly higher risk of autism.[13] There is much debate over this suggestion, and in reality, there may be no link at all. Nevertheless, the controversy provides more reason to build up your B12 stores while trying to conceive so you can take a lower dose during pregnancy (such as that found in a prenatal multivitamin), allowing your body to pull from your liver's reserves as needed. This is effectively relying on the body's own mechanisms to regulate the level of this important vitamin; you just need to replenish long-term stores of B12 in advance to allow this to occur.

Surprising Factor 2: Vitamin D

Optimal range: at least 40 ng/mL (100 nmol/L)

The more discoveries are made about vitamin D, the more puzzling it is that one compound could have such wide-reaching impacts. In the past few years, studies have shown that a sufficient level of vitamin D can significantly reduce the risk of developing breast cancer and a litany of autoimmune diseases while also protecting against infections.[14] A higher vitamin D level was found to almost halve the chance of being hospitalized or dying from COVID-19.[15] Although the research on vitamin D and fertility has only just begun and is somewhat inconsistent, several studies indicate that vitamin D may also play an important role in protecting fertility.[16]

In one of the most compelling studies, researchers at Columbia University and the University of Southern California (USC) measured vitamin D levels in nearly two hundred women undergoing IVF. Of the Caucasian women in the group, the odds of pregnancy were four times higher for women with high vitamin D levels compared to those who were deficient.[17]

An earlier study also found that in a group of women with the highest vitamin D levels, 47% became pregnant, whereas among women with low vitamin D levels, the pregnancy rate was only 20%.[18] Another more recent IVF study revealed a higher fertilization and implantation rate in a group of women with higher vitamin D levels.[19]

Although these positive results need to be balanced against the studies finding no impact of vitamin D on fertility rates, the evidence generally suggests higher odds of fertilization, implantation, and successful pregnancy in women with higher vitamin D levels or those taking vitamin D supplements.[20]

Researchers suspect one of the main effects of vitamin D is making the uterine lining more receptive to pregnancy.[21] It also plays a key role in hormone signaling in the ovaries.[22] This could explain why women with markers of low ovarian reserve (such as low AMH) often see an improvement in those markers when they are able to improve their vitamin D level.[23]

As will be explained in more detail in chapter 15, vitamin D may be particularly helpful if you have unexplained infertility or a history of unsuccessful embryo transfers, because these issues often involve immune system imbalances or silent infections. Because vitamin D can both strengthen the ability to fight infection and reduce unwanted inflammation, optimizing your vitamin D level can be very helpful when tackling these issues.

Vitamin D and miscarriage

Vitamin D is also important for preventing miscarriage.[24] In one clinical study that involved frozen embryo transfers with genetically normal embryos, the miscarriage rate was 27% in women with a deficiency but just 7% in women with adequate vitamin D.[25]

This stark difference may again relate to the impressive ability of vitamin D to regulate the immune system. Although many early miscarriages are due to chromosomal errors, when a miscarriage occurs with a genetically normal embryo, the most likely culprit is immune activity. This immune activity may be due to an infection or autoimmune antibodies, or may have no identifiable cause. Research has shown that vitamin D can help reduce the immune factors often involved in recurrent miscarriage, such as natural killer cells, autoimmune antibodies, and markers of systemic inflammation.[26]

Importantly, the critical time frame in which vitamin D is needed in order to reduce the risk of miscarriage is *before* pregnancy. Researchers at the National Institutes of Health and Johns Hopkins University found that having sufficient vitamin D before pregnancy was associated with lower odds of pregnancy loss, whereas the level of vitamin D at eight weeks of pregnancy had little impact.

This preconception time frame is also important for reducing the risk of pregnancy complications, including preterm birth and preeclampsia. Preeclampsia is a serious complication involving high blood pressure during pregnancy. It can be quite dangerous for both mother and baby. The evidence is growing that having adequate vitamin D is one of the most effective ways to prevent both preeclampsia and preterm birth, but the timing matters. If you wait until you are pregnant to address a deficiency, it may be too late.

According to Dr. Bruce Hollis and Dr. Carol Wagner, two leading vitamin D researchers at the Medical University of South Carolina, "Vitamin D needs to be administered as early in gestation as possible. In fact, it appears to be critical to provide vitamin D in the preconception period to have the maximum protective effect with respect to Preeclampsia."[27]

Optimal Vitamin D levels and supplement dosing

Although there is now much greater awareness of the role of vitamin D in fertility and pregnancy health, the standard advice still falls short because two important points are often neglected.

First, the optimal level of vitamin D when trying to conceive is significantly higher than the level considered "normal." The conventional benchmark of a normal vitamin D level, at 20 ng/ml, is based on the amount needed to prevent rickets, a bone disease caused by severe vitamin D deficiency. According to Dr. Hollis and Dr. Wagner, the role of vitamin D in bone health has blinded researchers for decades to the other essential functions of vitamin D, including regulating hormones and the immune system. They explain that "on the very top of this list would be vitamin D's ability to greatly improve birth outcomes."

To reduce the risk of miscarriage, preterm birth, and preeclampsia, the research of Dr. Hollis, Dr. Wagner, and others demonstrates that we should be aiming for a vitamin D level over **40 ng/mL (100 nmol/L)**.[28]

The vast majority of women in developed countries are far below this level. It is usually only reached with daily sun exposure or a supplement of at least **4,000 IU** per day.[29] Randomized clinical studies have reported no adverse effects from taking this dose during pregnancy.[30]

Taking an even higher dose while trying to conceive could be helpful if you have any condition associated with inflammation or autoimmunity, such as thyroid disease, endometriosis, or a history of recurrent miscarriage. To regulate the immune system in these conditions, an optimal level may be at least 60ng/mL, which typically requires a dose of at least 5,000–6,000 IU per day.

To obtain the most benefit from a vitamin D supplement, it is best to choose vitamin D3 in an oil-based formulation (whether as drops or a soft-gel capsule) rather than a solid tablet, and to take it with both vitamin K2 and a meal containing some fat. These measures significantly improve vitamin D absorption because it is a fat-soluble vitamin.[31] (For recommended brands, see itstartswiththeegg.com/supplements)

Surprising Factor 3: Thyroid Function

Most doctors now recognize that it is important to check thyroid function in anyone trying to conceive, but they will often test only one value—thyroid stimulating hormone (TSH)—and stop there if it is normal. If you have unexplained infertility, pregnancy losses, or diminished ovarian reserve at a young age, it can be helpful to get a more complete picture of thyroid health by testing for active thyroid hormones and thyroid antibodies.

TSH increases as thyroid function drops, so a TSH above the optimal range indicates an underactive thyroid. This is most often caused by autoimmune antibodies that bind to one or more proteins in the thyroid. Some endocrinologists consider a TSH below 4.5 mIU/L to be normal, but the data shows that it is best to be under 2.5 mIU/L when trying to conceive.[32] Some fertility specialists go further and argue that closer to 1 mIU/L is ideal, on the basis of research showing that this provides a buffer for the decline in thyroid function that often occurs during early pregnancy.[33]

Free T4 and free T3 represent circulating thyroid hormones. When either is below the optimal range, it can indicate an underactive thyroid. These values are particularly useful to know if TSH is borderline. Sometimes T3 and T4 values can be low even when TSH is normal or close to normal.

If any of your thyroid hormones suggest an underactive thyroid, it may be worth discussing medication with your doctor.[34] Even a mild reduction in thyroid function appears to contribute to infertility and miscarriage, particularly when thyroid antibodies are present.[35]

The typical medication for underactive thyroid is levo-thyroxine, known by the brand name Synthroid, which the body converts to active thyroid hormone. In a small study of women with underactive thyroid who had been trying to conceive for an average of almost three years, 84% got pregnant when treated with Synthroid.[36] Thyroid treatment can also improve success rates in IVF and may reduce the chance of miscarriage.[37]

If your thyroid hormone levels are normal but you have thyroid antibodies, it is open to debate whether medication is worthwhile.[38] The earlier studies on this question indicated that Synthroid could reduce miscarriages and pregnancy complications in women with thyroid antibodies but normal thyroid hormones.[39] Now the picture is becoming less clear. Several large, randomized studies have reported that thyroid hormone medication is not helpful for preventing miscarriage when antibodies are positive but hormone levels are normal.[40]

The American Thyroid Association has recognized the inconsistencies in the data but endorsed treatment anyway, stating that given the safety of Synthroid, "its use among patients with recurrent pregnancy loss may be reasonably considered in the setting of early gestation, especially when no other known cause of prior pregnancy loss has been identified."[41]

If you have thyroid antibodies and continue to struggle with unexplained infertility, low ovarian reserve, or pregnancy loss, addressing the issue from an immune perspective can be very helpful. This is discussed further in chapter 15, which focuses on immune factors. In addition, it is particularly important to have your DHEA-S and testosterone levels tested because women with thyroid autoimmunity are more likely to have a low level of the hormone DHEA.[42] Correcting the problem by supplementing with DHEA (as discussed in chapter 9) can significantly improve ovarian function for some women with thyroid autoimmunity and may also help lower thyroid antibodies.[43]

Optimal ranges for thyroid lab values:

- TSH: 0.5–2.5 mIU/L
- Free T4: at least 1.1 ng/dL
- Free T3: at least 3.2 pg/mL
- Reverse T3: less than a 10:1 ratio of reverse T3 to TSH
- Thyroid peroxidase antibodies: less than 9 IU/mL or negative
- Thyroglobulin antibodies: less than 4 IU/mL or negative

Action Steps

When trying to conceive, it is common for important lab tests to be overlooked, and for values to be compared to standard reference ranges that are inadequate for fertility. To rule out simple factors that can stand in the way of getting pregnant and having a healthy pregnancy, consider getting tested for

- vitamin B12 deficiency
- vitamin D deficiency
- thyroid function, including active hormone levels and thyroid antibodies

It also helpful to compare your value to the optimal range for fertility, rather than the normal range.

Download a printable guide to optimal lab values at **itstartswiththeegg.com/testing**

Chapter 4

Hormone Lab Tests

"To control your hormones is to control your life."
— BARRY SEARS

ORMONES AND EGG quality are intricately linked. A range of hormones is produced by the brain, the ovaries, and the adrenal glands in order to orchestrate the complex process of egg development. Testing these hormones can not only reveal how well your ovaries are functioning but also provide important clues as to the supplements and other strategies that are most likely to improve your egg quality.

In an ideal world, a knowledgeable doctor would order these tests and help you interpret the results. But not everyone has access to such guidance. It is common to have a long wait for an appointment with a fertility clinic. It is also common for clinics to order labs without explaining what the results mean. This chapter is to help provide an initial understanding of where you may fit into some of the common patterns of hormonal imbalances and how these patterns relate to the supplements discussed in the book.

If you do not have a provider assisting you with testing, in most locations you can order these tests yourself through various online services. You can then compare your values to the optimal values discussed in this chapter and included in the printable guide at itstartswiththeegg.com/testing.

Anti-Mullerian Hormone (AMH)

Optimal range: 1.0 to 3.5 ng/mL (7 to 25 pmol/L)
When to test: any day of the cycle

AMH reflects the number of immature follicles in the early stage of developing into a mature egg. In fertility clinics, AMH is used as one of the key pieces of information to predict the chance of success with IVF. If AMH is low, it suggests the number of eggs that could be retrieved is low, which reduces the chance of success.

Outside the IVF context, AMH is not as useful for predicting your chance of getting pregnant.[1] That is because natural conception does not depend on having a large pool of eggs available at any one time. All it takes is one good egg, and if the egg chosen for ovulation that month is of good quality, there is a high chance of getting pregnant, even with a low AMH.

Nevertheless, AMH testing is helpful even if you are not pursuing IVF because a low AMH (below 1 ng/mL) can suggest that the strategies in this book directed at diminished ovarian reserve or age-related infertility are likely to be the most helpful.

On the other hand, if testing reveals that AMH is higher than normal, that can indicate PCOS or potential hormonal imbalances similar to PCOS. If your AMH is above the normal range, the strategies in the book directed to addressing insulin resistance and PCOS are likely to be the most helpful.

Monitoring your AMH over time can also show that you are on the right path and the strategies are working. Many women who start with low AMH and follow the advice in this book see their AMH steadily increase over time. This is particularly pronounced for those who start with deficiencies in vitamin D and DHEA.[2]

Those who start with higher-than-normal AMH can also see their level normalize, particularly after supplementing with myo-inositol and vitamin D, and making dietary changes to address insulin resistance.[3]

It is worth noting that AMH does fluctuate from month to month, so a single measure is not always meaningful. AMH can also be temporarily suppressed by long-term use of hormonal birth control.

Follicle Stimulating Hormone (FSH)

Optimal range: under 10 mIU/ml
When to test: day 3 of cycle

Another hormone commonly used to assess ovarian function is follicle stimulating hormone (FSH). As the name suggests, it stimulates your follicles to grow. A surge of FSH is released by the pituitary gland during the early part of your cycle to encourage follicles to mature and prepare for ovulation.

Unlike AMH, which declines with age, FSH increases with age as follicles become more and more resistant to FSH and the pituitary needs to produce a larger amount of FSH to make follicles grow. A high FSH level therefore indicates that either fewer ovarian follicles are ready to grow or they are not responding well to FSH.

FSH is typically tested around day 3 of your cycle, when it is ideally under 10 mIU/ml. When FSH is between 10 and 20 mIU/ml, there is still a reasonable chance of success in IVF. If your FSH is over 20 mIU/ml, the odds depend on your age, because age has more impact than FSH.[4] Women over 38 with an FSH over 20 mIU/ml have a fairly low chance of getting pregnant in IVF, but keep in mind that FSH often improves after implementing the strategies covered in this book.

FSH is typically tested in combination with luteinizing hormone (LH), inhibin B, and estrogen because the level of these hormones can help interpret FSH results.

FSH used to be the primary test used for assessing ovarian reserve, but doctors have come to rely more heavily on AMH since research has shown that AMH is better at predicting chances of success in IVF cycles. Typically, low AMH and high FSH go hand in hand. If both suggest age-related decline in ovarian reserve or premature ovarian aging, the odds of success in IVF are lower. But if there is a discrepancy and only one number is abnormal, studies have shown that AMH is the more reliable indicator of your chance of becoming pregnant through IVF.[5]

Estradiol (Estrogen)

Optimal range: 20 to 75 pg/mL
When to test: day 3 of cycle

Estradiol is the major form of estrogen produced by the ovaries. A high estradiol level on day 3 can indicate lower ovarian reserve. High estradiol can also artificially suppress your FSH level, so if your FSH is reported as normal but estradiol is high, your ovarian function may in fact be lower than indicated by the FSH value.

Testosterone

Normal range: 10 to 55 ng/dL (total testosterone)
Optimal range: 25 to 45 ng/dL (total testosterone)
When to test: first half of cycle, but can be tested at any time

Although typically considered a male hormone, testosterone also plays an important role in female fertility. It is produced by the cells surrounding each egg and helps immature eggs make it through the initial stages of development. If testosterone is too low, many of these early-stage follicles will die off prematurely. The follicles that do survive will also be less receptive to the message from FSH to grow and mature. This can present as diminished ovarian reserve, with a low AMH.

On the other hand, if testosterone is too high, many eggs will begin maturing each month, but the final stage of egg development may be blocked, preventing ovulation. This leads to a high AMH and reflects a common pattern seen in PCOS. The cause of this high testosterone is often insulin resistance.[6]

If AMH is high but testosterone is normal or low, that can reflect a newly recognized form of "lean" PCOS in which testosterone starts out very high but suddenly drops at a certain age, along with a drop in DHEA.[7]

In women, testosterone is produced by both the adrenal glands and the ovaries. By testing the level of other hormones produced by the adrenals, particularly DHEA-S, it is possible to determine whether low testosterone is likely caused by poor adrenal function or poor ovarian function.

If testosterone and DHEA-S are both low, that suggests the issue is with the adrenal glands, and supplementing with DHEA may help. If testosterone is very low but DHEA-S is normal or high, it may instead be due to poor ovarian function, which is harder to correct. Some fertility doctors are now attempting to address the problem by prescribing testosterone gel in preparation for IVF, with promising results in certain patients.[8]

In the bloodstream, some testosterone is bound to proteins, and the remainder is known as "free" testosterone. A comprehensive analysis by a fertility clinic will typically measure several of these different forms—testing total testosterone, bioavailable or free testosterone, and sex-hormone binding globulin. If you are testing just one form, total testosterone appears to be the most informative.[9] It is more accurate to measure testosterone with a method called mass-spectroscopy (abbreviated LC-MS/MS) rather than immunoassay.

DHEA-S

Optimal range: 95 to 270 mcg/dL, ideally around 180 mcg/dL

When to test: any day of cycle

DHEA is a hormone made by the adrenal glands and used by the ovaries to produce estrogen and testosterone. With age or various autoimmune conditions, the adrenals may stop making enough DHEA, which impairs the ability of the ovaries to produce the testosterone and estrogen needed for proper egg development. If your testosterone is low, the underlying reason may be too little DHEA.

To accurately assess your DHEA level, it is necessary to test a form called DHEA-sulfate (DHEA-S), which is the major form in the blood and is not subject to short-term fluctuations. As will be discussed in chapter 9, if your level is low, supplementing with DHEA may significantly improve fertility.

In one study, women who started with a DHEA-S level below 95 mcg/dL and took DHEA for three months saw an increase in the number of eggs retrieved in IVF, a doubling in the percentage of eggs able to progress to a day-5 embryo, and a doubling in the chance of a live birth.[10]

Conversely, the same study showed that egg quality can also be compromised if DHEA-S is too high. Specifically, lower egg quality was evident in women starting with DHEA-S over 270 mcg/dL, which is often seen in those with insulin resistance or PCOS. The poor egg quality in these women was reflected in a low proportion of eggs able to fertilize and grow to a day-5 embryo and very few live births. Interestingly, egg quality improved dramatically when the women were given Metformin. This medication is commonly given to women with PCOS to address insulin resistance. In this study, it was able to reduce DHEA-S levels to within the optimal range.

Progesterone

Optimal range: at least 10 ng/ml (32 nmol/L) blood test or a positive urine PdG test

When to test: approximately day 21, or days 7, 8, 9, and 10 after ovulation

If you are trying to conceive naturally, it can be helpful to monitor your progesterone in the last week of your cycle to ensure that you are making enough progesterone to support implantation. (In IVF, your natural progesterone level is less relevant because large doses of progesterone are given to prepare for embryo transfer and throughout early pregnancy.)

Progesterone is produced by the cells of an empty ovarian follicle after an egg is released. It acts to prepare the uterine lining for pregnancy by stimulating the growth of blood vessels and the release of nutrients needed for a developing embryo.

Just as age, oxidative damage, high insulin, and other conditions can compromise egg quality, these factors can also compromise the quality of the cells surrounding the egg, reducing their ability to make enough progesterone.

This is problematic because progesterone needs to reach a certain minimum level and then stay elevated for a sufficient time after ovulation to allow for implantation. If the amount of progesterone is too low, or if it drops too soon, the uterine lining will not be primed for implantation and will not be able to nourish a newly implanted embryo. This is known as a luteal phase defect or luteal phase deficiency. Signs of a luteal phase defect include cycles shorter than 28 days, fewer than 7 days between ovulation and your period, and spotting mid-cycle.

Diagnosing low progesterone levels in the luteal phase can be difficult with standard blood tests because progesterone is released in pulses during the day. As a result, the amount in the bloodstream can fluctuate significantly from one hour to the next, and any one blood test is not that reliable. Nevertheless, a blood level below 10 ng/mL or a sum of three days' tests below 30 ng/mL around day 21 of the cycle has been reported to suggest a luteal phase defect.[11]

A newer approach is to use test kits that measures a marker of progesterone in the urine. These kits are sold online for use at home, by companies such as Proov. The kits work by measuring a metabolite called PdG. After progesterone circulates in the bloodstream, it is metabolized by the liver and excreted in urine as PdG. The level of PdG in first-morning urine is correlated to the average progesterone level over the course of the previous day, providing a useful way to determine whether progesterone is sufficient to support a pregnancy.

Dr. Amy Beckley, a biochemist and the founder of Proov, recommends testing PdG on days 7, 8, 9, and 10 after peak fertility (indicated by a positive LH ovulation test strip or egg-white cervical mucus). If this testing shows that progesterone is too low or declines too soon, it is worth discussing with a fertility specialist. Your doctor may recommend additional progesterone, typically in the form of a prescription vaginal gel or suppository during the week following ovulation. (In the United States, progesterone oils and creams are also available over the counter, but prescription forms may have more accurate dosing.)

Although we do not yet have clear evidence that supplementing with progesterone can help women get pregnant, it is considered very low risk, and many doctors will prescribe progesterone to women with unexplained infertility in case it helps.

If your progesterone is low, it can also be helpful to test your fasting insulin level, because high insulin appears to suppress the production of progesterone in the luteal phase.[12] The optimal range for fasting insulin is below 10 mIU/mL. You can lower insulin through the diet strategies covered in chapter 12 and by supplementing with myo-inositol, discussed in chapter 8.

Another complementary approach is to use the strategies discussed in this book to help support the cells in the ovaries that make progesterone. It appears that one of the major drivers of low progesterone in the luteal phase is oxidative damage to the collection of cells in the ovarian follicle that make progesterone, known as the corpus luteum. Studies have found that antioxidants discussed in chapter 7, such as melatonin and vitamin C, can improve the ability of ovarian cells to produce progesterone.[13]

Progesterone may also have a role to play in addressing recurrent miscarriage, but this is more controversial. There was initially great optimism around using progesterone to prevent miscarriage, but these hopes were dashed by a large clinical trial finding that it made little difference.[14] One possibility is that progesterone was given too late in that study—starting at the time of a positive pregnancy test—and that a more significant difference would be seen if progesterone was started around the time of implantation.

The study may have also failed to identify the women who could benefit most from progesterone supplementation. Follow-up research indicates that giving progesterone during pregnancy reduces the risk of miscarriage only in very specific circumstances, namely in women who either have bleeding during pregnancy or a history of at least three prior miscarriages.[15]

Action Steps

To understand your starting point and where to focus your efforts, it can be helpful to test the level of various hormones that can provide an insight into your fertility. The highest priorities to test are

- AMH
- DHEA-S
- Total testosterone
- Progesterone (if trying to conceive naturally)

Download a printable guide to optimal lab values at **itstartswiththeegg.com/testing**.

PART 2

HOW TO CHOOSE THE RIGHT SUPPLEMENTS

Chapter 5

What to Look for in a Prenatal

"The more original a discovery, the more obvious it seems afterwards."

— ARTHUR KOESTLER

Recommended for
Basic, Intermediate, and Advanced Fertility Plans

T AKING A PRENATAL multivitamin every day is one of the most important things you can do to prepare for pregnancy. And it is never too early to start. Vitamins such as folate are not only critical to preventing birth defects but may also make it easier to get pregnant by restoring ovulation and boosting egg quality. Some vitamins can also help reduce the risk of miscarriage. For all these reasons, it is important to start taking a good-quality prenatal vitamin early—ideally at least three months before trying to conceive.

Folate

Folate is a B vitamin needed throughout the body for hundreds of different biological processes. Folic acid is the synthetic form of folate used in supplements. This important vitamin is traditionally known for its role in preventing serious birth defects such as spina bifida, but recent research has also uncovered new evidence that folate plays a significant role even earlier—during the development of the egg. Because eggs begin maturing three to four months before ovulation, this suggests that the earlier you can start taking folate, the better.

It is not at all surprising that folate impacts egg quality because it is important for making new DNA and proteins. It also helps break down toxic metabolites that can damage eggs and embryos. Before delving into the research showing just how much impact folate has on fertility, it is useful to understand the broader context of how this vitamin came to be such an important part of planning for pregnancy.

Folic acid supplementation has now been hailed as one of the greatest public health achievements of the late twentieth century.[1] Yet it was not always so, and early research into the role of folic acid in preventing birth defects was marred by controversy. This controversy furnishes interesting background information for the other supplements discussed in this book because it provides an example of why there is often a huge gap between research findings and medical practice.

Until the 1990s, doctors had very little understanding of what could be done to prevent neural tube defects. These birth defects were unfortunately common and resulted in stillbirth, death shortly after birth, or lifelong paralysis.

The world changed in 1991, when researchers in England published the results of a large study showing that 70–80% of neural tube defects could be prevented by taking a folic acid supplement immediately before pregnancy.[2] The beneficial effects of folic acid were so clear that the study was halted early so more women could benefit from the findings.

Yet this large study was not the first to reveal that folic acid supplements could prevent neural tube defects. An earlier study showing the same thing,[3] published in 1981, generated many years of hostile criticism.[4]

The criticism mainly centered on the design of the trial because folic acid was given to all women presenting with a history of a previous pregnancy affected by neural tube defects, and the control group consisted of women who were already pregnant at the time they came to the doctors running the study. This is a departure from the ideal study design, in which a group of women are randomly assigned to receive either folic acid or a placebo, and the doctor and patient are "blind" as to which pill is being taken until the data are analyzed. This is referred to as a "gold standard" clinical trial and is designed to minimize the effect of bias.

In the case of folic acid, it was another 10 years before the results of the 1991 randomized, double-blind, placebo-controlled trial were available to confirm the initial research findings. In the meantime, the authors of the first study claimed that their results were persistently ignored while the possibility of a bias was overemphasized.[5] The practical impact of this controversy is that between 1981, when there was very good evidence of the protective effects of folic acid, and 1991, when a double-blind, placebo-controlled study finally satisfied the skeptics, 10 years passed, during which many women who should have been taking folic acid supplements were not, likely resulting in countless tragic outcomes that could have been prevented.

This serves as a cautionary tale that we should not overlook the best available evidence while we wait for the perfect clinical study—a philosophy echoed throughout this book. The philosophy of acting on the "best evidence" does of course need to be limited by safety concerns. If the benefit of a supplement is clear but we do not yet have reliable evidence of safety, it is necessary to wait for further research. But if safety has been firmly established in good-quality studies and there is good, but not perfect, evidence of a very significant benefit, we have every reason to act rather than wait for a perfect clinical study that may never happen.

This is particularly true in the fertility context, in which women may have only one or two chances to conceive with IVF before running out of financial (or emotional) resources, and there is often no time to wait. That is the background for the supplement recommendations in the rest of this book: weighing all the available evidence for each supplement rather than waiting for medical practice to catch up with research.

Returning to the specific example of folic acid, we now know that taking this supplement before pregnancy dramatically cuts the risk of spina bifida and other neural tube defects.[6] The US Centers for Disease Control (CDC), the UK Department of Health, and many other public health authorities recommend that to prevent neural tube defects, all women thinking of having a baby should take a 400-mcg folic acid supplement every day, in addition to natural dietary sources of folate.[7]

This should be considered a minimum, and some authorities recommend at least 800 mcg for all women trying to conceive. As is discussed further, the science has now advanced and suggests it is preferable to choose a prenatal multivitamin that contains folate in a natural form, such as methylfolate, rather than synthetic folic acid.

Although the early research on folate focused on preventing birth defects, that is not the only benefit. The latest research clearly establishes that folate is important for every stage of fertility, from egg development to ovulation to fetal growth.[8]

Folate and ovulation

Doctors have long suspected that vitamin deficiencies could play a role in ovulation problems in some women. This idea was supported by the results of the Nurses' Health Study, which followed tens of thousands of nurses over many years, including a subgroup of more than 18,000 who were trying to conceive or who became pregnant over the course of eight years.

When researchers at the Harvard School of Public Health analyzed the data from the Nurses' Health Study, they found that the women who took a daily multivitamin were much less likely to have infertility due to ovulation problems. Taking a multivitamin just a few times per week was associated with a one-third lower chance of ovulatory infertility, and women who took a multivitamin every day had an even lower risk.[9] The researchers suggested that this was probably due to folic acid and other B vitamins.

The findings of this large population-based study are consistent with other double-blind, placebo-controlled studies reporting higher pregnancy rates in women taking a multivitamin.[10] Researchers have also found higher levels of progesterone and lower risk of ovulation disorders in women with a higher intake of folate from food.[11]

In the IVF context, folate appears to improve egg quality and overall success rates. In one study, women with a twofold higher level of folate in ovarian follicles were three times more likely to become pregnant.[12]

Synthetic folic acid versus methylfolate

There is an ongoing debate over the optimal form of folate and the impact of genetic variations in folate metabolism. A 2016 study by researchers at Oxford University found that women with certain variants in a folate metabolism gene, called MTHFR, were more likely to have chromosomally abnormal embryos and implantation failure and were much less likely to become pregnant following IVF.[13] These genetic variants have long been associated with recurrent miscarriage,[14] although some recent studies have questioned the link.[15]

The enzyme encoded by the MTHFR gene is responsible for converting other forms of folate to the biologically active form, methylfolate. Methylfolate has many key roles, but perhaps its most important is detoxification. The body uses methylfolate to detoxify unwanted byproducts of normal metabolism, such as homocysteine.

Common variations in the MTHFR gene reduce the activity of the enzyme that produces methylfolate from other forms of folate. This reduces the amount of methylfolate available for detoxification functions, which allows homocysteine to accumulate. It is in fact an excess of homocysteine that is thought to contribute to infertility and possibly miscarriage risk in those with MTHFR mutations.[16] High homocysteine not only contributes to DNA damage but may also increase the risk of blood clots.

The two most common variants in the MTHFR gene are known as A1298C and C677T. Approximately 40% of the population has one copy of A1298C, but this causes only a mild reduction in the ability to process folate (a 20–40% reduction in enzyme activity). Having two copies of this variant, or having one or two copies of the C677T variant, has a much more significant impact, reducing the activity of the enzyme by up to 70%. These more significant mutations affect approximately 10% of the population and are associated with higher homocysteine levels.[17]

There is currently a heated debate on the extent to which these mutations contribute to recurrent miscarriage. Some studies have found a connection, whereas others have not.[18] The good news is that if MTHFR variants do indeed increase the risk of miscarriage, it appears that much of this risk can be mitigated with the right supplements.

If you would like to know which forms of the MTHFR gene you have, your doctor can order an MTHFR blood test, or you can order DNA analysis yourself through 23andme.com and then upload your data to the free website GeneticGenie.org. Testing is not essential, though, because you can simply choose to supplement as you would if the mutations were present.

Historically, doctors have recommended that women with an MTHFR mutation should take a much higher dose of folic acid (up to 4,000 mcg per day) to make up for the reduced efficiency of processing folic acid to methylfolate. It is now known that at high doses, unmetabolized folic acid builds up in the bloodstream, which appears to interfere with the ability of cells to take up methylfolate.[19] A much more effective approach is to supplement directly with methylfolate.[20] (Recommended prenatals that contain folate in this form are listed at www.itstartswiththeegg.com/supplements)

If you have not yet had any genetic testing but you have a history of recurrent miscarriage or failed IVF cycles, the most cautious approach is to take a prenatal that contains methylfolate just in case you do have a mutation that compromises folate metabolism. It may also make sense for your partner to take a methylfolate supplement because new research indicates that when a father has defects in folate metabolism, this may also contribute to miscarriage, likely by increasing DNA damage within sperm.[21]

The typical recommended dose of methylfolate is 800–1,000 mcg per day, even for those with MTHFR variants. In rare cases, methylfolate causes side effects such as muscle pain or anxiety. If these side effects bother you, an alternate natural form that is preferable to synthetic folic acid is folinic acid.

Although synthetic folic acid can be poorly metabolized in humans, other versions of folate naturally found in foods, such as folinic acid, are quickly converted into usable methylfolate.[22]

Supplementing with additional vitamin B12 may also reduce the side effects of methylfolate and has the advantage of further reducing homocysteine levels. As a result, initial studies have suggested that this vitamin may be just as important as folate in preventing miscarriages associated with MTHFR variants.[23]

The latest controversy over methylfolate

Some health bodies have recently released public statements recommending that women trying to conceive should only supplement with synthetic folic acid and not methylfolate, claiming that only folic acid has been shown to prevent neural tube defects. That argument is based on a fundamental misunderstanding of the science.

Studies have clearly demonstrated that what matters for preventing neural tube defects is having a high enough red blood cell (RBC) folate level.[24] More than 90% of the folate present in red blood cells and measured in RBC folate lab tests is in the form of methylfolate.[25] Studies have also demonstrated that supplementing with methylfolate is much more effective at raising RBC folate than supplementing with synthetic folic acid.[26] In addition, the way in which folate helps prevent neural tube defects is by lowering homocysteine.[27] Methylfolate has a much greater ability to lower homocysteine than folic acid.[28] In short, there is no rational basis to believe that supplementing with synthetic folic acid is uniquely able to prevent neural tube defects. To the contrary, supplementing with methylfolate is likely to be far more effective.

For current prenatal recommendations, see **itstartswiththeegg.com/supplements**

Other Vitamins and Fertility

A good prenatal multivitamin should also include several other key vitamins and minerals. As mentioned earlier, one vitamin that plays a critical role in egg quality and fertility is B12.[29] That is likely because vitamin B12, like folate, decreases homocysteine.[30]

Another specific vitamin critical to fertility is B6. Studies have reported that women with sufficient vitamin B6 are much more likely to get pregnant and less likely to miscarry than women who are deficient.[31] That said, some prenatals contain more B6 than necessary because it is used in higher doses to treat morning sickness. If you suspect your prenatal is causing headaches or insomnia, look for a brand with a lower dose of B6. Some people may also respond better to the biologically active form of B6, known as pyridoxal 5'-phosphate.

The minerals found in prenatal multivitamins are also helpful for egg quality and fertility. Zinc and selenium are especially important because they play key roles in antioxidant defenses. Selenium, for example, is essential for the function of key enzymes that protect against oxidative damage to ovarian cells. Studies indicate that 200 mcg per day of selenium can be especially helpful for those with autoimmune thyroid conditions or low ovarian reserve.[32] If your prenatal falls short, you can make up the difference by adding a small number of Brazil nuts to your diet each week. A single Brazil nut provides around 90 mcg of selenium.

Iron can also play a role in prenatals, both positive and negative. If you experience digestive problems from your prenatal, look for a brand without iron or with iron in the form of ferrous bisglycinate. If you struggle with significant fatigue, weakness, or joint pain and have unexplained infertility, it may be worth testing for both iron deficiency and iron overload. Both high and low levels of iron can cause severe fatigue and potentially contribute to infertility. Iron deficiency is usually evident from low ferritin levels, whereas iron overload is diagnosed by testing transferrin saturation.

An introduction to other supplements

The next several chapters will describe further specific supplements that may help improve egg quality. If you are going to add just one other supplement, make it coenzyme Q10 (CoQ10 for short). As explained in the next chapter, the latest research suggests that taking CoQ10 increases egg and embryo quality by increasing the supply of cellular energy available to eggs.

The subsequent chapters discuss additional supplements that may improve egg quality for those with specific fertility challenges or a history of pregnancy loss. By way of general overview, chapter 6 on CoQ10 and chapter 7 on antioxidants are generally applicable to anyone trying to conceive. Chapter 8 on myo-inositol is more relevant to women with PCOS, irregular ovulation, or a history of miscarriage and insulin resistance. Chapter 9 on DHEA is relevant for women with diminished ovarian reserve, autoimmunity, age-related infertility, or a history of miscarriage. Chapter 10 discusses why some so-called "fertility supplements" are best avoided, and chapter 11 provides an overview of the various supplement plans. Chapter 14 covers supplements that may be useful while preparing for frozen embryo transfer. If you have severely diminished ovarian reserve and want to consider every possible avenue, chapter 16 discusses some additional supplements that may be helpful but are still considered somewhat experimental because they have not been studied extensively.

Action Steps

To optimize egg quality, it is important to take a good-quality prenatal multivitamin. Look for a brand that includes at least 800 mcg of methylfolate. Other important vitamins that can help improve egg quality include B6, B12, zinc, and selenium.

Chapter 6

Energize Your Eggs with CoQ10

"Energy and persistence conquer all things."
— BENJAMIN FRANKLIN

Recommended for
Basic, Intermediate, and Advanced Fertility Plans

COENZYME Q10, OR CoQ10 for short, is a small molecule found in just about every cell in the body, including your eggs. Recent scientific research has revealed just how important this molecule is to preserving egg quality and fertility. Along with many other benefits, adding a CoQ10 supplement may have the potential to prevent or even reverse some of the decline in egg quality that comes with age.

Anyone trying to conceive can likely benefit from adding a CoQ10 supplement, but it is particularly helpful if you are in your mid-thirties or older, or have fertility problems such as diminished ovarian reserve.

What Does CoQ10 Do?

CoQ10 has long been a favorite nutritional supplement of marathon runners and Olympic athletes.[1] It is also commonly used to prevent the muscle pain associated with statins and in conditions such as heart failure and Parkinson's. But research shows yet another likely benefit of CoQ10: improved egg quality.

How is it that one tiny molecule can do so much? It is likely because CoQ10 plays an important role in making energy throughout the body—in muscles, the brain, and developing eggs. CoQ10 is in fact critical for energy production by mitochondria, the power plants inside our cells.

CoQ10 is a vital part of the reaction that creates electrical energy inside mitochondria. Mitochondria then harness this electrical energy to make energy in the form of ATP. Cells then use ATP to power just about every biological process.

CoQ10 is also an antioxidant that can recycle vitamin E and perform many other roles inside cells,[2] but it is the role this molecule plays in mitochondria that is most interesting for improving egg quality.

Energy for eggs

As we age, mitochondria become damaged and less efficient at producing energy, much like an old, damaged power plant.[3] This is thought to play a key role in the aging process.[4] A decline in mitochondrial function happens throughout the body as we age, but particularly in eggs. Studies have specifically shown that in eggs from women over 40, structural damage to mitochondria is much more common.[5] Aging eggs also accumulate genetic damage in mitochondria,[6] and even the number of mitochondria declines in the follicle cells that surround each egg.[7]

As a result, eggs from older women make less energy—that is, less ATP.[8] The inability to make enough ATP is a big problem for egg quality and is likely a major way in which age negatively affects egg quality.[9] There is also evidence of poor mitochondrial function in women with other fertility concerns, such as premature ovarian failure or a poor response to stimulation medication in IVF.[10]

In 1995, a pioneer in this research, Dr. Jonathan Van Blerkom, was first to suggest the link between the ATP level in an egg and that egg's potential to mature properly and become a high-quality embryo.[11] This has since been confirmed by several researchers who have demonstrated that an egg's ability to produce a spike of ATP in the specific time and place needed for major developmental tasks is critical for proper egg development.[12]

The ability to make energy when needed may be the single most important factor in determining the competence of eggs and embryos.[13] The more easily an egg can produce energy, the more likely it is to mature and successfully fertilize.[14]

An egg with good mitochondrial function is also more likely to mature with the correct number of chromosomes. This is because the process of separating and ejecting chromosomes is very energy-intensive.[15] Scientists have actually seen the mitochondria cluster together and suddenly produce a burst of ATP at the precise time and place needed to form the structure that separates the chromosomes.[16]

If an egg does not have enough energy to neatly organize the chromosomes and separate the copies that are to be pushed out, it may end up with an extra copy of a chromosome, or a missing copy.

Just as we would expect, research has found that eggs and embryos with poorly functioning mitochondria are more likely to have chromosomal errors.[17] As discussed in earlier chapters, these errors are a major contributor to infertility and pregnancy loss.[18]

The role of energy supply does not end when an egg is fertilized—mitochondria from the egg also provides the fuel for a growing embryo. Problems with energy production in an egg can manifest later in embryo development because ATP is needed for all the work an embryo must do to grow and successfully implant.[19] Dysfunctional mitochondria in eggs are thought to be especially problematic for early embryo survival.[20]

CoQ10 to improve egg quality

Based on the critical role of mitochondria to egg and embryo quality, it stands to reason that anything we can do to help eggs produce more energy will improve egg quality and embryo viability. Research has found that CoQ10 does just that.

As explained by Dr. Yaakov Bentov, a fertility specialist who has pioneered the use of CoQ10 to improve egg quality, "our thought is that it's not the egg that's different [in older women]; it's the ability of the egg to produce the kind of energy needed to complete all the processes that are involved with maturing and being fertilized. That's why we're recommending that women use all these supplements like co-enzyme Q10."[21]

CoQ10 has powerful benefits because it is an essential raw ingredient needed for energy production by mitochondria.[22]

Many studies have shown that adding CoQ10 to cells grown in the laboratory increases the production of ATP.[23] It has also been found to protect mitochondria from damage.[24]

CoQ10 is naturally found in ovarian follicles, where it performs this important role of supporting energy production and protecting mitochondria. Researchers have even measured the amount of CoQ10 naturally present inside follicles, and they found a higher level in higher-quality eggs that are more likely to lead to pregnancy.[25]

By taking a CoQ10 supplement to increase the supply of this important nutrient, we can increase the energy supply needed to fuel egg development. This in turn helps prevent chromosomal errors and increase egg and embryo viability.

Controlled studies have confirmed that taking CoQ10 for one or two months before IVF can significantly boost egg quality.[26] CoQ10 increases the proportion of eggs that fertilize and develop into good-quality embryos. It also reduces the chance of a cycle being cancelled due to poor egg development. A double-blind, placebo-controlled study by Dr. Bentov and Dr. Casper also found a lower rate of chromosomal abnormalities in embryos from women taking CoQ10.[27]

Supplementing With CoQ10

CoQ10 is made in just about every cell in the body, but as we age, the body may not be able to make enough CoQ10 to keep up with the demands to make cellular energy. It is extremely difficult to obtain significant amounts from food, so adding a supplement is the best solution.

In the clinical trials conducted so far, the dose ranged from

400–600 milligrams (mg) per day of CoQ10, starting one or two months before IVF. This is actually a fairly conservative dose, with studies outside the fertility context reporting safety of much higher doses. A recent double-blind study reported no safety concerns with 2,400 mg taken daily for five years.[28]

To benefit egg quality, the minimum dose likely depends on the precise form of CoQ10 used. The standard form in supplements is called ubiquinone. This form is not very soluble, so much of it is not absorbed. What does get absorbed is then converted to the active antioxidant form, ubiquinol.[29]

To get around the problem of poor absorption, there are two solutions. The first is to buy a supplement already in the form of ubiquinol. Even though ubiquinol is typically more expensive than traditional CoQ10, it may still offer better value because you can take a lower dose and will absorb significantly more of the active ingredient.[30]

The second solution is to choose a special formulation of ubiquinone that is designed to be more readily absorbed. A variety of formulations have been developed to increase absorption of ubiquinone, such as suspending it in tiny droplets.[31] Studies have shown that some of these high-tech formulations are absorbed significantly better than traditional ubiquinone supplements.[32] One brand with particularly clear data is Bio-Quinon by Pharma Nord.

A study published in the journal *Nutrition* in 2019 tested seven different supplement formulations containing 100 mg of CoQ10 in 14 young, healthy individuals.[33] They found that the two formulations that were best at raising CoQ10 levels in the body were ubiquinol Kaneka QH (found in Jarrow's Ubiquinol, for instance) and a particular soft-gel version of ubiquinone in a soy oil matrix, made by Pharma Nord.

This second version is sold under the name Myoqinon in Europe and Bio-Quinon Q10 Gold in the United States. Participants absorbed more than twice as much CoQ10 from these formulations compared to the other supplements. If these supplements are not available to you or are outside your price range, another solution is to take a higher dose of standard CoQ10.

If you are just beginning the process of trying to conceive and have no reason to expect fertility problems, a dose of 200 mg of ubiquinol or Bio-Quinon is probably sufficient.

The recommended dose for those with any fertility challenges or history of pregnancy loss is 400 mg of ubiquinol or a high-absorption form of CoQ10. Alternatively, you may decide to take 600 mg of standard CoQ10, although this may still be less effective than the recommended formulations. Some IVF clinics now take an even more aggressive approach and recommend 600 mg of Bio-Quinon or ubiquinol. There is likely little downside to this higher dose other than additional cost.

In addition to choosing one of the preferred forms of CoQ10, you can also maximize the benefit by dividing the dose. That is because there is a limit to how much can be absorbed at a time, with the percentage absorbed beginning to drop when the dose is above 200 mg. If you are taking 400 mg per day, it is therefore helpful to take the supplement in two separate doses—one 200 mg capsule with breakfast and another capsule with lunch.[34] (Some people experience trouble sleeping when CoQ10 is taken at night.) CoQ10 is fat soluble and therefore best absorbed with meals.

Safety and side effects

Because CoQ10 holds promise in treating a range of diseases associated with impaired mitochondrial function, it has been studied extensively in large clinical trials. As part of these double-blind, placebo-controlled clinical studies, thousands of people have taken ubiquinone CoQ10 at high doses over many years and have been carefully observed. Researchers have reported no safety concerns, even at doses as high as 3,000 mg/day.[35] At the time of writing, the only significant side effect reported in clinical studies is mild gastrointestinal symptoms in a small number of people.[36]

Although rare, there have been anecdotal reports of CoQ10 or ubiquinol delaying ovulation by several days for some people. There is no scientific research on this issue, so it is difficult to know the mechanism or whether this provides a reason to reduce the dose if your cycle length changes. The research as a whole suggests that the benefits of CoQ10 for egg quality likely outweigh the potential for slight disruption of cycle length.

A small number of people may also experience low blood pressure or headaches with ubiquinol or CoQ10. This problem can usually be solved by switching from ubiquinol to CoQ10 (or vice versa), switching to a brand that uses fewer inactive ingredients, or lowering the dose.

One final possible effect of CoQ10 to be aware of is that it may gradually improve blood sugar control in people with type 2 diabetes, so your medication may need to be adjusted.[37]

When to start and when to stop

Whether you are trying to conceive naturally or with the help of IUI or IVF, it is best to start taking CoQ10 as early as possible, ideally at least three months before a planned IUI or IVF cycle. Because it takes approximately three months for eggs to fully develop, supplementing throughout this window of time allows the eggs to mature in an optimal environment, with a good supply of energy to process chromosomes correctly. Nevertheless, the most recent clinical studies show that even taking CoQ10 for one or two months before IVF can be very helpful.

It is typical to continue taking CoQ10 until you get a positive pregnancy test. In the context of IVF, many clinics recommend stopping CoQ10 and other egg-quality supplements the day before egg retrieval because the supplements are no longer needed. But continuing to take CoQ10 after egg retrieval could also potentially help prepare the uterine lining for embryo transfer, as discussed in chapter 14.

The general recommendation is to stop taking CoQ10 during pregnancy, simply because there is a lack of data demonstrating safety during pregnancy, and there is good reason to be conservative with supplements during this time. Yet there is little reason to expect that taking CoQ10 while pregnant is harmful. On the contrary, research so far indicates that a low dose of CoQ10 during pregnancy may reduce the risk of complications such as preeclampsia.[38] It may also reduce the risk of miscarriage.[39]

Although the main role of CoQ10 in preventing miscarriage is reducing chromosomal errors in eggs, research suggests another link that goes beyond egg quality. Specifically, CoQ10 appears to reduce the immune and clotting mediators involved in antiphospholipid syndrome, a common cause of miscarriage. In a randomized, placebo-controlled study, 36 patients with antiphospholipid syndrome were randomized to receive 200 mg/day of ubiquinol or a placebo.[40] After one month, there was a significant reduction in the immune and clotting mediators involved in antiphospholipid syndrome. We do not know how this would translate to miscarriage, but it is a promising avenue of research.

Action Steps

CoQ10 can protect energy production in developing eggs, providing the fuel for chromosome processing and embryo development. This likely translates into fewer chromosomal abnormalities and embryos with a greater potential to develop into a healthy pregnancy.

Whether you are trying to conceive naturally or through IVF, and whether you face any specific fertility challenges or are merely looking to support your preconception health, CoQ10 is one of the most useful supplements to take when trying to conceive.

The best forms are ubiquinol and high-absorption ubiquinone.

Basic Plan

200 mg, once per day

Intermediate and Advanced Plan

400–600 mg, ideally divided into two doses

Chapter 7

Melatonin and Antioxidants

*"All truth passes through three stages: First,
it is ridiculed; second, it is violently opposed;
third, it is accepted as self-evident."*
— ARTHUR SCHOPENHAUER

Recommended for
Intermediate and Advanced Fertility Plans

OVARIAN FOLLICLES NATURALLY contain a whole host of antioxidant vitamins and enzymes that serve to protect developing eggs from oxidative damage. Unfortunately, these antioxidants decline with age and are often diminished in women with fertility problems. The good news is that we have the opportunity to improve egg quality and avoid some of the damage to eggs by restoring the antioxidant defense system.

What are antioxidants?

The process of oxidation can be seen in everyday life, such as when metal rusts or silver tarnishes. Analogous chemical reactions constantly occur inside cells. If not kept in check, oxidation can damage DNA, proteins, lipids, cell membranes, and mitochondria. But that is where antioxidants come in— they can be considered protectors against this chemical reaction of oxidation, analogous to using lemon juice to prevent an apple turning brown.

Antioxidants work by neutralizing free radicals. We produce free radicals continuously as a byproduct of normal metabolism, and these highly reactive and unstable molecules steal electrons from other molecules they encounter, causing damage in the process. Antioxidants can donate a spare electron to a free radical, neutralizing it and preventing oxidative damage.

Each cell has an army of antioxidant defenses, including specialized antioxidant enzymes and vitamins, such as vitamins A, C, and E. In developing eggs, these antioxidants play a critical role in preventing oxidative damage.

How do antioxidants impact egg quality?

As we age, oxidative damage causes more and more problems for eggs.[1] This is in part due to a weakened antioxidant enzyme defense system. In eggs from older women, the production of antioxidant enzymes dwindles, which leaves more oxidizing molecules free to cause damage.[2] Unfortunately, eggs from older women also have a greater need for antioxidants because aging or damaged mitochondria release more free radicals.[3]

If the antioxidant defense system cannot keep up, damage to mitochondria reduces their ability to produce cellular energy in the form of ATP—energy that is critically important to egg development and embryo viability. Oxidative damage to mitochondria is now thought to be one of the major ways that aging impacts egg quality. [4]

This oxidative damage is not limited to eggs from older women. Researchers have also found higher levels in women with unexplained infertility, recurrent miscarriage, pre-eclampsia, and endometriosis.[5] For example, two studies found higher levels of oxidative damage in the follicles of women with endometriosis, and this was associated with a lower chance of an egg making it to the blastocyst stage.[6]

In women with PCOS, the role of oxidative stress is even more pronounced. PCOS often involves insulin resistance and high blood sugar. As a result of this high blood sugar, the body produces more reactive oxygen molecules, which increases oxidative stress.[7]

Fortunately, antioxidants may be able to prevent some of this damage, with the net effect of improving fertility.[8] Researchers have found that women with higher total antioxidant levels during IVF cycles have a greater chance of becoming pregnant.[9] A large study of women undergoing fertility treatment in Boston found the use of antioxidant supplements was associated with a shorter time to pregnancy.[10]

Although there is still much more to investigate and many conflicting results so far, the balance of the current evidence suggests that having well-armed antioxidant defenses can protect eggs and improve fertility.

The specific antioxidant supplements most useful for fertility are melatonin, vitamin E, vitamin C, alpha-lipoic acid, and N-acetylcysteine. Each of these supplements serves slightly different purposes and may suit different situations, as the remainder of this chapter explains.

Melatonin

Melatonin is a hormone secreted at night by a small gland deep inside the brain, the pineal gland. It is used as a supplement to help with sleep because melatonin regulates circadian rhythms, telling the body to go to sleep at night and wake up in the morning. It is so important in regulating sleep that exposure to bright light at night, which suppresses melatonin production in the brain, can compromise sleep quality and cause insomnia.

Melatonin is not just a sleep regulator, though; it is also involved in fertility. In some species, melatonin is involved in regulating seasonal fertility to ensure that lambs, calves, and other baby animals are born in spring.[11] Melatonin also plays a surprisingly important role in human fertility.

One clue that melatonin is important to human fertility is that particularly high levels of melatonin are found in the fluid of ovarian follicles.[12] In addition, the amount of melatonin increases as the follicles grow, and this is thought to play an important role in ovulation.[13]

Melatonin and fertility

Melatonin has traditionally been regarded as a hormonal messenger molecule that works by binding to specific receptors and thereby sending a message to cells. In other words, it was thought of as a molecule that merely communicates rather than having a direct biological effect. But in 1993, it was discovered that melatonin is also a powerful antioxidant that directly neutralizes free radicals.[14] This has since been confirmed by many different studies.[15]

Melatonin levels decline with age and as a result, the ovaries start to lose this natural protector against oxidative stress.[16] This likely plays a role in declining ovarian reserve.[17] Studies have found that women with higher melatonin levels tend to have a higher AMH level and a higher follicle count. [18] There is also a correlation between melatonin levels and the results of IVF cycles, with higher melatonin levels corresponding to a greater number of eggs retrieved and more high-quality embryos after IVF.[19]

A reduction in melatonin could therefore be one contributor to age-related infertility, but it is also a factor that can be changed. There is clear evidence that melatonin supplementation can restore antioxidant defenses inside eggs and improve egg quality.

Over the past 20 years, an array of studies has demonstrated that melatonin helps eggs mature properly and develop into good-quality embryos.[20] In one of these studies, women were given melatonin from the beginning of an IVF cycle, and their egg quality was compared with the previous cycle. After treatment with melatonin, there was a dramatic improvement, with an average of 65% of their eggs giving rise to good-quality embryos, compared to just 27% in the previous cycle.[21] A larger follow-up study demonstrated that supplementing with melatonin before IVF improved the percentage of eggs that fertilized and nearly doubled the chance of becoming pregnant.[22]

The ability of melatonin supplements to improve egg quality in IVF has now been observed in a range of other studies, including double-blind, placebo-controlled trials.[23] The benefits are often particularly clear for women undergoing IVF who have had failed IVF cycles due to poor egg quality or diminished ovarian reserve.

As a side benefit, melatonin can also improve sleep and help reduce pain associated with chronic migraine and endometriosis.[24]

Adding a melatonin supplement before IVF

In the United States, melatonin is available over the counter in supplement form. In many other countries, a prescription is normally required, although it can also be ordered online from overseas.

The optimal timing of when to start a melatonin supplement before IVF is still an open issue. Even starting a few weeks or a month before egg retrieval is beneficial, improving fertilization rates and the proportion of good-quality embryos.[25] In a 2017 double-blind study, melatonin was started about one month before IVF, and the women taking melatonin were twice as likely to have top-quality embryos compared to those in the placebo group. [26]

Yet it is likely to be more effective when started earlier, to give ovarian follicles the protective benefit of melatonin throughout the final three months of the egg development cycle.

The typical dose used in IVF studies when melatonin is taken for up to one month is 3 mg per day, taken shortly before bed. This dose is fairly high when compared to how much melatonin the body naturally produces. More recent research reported positive results from a dose of 1 mg per day for three months, but it is possible an even lower dose is effective when taken for this length of time.

Melatonin outside the IVF context

Traditionally, melatonin has only been recommended for women trying to conceive through IVF, not those trying to conceive naturally or through IUI. It was thought that melatonin could alter the production of hormones that control the ovulation cycle and thereby disrupt ovulation.[27]

It may be time to question that thinking, given recent studies finding that melatonin can help improve ovulation in the context of Clomid treatment.[28] It can also help regulate ovulation in women with PCOS, with one study reporting a normalization in menstrual cycles in 95% of women with PCOS who took melatonin for six months. [29]

In addition, the original research suggesting that melatonin disrupts ovulation involved a very high dose; 100 times greater than the 3 mg typically used as a supplement. Many women regularly take 1–3 mg of melatonin for insomnia, and there is little evidence that this disrupts ovulation. To the contrary, one study found that when women in their forties and fifties took 3 mg of melatonin each night for 6 months, there was a slight improvement in LH and FSH levels and some menopausal women resumed normal menstrual cycles.[30]

Even so, a conservative option if you are trying to conceive naturally is to take an even lower dose to replicate our normal biology more closely. The amount of melatonin the body produces naturally is just 0.1–0.3 mg (100–300 mcg) per day. By supplementing with around 300 mcg per day, we would be effectively restoring the level of melatonin seen in young women and correcting the decline in melatonin that naturally occurs with age. Although more research is needed on whether this low dose can improve fertility, it may be just enough to provide antioxidant support to developing eggs.

Other Fertility-Boosting Antioxidants

Vitamin E

Vitamin E is a fat-soluble antioxidant found in nuts, seeds, and oils. It is an important part of our natural antioxidant defense system, particularly in ovarian follicles.[31] The chemical name for vitamin E, tocopherol, is based on this important role, coming from the Greek words *tocos*, meaning "childbirth," and *phero*, meaning "to bring forth."[32]

Researchers have seen that when there is sufficient vitamin E in ovarian follicles, egg quality is typically higher, with a higher percentage of mature eggs and a lower percentage of degenerated, abnormal, or immature eggs.[33] Although further research is needed, experts now believe that vitamin E may compensate for some of the decline in antioxidants that naturally occurs as women age.[34] Vitamin E seems to be particularly useful for women with age-related infertility, unexplained infertility, or endometriosis.[35]

In a study of women with unexplained infertility, researchers found that women who had a greater intake of vitamin E through supplements were likely to get pregnant sooner.[36] Another study found that supplementing with both vitamin E and selenium could increase markers of ovarian reserve, including AMH and the number of developing follicles visible on ultrasound.[37]

The commonly recommended dose for vitamin E is 200 IU per day. Check with your doctor before adding vitamin E if you are taking Warfarin, Lovenox, or high-dose aspirin, because the combination may enhance the anti-clotting effects of these medications. This is not thought to be a concern with low-dose aspirin.

As will be discussed in chapter 14, vitamin E also appears to be helpful for supporting the development of the uterine lining in preparation for embryo transfer.

Vitamin C

It has been known since the 1950s that ovarian follicles accumulate a large amount of vitamin C.[38] It was suspected that this vitamin C was there for a reason—perhaps playing a role in hormone production. It has now become clear that vitamin C not only helps prevent oxidative damage in the ovaries but also supports the production of progesterone after ovulation.

In one of the most interesting studies, women with low progesterone were randomly assigned to either vitamin C supplementation or no treatment and were tracked for six months or until they got pregnant.[39] Women were eligible for the study if their progesterone level was less than 10 ng/mL at five, seven, or nine days after ovulation. The study revealed that more than half the women taking vitamin C had their progesterone increase to a normal level, with the average going from 8 ng/mL to 13 ng/mL. The women taking vitamin C were also twice as likely to get pregnant as the women not taking vitamin C.

The amount of vitamin C provided by a healthy diet and a good-quality prenatal multivitamin may be sufficient for most women, but supplementing with additional vitamin C is likely to be helpful for those with low progesterone or a condition associated with increased oxidative damage, such as PCOS or endometriosis.

In a randomized trial of women with endometriosis who were trying to conceive through IVF, supplementing with 1000 mg of vitamin C per day for two months before IVF led to a significantly higher number of good-quality embryos and a slightly higher chance of pregnancy.[40]

If you choose to add a vitamin C supplement, the typical dose is 500 mg per day, or 1000 mg per day for those with endometriosis.

Alpha-lipoic acid

Alpha-lipoic acid is a key antioxidant that plays a variety of roles in the body. It helps recycle CoQ10, vitamin C, and vitamin E back into their active antioxidant forms while also increasing the level of another critical antioxidant called glutathione. Perhaps most importantly for our purposes, alpha-lipoic acid is found naturally in mitochondria, where it assists with energy production.[41] Supplementing with alpha-lipoic acid appears to help protect mitochondria from the effects of aging.[42]

We are still waiting for clinical trials to confirm the benefits of alpha-lipoic acid for age-related infertility, but studies have demonstrated clear benefits for male fertility and women with PCOS.

In PCOS, supplementing with alpha-lipoic acid results in a higher number of good-quality embryos after IVF.[43] It can also help address the hormonal imbalances characteristic of PCOS and restore normal ovulation.[44] As will be discussed in chapter 13 on male fertility, clinical studies have found that supplementing with alpha-lipoic acid also significantly improves sperm count, concentration, and motility.[45]

In addition, alpha-lipoic acid reduces inflammation and may therefore have particular benefit for those with endometriosis or recurrent miscarriage, two conditions in which inflammation is thought to play a major role.[46]

Even though more research is needed, the ability of alpha-lipoic acid to protect mitochondrial function and support the entire antioxidant system suggests it is likely to be helpful whenever egg quality is an issue.

Alpha-lipoic acid and hypothyroidism

It has been suggested that alpha-lipoic acid may lower thyroid hormones by reducing the conversion of T4 to the active hormone T3.[47] That did not seem to occur in a study of women with subclinical hypothyroidism taking alpha-lipoic acid for three weeks,[48] but if you have an underactive thyroid, it may be better to choose an alternative antioxidant or monitor your thyroid function regularly. Alpha-lipoic acid may also improve blood sugar levels in diabetics,[49] necessitating an adjustment to medication.

Dosage and form of alpha-lipoic acid

The typical dose is 400–600 mg per day of standard form alpha-lipoic acid, or 200–300 mg per day of the more purified form, called R-alpha lipoic acid or R-lipoic acid for short. Alpha-lipoic acid is somewhat better absorbed on an empty stomach, but this can cause nausea or heartburn for some people, and it will still be effective if taken with food.

N-acetylcysteine

N-acetylcysteine (NAC) is an amino acid derivative that not only directly reduces oxidative damage but also helps replenish one of the most important antioxidants found in virtually every cell in the body: glutathione. [50] NAC can also help reduce damage caused by environmental toxins such as BPA,[51] along with improving mitochondrial function in developing eggs. [52]

There have only been a few studies of NAC in women with unexplained or age-related infertility, but the results have been promising. In women with unexplained infertility, supplementing with NAC before a cycle of Clomid and IUI significantly improved egg development, increasing the number of good-size follicles and increasing the pregnancy rate.[53] Similarly, in a randomized study in women preparing for IVF, those taking NAC ended up with more eggs retrieved and a higher chance of getting pregnant (74% versus 50%). There was also a much lower level of the toxin homocysteine in ovarian follicles.[54]

If N-acetylcysteine can reduce homocysteine levels in ovarian follicles, that has wide implications for a range of causes of infertility. Homocysteine is incredibly damaging for developing eggs because it damages mitochondria. One of the main ways in which folate boosts fertility is by detoxifying homocysteine. It is clearly helpful to have yet another tool to assist with this important detoxification work and thereby support energy production in developing eggs.

N-acetylcysteine may therefore be particularly important for those with risk factors associated with high homocysteine levels, such as genetic variations in folate metabolism genes (including MTHFR) and those with premature ovarian failure or a history of recurrent miscarriage.

N-acetylcysteine and PCOS

The clearest evidence demonstrating the ability of N-acetylcysteine to improve fertility comes from clinical trials in PCOS. A series of randomized, double-blind, placebo-controlled studies have now found that in women with PCOS, supplementing with N-acetylcysteine restores ovulation, improves egg and embryo quality, increases the chance of pregnancy, and reduces miscarriage rates.[55] This has been seen in women trying to conceive naturally, those taking medications such as Clomid or letrozole, and those trying to conceive through IVF.

The difference that N-acetylcysteine makes is perhaps most dramatic in the women with PCOS who have been struggling with infertility the longest. In one clinical trial, women with PCOS who on average had suffered from infertility for more than four years took N-acetylcysteine and the ovulation-stimulating drug Clomid for five days. After treatment, 21% of the women taking N-acetylcysteine became pregnant compared to 9% of women taking the placebo.[56]

Preventing miscarriage with N-acetylcysteine

Just as we would expect from its ability to reduce inflammation and homocysteine, N-acetylcysteine also appears to reduce miscarriage risk.

When compared with folic acid alone, the combination of NAC and folic acid has been associated with a significant decrease in the chance of miscarriage. In one study, the women taking N-acetylcysteine were twice as likely to take home a baby.[57] Other studies have also shown that N-acetylcysteine decreases the miscarriage rate by 60% in women with PCOS.[58]

N-acetylcysteine and endometriosis

N-acetylcysteine may also be particularly helpful for those with endometriosis. In a recent laboratory study, researchers demonstrated that this antioxidant can help counteract the negative influence of endometriosis on egg quality.[59] In addition, a clinical study in Italy found that in women with endometriosis, taking N-acetylcysteine can reduce the pain and cysts associated with this condition.[60] After three months of treatment, one-third of the patients taking N-acetylcysteine showed sufficient improvement that their surgery was canceled. In the words of the study authors, "We can conclude that NAC actually represents a simple, effective treatment for endometriosis, without side effects, and a suitable approach for women desiring a pregnancy."

Safety and side effects of N-acetylcysteine

N-acetylcysteine is widely recommended by doctors for a variety of conditions,[61] but allergies and side effects sometimes occur. Rarely, allergic reactions have occurred after the use of high doses of intravenous N-acetylcysteine to treat pain-killer overdose.[62] In some people, N-acetylcysteine also causes nausea, diarrhea, or abdominal pain. If you experience these side effects, it likely makes sense to stop the supplement and focus on the other antioxidants discussed in this chapter.

Dosage of N-acetylcysteine

The typical dose of N-acetylcysteine used in clinical trials is 600 mg per day.

N-acetylcysteine versus acetyl-L-carnitine

Acetyl-L-carnitine is another supplement that is often confused with N-acetylcysteine. They are entirely different molecules that cannot be substituted for one another, but both have beneficial effects.

N-acetylcysteine is made from the amino acid cysteine. In contrast, carnitine is made from the amino acid lysine. Carnitine exists in two common forms, as L-carnitine or acetyl-L-carnitine. It is often taken as a sports and weight loss supplement because it aids the conversion of fat into cellular energy. Research shows that this supplement is also likely to benefit sperm quality because it is an antioxidant that participates in energy production in the mitochondria. Yet the effect on egg quality is still quite uncertain.

In the context of female fertility, most of the research to date has focused on the L-carnitine form, specifically in the context of PCOS. Randomized clinical trials have found that in women with PCOS, L-carnitine supports weight loss, regulates insulin levels, restores ovulation, helps eggs develop to maturity, and improves pregnancy rates.[63] These studies fit together with the finding that L-carnitine levels are often significantly lower in women with PCOS.[64] If you have PCOS, consider adding L-carnitine at a dose of 3 g per day. It is not recommended if you are hypothyroid.

For women without PCOS, there is not enough evidence at this stage to support the use of either L-carnitine or acetyl-L-carnitine. The majority of animal studies have found beneficial effects for female fertility, but others have reported the opposite.[65] One IVF study found that although L-carnitine does not increase the number of eggs retrieved or their ability to fertilize, it may increase the proportion of fertilized eggs that become a good-quality embryo on day five.[66] It is still too early to know for sure whether this supplement is beneficial for women, but it could be considered if you have had previous IVF cycles in which many embryos stopped growing between fertilization and day five. For men, the evidence supporting this supplement is much stronger, as discussed in chapter 13.

Conclusion

Many experts believe that oxidative damage to mitochondria is a major mechanism underlying ovarian aging.[67] To support energy production in developing eggs, oxidative damage must be continuously kept in check by the eggs' natural antioxidant defense system. In women with age-related infertility, endometriosis, PCOS, or unexplained infertility, these defenses may be compromised, allowing damage to go unchecked. Antioxidant supplements can help address this problem, giving immature eggs a healthy and protective environment in which to develop.

Action Steps

How many and which antioxidants you should add to your supplement regime depends on the fertility challenge you are facing, but it is reasonable to choose two or three supplements within this category. For specific examples of supplement plans, see chapter 11.

The most helpful antioxidants are usually melatonin, N-acetylcysteine, and alpha-lipoic acid, but if you have a sensitive stomach, a combination of melatonin and vitamin C and E may work better for you. The typical doses are:

- Melatonin: 1–3mg for IVF or PCOS or 0.3–1 mg in other cases
- Vitamin E: 200 IU
- Vitamin C: 500 mg
- Alpha-lipoic acid: 200-300 mg of R-lipoic acid, or 400-600 mg of standard form
- N-acetylcysteine: 600 mg

Chapter 8

Restoring Ovulation with Myo-Inositol

"Sometimes the questions are complicated and the answers are simple."
— Dr. Seuss

Recommended for
Intermediate and Advanced Fertility Plans

MYO-INOSITOL IS MOST helpful for improving egg quality in women with PCOS or insulin resistance. In some cases, it may also be helpful if you have had a previous IVF cycle in which many eggs were immature or failed to fertilize, you have high FSH, a history of unexplained recurrent miscarriage, or you are not ovulating regularly.

What is myo-inositol?

Myo-inositol is a type of sugar molecule naturally found in a variety of foods, such as fruits, vegetables, grains, and nuts.

It is generally regarded as a type of B vitamin (vitamin B8), but it is not truly considered an essential vitamin, because the body can produce it from glucose. Myo-inositol performs a variety of important functions, including playing a key role in glucose transport into cells, the conversion of testosterone into estrogen, and transmitting the signal from FSH that tells ovarian follicles to develop.

In the fertility context, myo-inositol is most often used to treat PCOS, because it is one of the most effective ways of addressing the specific hormonal imbalances characteristic of that condition. Yet there is a growing interest in using myo-inositol in the absence of PCOS to improve the number and quality of eggs in IVF and address recurrent miscarriage caused by insulin resistance.

Myo-inositol for IVF

For women without PCOS or insulin resistance, the value of myo-inositol is still uncertain, but there have been some promising results in recent studies.[1] Overall, the most consistent finding in the research is that in women without PCOS who are trying to conceive through IVF, myo-inositol may not make much difference to overall success rates, but it can increase the percentage of eggs that are mature and increase the percentage that fertilize.[2]

This limited evidence probably does not justify adding this supplement under ordinary circumstances, but myo-inositol may be worth considering if

- in previous IVF cycles, many eggs were immature or failed to fertilize

- you have insulin resistance or high fasting insulin
- you have irregular or long cycles (more than 30 days)
- you have hormonal disruptions commonly associated with PCOS (such as high testosterone or high AMH)

In addition, because myo-inositol plays a role in FSH signaling, it has been suggested that this supplement could improve egg development in women who have high FSH and have poor egg growth in response to stimulation medication in IVF.

As will be discussed later in this chapter, myo-inositol may also play a role in preventing miscarriage in some cases.

Myo-inositol and PCOS

Myo-inositol is one of the most effective ways of improving fertility in women with PCOS because it can help correct the hormonal imbalances characteristic of this condition, including insulin resistance and high testosterone.

Doctors have known for more than 30 years that PCOS is associated with a high level of insulin.[3] This insulin can directly compromise fertility by raising the level of testosterone in the ovaries, which can inhibit the final stages of egg development.[4] High testosterone results in a large number of immature eggs that may never mature enough to reach the stage of ovulation.

One of the potential causes of both high insulin and high testosterone in PCOS is a defect in the processing of molecules in the inositol family. These important molecules, which include myo-inositol and D-chiro inositol, are involved in both the function of insulin and the conversion of testosterone to estrogen. In PCOS, there is often an excess of D-chiro inositol and not enough myo-inositol. Supplementing with myo-inositol can therefore address the underlying cause of infertility in PCOS by restoring insulin function and removing the block on conversion of testosterone into estrogen.[5]

Many studies have now consistently shown that taking a myo-inositol supplement is beneficial in women with PCOS. One of the first studies reported that over the course of six months taking myo-inositol, 72% of women began ovulating normally again.[6] More than half then became pregnant. Other researchers have reported the same pattern.[7]

In IVF studies, myo-inositol has been found to increase the proportion of mature eggs retrieved and decrease the number of immature and degenerated eggs.[8] When it is taken for at least three months before IVF, it can also increase the proportion of eggs that develop into good-quality embryos.[9]

In short, myo-inositol seems to improve egg development and embryo quality in women with PCOS, along with lowering insulin and improving blood sugar control. And it is not just women with poor insulin sensitivity who can benefit. A study conducted in Italy found that even in PCOS patients with a normal insulin response, myo-inositol treatment improved egg and embryo quality during IVF, likely because it also plays a role in the conversion of testosterone to estrogen.[10]

The fertility benefits of myo-inositol may be even more pronounced when it is used in combination with other supplements, particularly melatonin. Researchers have found that when women with PCOS take both melatonin and myo-inositol, the result is better than either alone, with a synergistic improvement in egg and embryo quality.[11]

PCOS and gestational diabetes

If you have PCOS, taking myo-inositol could have another added benefit: reducing your risk of gestational diabetes. This condition, which involves high blood sugar levels during pregnancy, is much more common in women with PCOS.

In 2012, researchers found that women with PCOS taking a myo-inositol supplement during their pregnancy had a much lower risk of gestational diabetes: just 17% compared to 54% in women not taking the supplement.[12] Several other clinical trials have now reported similar positive results. In 2015, the Cochrane Organization reviewed the trials available at that time and concluded that myo-inositol does show a potential benefit for reducing the incidence of gestational diabetes.[13] If you have PCOS or other risk factors for gestational diabetes, you should therefore ask your doctor whether to continue taking myo-inositol during pregnancy.

Myo-inositol and miscarriage

Myo-inositol may also play a role in preventing miscarriage. One of the common culprits behind recurrent miscarriage is insulin resistance.[14] Insulin resistance occurs when cells in your muscles, fat, and liver stop responding well to insulin's message to take up glucose. This results in high blood glucose and even higher insulin levels. Symptoms include excessive thirst or hunger, fatigue, and frequent infections.

In one study, insulin resistance was more than twice as common in women with a history of multiple miscarriages.[15] There are many potential explanations for the link, but researchers have recently found that insulin can directly damage cells in the placenta.[16]

As a result, if you have a history of miscarriage, it can be useful to test your fasting insulin level. If it is above 10 mIU/L, treatment to lower your insulin level could also reduce your chance of another miscarriage.

Myo-inositol is one of the most effective ways of addressing high insulin levels because it plays a key role in insulin signaling and helps cells soak up glucose. It is as effective as the insulin-sensitizing drug Metformin, which is typically used to treat diabetes.[17]

Safety, side effects, and dose

Myo-inositol is a natural compound found in food and made in the body in significant amounts each day. Supplementing with additional myo-inositol has been described as very safe, with only high doses of 12 g per day causing mild gastrointestinal symptoms such as nausea.[18] Myo-inositol should be used with caution if you have schizophrenia or bipolar disorder because there is a theoretical risk of exacerbating manic episodes.[19]

The typical recommended dose, shown to be effective in clinical studies, is 4 g per day, divided into two doses: half in the morning and half at night. This is similar to the amount of myo-inositol naturally produced in the body each day. Ideally, myo-inositol should be taken for at least three months before IVF. Talk to your doctor about when to stop the supplement. Many doctors recommend that women with PCOS or insulin resistance continue myo-inositol through pregnancy to prevent gestational diabetes.

What about d-chiro inositol?

A similar-sounding and related compound, D-chiro inositol, is often used by women with PCOS in the hope of improving their fertility, but in large doses it may have just the opposite effect: reducing the number and quality of eggs.[20] This negative effect is unfortunately not widely known. The early studies showing a possible benefit of D-chiro inositol have overshadowed more recent studies showing that the supplement simply does not work or may do more harm than good.[21] As just one example, one study found that women with PCOS who were given D-chiro inositol rather than a placebo had fewer eggs and fewer good-quality embryos.[22]

Researchers are now beginning to understand why D-chiro inositol is so unhelpful in PCOS. In the body, an enzyme converts a small proportion of myo-inositol to D-chiro inositol to maintain the proper ratio for different parts of the body. In the liver and muscles, the normal ratio is approximately 40:1, with 40 parts myo-inositol to 1 part D-chiro inositol. In the ovaries, the normal proportion of myo-inositol is even greater, with a ratio of approximately 100:1.

The two closely related molecules actually have distinct jobs to do in the ovaries. Myo-inositol supports the function of follicle-stimulating hormone (FSH), whereas D-chiro inositol supports testosterone production.[23] It appears that PCOS may involve overactive conversion of myo-inositol into D-chiro inositol, depleting normal levels of myo-inositol and causing excess testosterone production.[24] This could in turn cause poor egg quality, which would explain why myo-inositol could improve egg quality, whereas supplementing with large amounts of D-chiro inositol could simply make the problem worse.

Some of the popular myo-inositol supplements marketed for fertility purposes, such as Ovasitol, include a small amount of D-chiro inositol. The idea behind this combination is mimicking the 40:1 ratio of myo-inositol to D-chiro inositol that is naturally found in the body. This combination supplement has been shown to improve metabolic function and ovulation in women with PCOS,[25] but it is unclear whether it has any advantage over the use of myo-inositol alone.

Action Steps

- If you have PCOS, insulin resistance, or irregular ovulation, consider adding a daily myo-inositol supplement to rebalance hormones.

- Myo-inositol may also be worth considering if you had a previous IVF cycle in which many eggs were immature or failed to fertilize, or you have high FSH and your follicles did not respond to stimulation medication.

- The typical dose is 4 g per day, half in the morning and half at night.

Chapter 9

DHEA for Low Ovarian Reserve

"Don't be discouraged. It's often the last
key in the bunch that opens the lock."

— UNKNOWN

Recommended for
Diminished Ovarian Reserve and Age-Related Infertility

DHEA IS A hormone precursor used by the ovaries to make estrogen and testosterone. Because it plays such a vital role in hormone production and often declines with age, correcting a deficiency may help address low ovarian reserve. It is most often used in preparation for IVF, but DHEA may also improve the odds of getting pregnant naturally. Supplementing with DHEA could also be helpful for a newly recognized form of PCOS characterized by low testosterone, although the research in that area is just beginning.

Not recommended for...

Even though DHEA is sold over the counter as a nutritional supplement, it is a hormone that can increase production of estrogen and testosterone. Before supplementing, it is important to check with your doctor and get lab testing to find out whether you are deficient. It is also important to have regular lab tests to ensure that your dose is not too high.

Starting DHEA in the month before IVF is not typically recommended because this supplement has the most benefit for early-stage follicles that are at least three months from ovulation. In addition, it can also take some experimentation to find the right dose. This is important because very high DHEA levels immediately before IVF can impair the final stages of egg development. In addition, DHEA can interact with some medications and is generally not recommended for those with high testosterone levels or a history of estrogen-sensitive cancer.

What Is DHEA?

DHEA stands for dehydroepiandrosterone. It is a hormone precursor made primarily by the adrenal glands, which sit above your kidneys, and in small amounts in the ovaries. The ovaries use DHEA to make estrogen and testosterone. Levels of DHEA typically decline with age, and this is thought to be one possible cause of age-related infertility.[1] DHEA levels may also be low in younger women with autoimmune conditions such as thyroid disease, rheumatoid arthritis, or antibodies that attack the adrenal glands. Autoimmunity is now understood to be a common cause of premature ovarian insufficiency, and studies have found that DHEA is often particularly low in women with both autoimmunity and poor ovarian function.[2]

If the adrenal glands cannot produce enough DHEA, the production of testosterone will drop, which impairs the early stages of egg development. As a result, fewer follicles are recruited to start maturing each month, and fewer survive to the stage at which they start producing AMH and become visible on ultrasound. The result is a low AMH and low follicle count, even if you have thousands of eggs remaining in the dormant stage ready to be recruited.

If testing shows that your DHEA levels are too low to support adequate testosterone production, correcting this deficiency could potentially increase both the number and quality of eggs available for retrieval in IVF or help you get pregnant naturally.[3] As discussed later in this chapter, DHEA may also reduce miscarriage risk by increasing the proportion of chromosomally normal eggs, although there is limited data on this point.

The Discovery of DHEA Boosting Fertility

The pioneers in the use of DHEA to increase fertility are the reproductive endocrinologists at the Center for Human Reproduction (CHR), a large IVF clinic in New York that specializes in treating older patients with low ovarian reserve. Their work on DHEA began with a single patient, a 43-year-old woman scouring the medical literature for anything that could help improve her egg numbers.

In her first IVF cycle, before taking DHEA, she produced just a single egg and embryo, and her doctors discouraged further attempts at IVF using her own eggs. Determined to have a child with her own eggs, she began her own search of the scientific literature for anything that could help.

During this research, she stumbled upon a publication from researchers at Baylor University suggesting a possible benefit of DHEA in IVF cycles.[4] The Baylor study described an increase in egg numbers in five women taking DHEA for two months, but it received very little attention until it was rediscovered and put to the test several years later by this individual patient in New York.

After reading the Baylor paper, she began taking DHEA supplements, unbeknownst to her doctors. In her second IVF cycle, she produced three eggs and embryos. Amazingly, as she continued taking DHEA, her egg and embryo numbers progressively increased.[5] She explains, "I was beginning to realize I was on to something."[6] The results were so astounding that her clinic quickly became pioneers in the use of DHEA to improve IVF outcomes. She ultimately produced 16 embryos in her ninth IVF cycle.[7]

This continuous improvement in egg numbers suggested that the beneficial effects of DHEA were cumulative. It is now understood that this longer-term effect is because DHEA has the greatest impact on survival of very early-stage follicles—those that are at least three or four months away from ovulation.

Who Can Benefit from DHEA?

Many fertility specialists now recommend DHEA to all their IVF patients who are diagnosed with diminished ovarian reserve, are over the age of 40, or have had an IVF cycle that produced very few eggs, regardless of hormone lab testing. A more nuanced approach that likely produces better results is to take DHEA only if lab tests show that your natural production of DHEA is low, resulting in low testosterone levels. When used in this way, DHEA may also be helpful for those trying to conceive naturally. These issues are explained in more detail in the sections that follow.

Correcting low DHEA in preparation for IVF

Most of the research on DHEA has focused on women with diminished ovarian reserve who are trying to conceive through IVF. This category includes women over 40 as well as younger women who have a low AMH or a low number of ovarian follicles visible on ultrasound.

Several randomized, controlled studies have reported that in women with diminished ovarian reserve, supplementing with DHEA for at least three months can improve pregnancy rates in IVF.[8] A controlled trial published in 2016, for example, found that women receiving DHEA before IVF were twice as likely to get pregnant.[9] A 2018 study showed similar results.[10]

Although these and other studies have reported encouraging results, some studies have found no significant benefit after supplementing with DHEA.[11] When researchers pool all the data from the various studies on DHEA in a so-called met-analysis, some researchers find a significant improvement in IVF pregnancy rates and others do not, depending on which trials are included or excluded from the analysis.[12]

One potential explanation for the mixed results is that in some cases DHEA was not given for long enough or to the right patients.[13] Only those who start with low levels of DHEA are likely to benefit.[14] It is also helpful to adjust the dose based on regular lab testing. But many of the clinical studies did not monitor DHEA levels before or during supplementation.

A lack of testing is problematic because when it comes to DHEA, more is not always better. If DHEA is either too low or too high, eggs are less likely to fertilize and less likely to develop into healthy embryos. One study elegantly revealed this "Goldilocks" effect by correcting both low and high DHEA levels to bring all patients into the normal range of 95–270 mcg/dL. Doing so significantly increased the number of eggs that fertilized and the pregnancy rate, for patients at both ends of the spectrum.[15] This explains why studies in which DHEA is prescribed across the board without testing or adjusting the dose may fail to show a benefit.

Overall, the research suggests that DHEA is likely to improve IVF success rates, but only when it is given for a sufficient time and only when it is used to bring low levels of DHEA and testosterone into the optimal range without raising levels too high.

Trying naturally with low ovarian reserve

Although most of the research on DHEA has focused on the IVF context, studies have also reported that it can improve pregnancy chances for those trying to conceive naturally or through IUI.[16] In the case of IUI, fertility specialists in Toronto reported positive results from treating women with DHEA for several months before a clomid-medicated IUI cycle. Compared to controls, DHEA-treated women showed higher follicle counts and improved pregnancy rates, with 30% conceiving versus 9% in the nontreated group, and a live birth rate of 21% versus 7%.[17]

Researchers have also reported surprising numbers of naturally conceived pregnancies in women taking DHEA.[18] A group of doctors in Italy were so intrigued by the number of their patients conceiving spontaneously while taking DHEA that they decided to conduct a study to investigate this phenomenon. The doctors reported that in a group of younger poor responders taking DHEA for three months before starting IVF, 25% became pregnant naturally before the IVF cycle began.[19] Amongst their patients over 40, the natural pregnancy rate among those taking DHEA was 21%, compared to just 4% in the control group.

This is an extraordinary finding that requires further confirmation, but it is in line with anecdotal reports from several other fertility clinics.[20] If correct, these results indicate that DHEA may improve fertility enough for many women with diminished ovarian reserve to conceive without the cost or risks of IVF.[21]

In rare cases, even women with severely compromised ovarian function have been able to conceive after supplementing with DHEA.[22] Several case reports have described women with either premature ovarian failure (POF) or premature ovarian insufficiency (POI) resuming normal cycles and conceiving naturally after several months of DHEA treatment.[23] This remarkable outcome appears to be relatively rare and a larger study reported disappointing results.[24] Nevertheless, if you fall into this category DHEA may be worth trying, even if the odds of success are low. Additional strategies for premature ovarian insufficiency are discussed in chapters 15 and 16.

DHEA and miscarriage

Although the evidence is still uncertain, it appears that DHEA may also reduce chromosomal abnormalities in eggs and thereby reduce the odds of miscarriage. A study of IVF patients reported a surprisingly low miscarriage rate in women taking DHEA.[25] Pregnancy loss was reduced by 50–80% in comparison to national averages, bringing the miscarriage rate down to just 15% of pregnancies.

Delving into the question a little further, the researchers then looked at data from women who underwent IVF and had their embryos screened for chromosomal abnormalities. The researchers found that women taking DHEA had a greater proportion of chromosomally normal embryos.[26]

Although more research is needed, these promising results suggest that DHEA may indeed reduce the rate of chromosomal abnormalities and therefore reduce the risk of miscarriage. This fits with early research that found a link between higher levels of DHEA and testosterone in ovarian follicles and a lower chance of chromosomal errors.[27]

A reduction in miscarriage rates has not been seen in every study on DHEA, but when researchers recently looked at all the data from the controlled trials, they found a general trend of lower miscarriage rates in women taking DHEA.[28] Here again, supplementing is only likely to be helpful if your DHEA is too low to support adequate testosterone production.

DHEA and endometriosis

Very little research has been done on the use of DHEA in women with endometriosis, and it cannot be ruled out that long-term use could worsen the condition by increasing estrogen levels. Nevertheless, some IVF clinics are beginning to recommend the short-term use of DHEA to women with endometriosis and low AMH, apparently with good results.

Several case reports have been published describing successful IVF cycles after DHEA supplementation in women with endometriosis, with a significant increase in the number of eggs retrieved.[29] In 2021, the first randomized trial of DHEA for endometriosis was published. It found that although supplementing with DHEA for 90 days before IVF did not increase the number of embryos, it significantly increased the chance of the embryos implanting and leading to a live birth.[30] It is unclear whether the embryos were more likely to implant and lead to a successful pregnancy because they were higher quality, or whether DHEA somehow makes the endometrial lining more receptive to pregnancy in women with endometriosis.

DHEA and PCOS

DHEA is generally not recommended for those with the classic form of PCOS, which involves high testosterone levels. Yet there is a subgroup of PCOS patients who may in fact benefit. These patients are characterized by the unusual combination of high AMH but low DHEA-S and low testosterone. Dr. Gleicher at CHR has reported that DHEA was able to improve IVF outcomes in these patients.[31]

Lab testing to assess your DHEA level

To determine whether you may benefit from a DHEA supplement, the first step is lab testing. The amount of DHEA in the bloodstream at any given time fluctuates widely, so it is necessary to test for the sulfated version, called DHEA-S. This reflects the stored form and changes less over time. It is also important to test for testosterone at the same time because the main reason for supplementing with DHEA is to support testosterone production.

Although normally considered a male hormone, testosterone performs important work in the ovaries, encouraging more early-stage follicles to develop each month. Supplementing with DHEA likely improves fertility in part by replenishing testosterone levels to support the earliest phase of egg development. That means if your DHEA level is relatively low but testosterone is normal, supplementing with DHEA may not help.

The precise DHEA-S and testosterone level at which supplementation is justified is not entirely clear, but the studies indicate that for fertility purposes, DHEA-S should be in the range of approximately **95–270 mcg/dL**, and ideally closer to **180 mcg/dL**.

The normal range for total testosterone in women is **8–60 ng/dL**, but the optimal range for fertility is likely **25–45 ng/dL**. Your testosterone value is likely more important than your DHEA-S value because the purpose of supplementing with DHEA is to bring testosterone to the preferred level. If your total testosterone is above 25 ng/dL, supplementing with DHEA is probably not necessary, even if your DHEA-S is somewhat low.

If your doctor recommends that you take DHEA, it is important to regularly monitor your DHEA-S and testosterone levels to ensure that you are taking the correct dose. Many women find that their testosterone rises above the preferred range and they need to reduce the dose.

Dosing

The dose of DHEA most often recommended by fertility clinics and used in studies is 75 mg per day, taken as 25 mg three times per day.[32] Because studies have so consistently used this dose, there is very little research about what dose is actually required to improve fertility, but it is likely much less.

If our goal is to mimic the amount of DHEA naturally produced each day by young women with healthy adrenal function, a more appropriate dose would be 25 mg per day. Even at this dose, it is important to test your DHEA-S and testosterone levels after four weeks to ensure that you are not taking more than you need, because some women have more pronounced increases in testosterone even at relatively low doses of DHEA.

Because DHEA works by supporting early-stage follicles that are several months from maturing, the time frame when it is most helpful is three to four months before IVF, IUI, or ovulation.[33] As egg maturation gets closer, DHEA becomes less helpful and it becomes even more important to ensure that your testosterone level is not too high. That is because testosterone is helpful to early-stage follicles, but excess testosterone can impair the final stage of egg development, resulting in immature eggs that are unable to fertilize. Some clinics therefore recommend stopping DHEA when you begin medication for IVF. If you are trying to conceive naturally or through IUI, DHEA is typically stopped once you get pregnant.

Supplementing with DHEA instead of testosterone

If the goal of taking DHEA is to correct low testosterone levels, this raises the question of why we would not just administer testosterone directly. Some doctors do in fact prefer to directly treat patients with testosterone, particularly if someone has difficulty converting DHEA into testosterone. The majority of trials investigating the use of testosterone before IVF have also reported positive results.[34]

In general, however, DHEA is thought to be a preferable starting point because it reduces side effects by allowing the body to produce testosterone only where it is needed rather than flooding the entire body with testosterone evenly.

Safety and side effects

Because DHEA increases testosterone, it may have side effects related to male hormones, including oily skin, acne, hair loss, voice changes, and facial hair growth, particularly if the dose is too high.[35] DHEA can also result in longer cycles.

The CHR group has reported that in over a thousand patients supplemented with DHEA, they have not encountered a single complication of clinical significance.[36] The randomized clinical studies have reported no significant side effects,[37] and additional studies outside the fertility context have reported that long-term use of DHEA is safe.[38]

DHEA can, however, interact with medications. For example, it can interact with diabetes medication and increase insulin sensitivity. DHEA is not appropriate for those with certain medical conditions, including bipolar disorder or a history of hormone-sensitive cancer, because DHEA can increase estrogen production.

It is also worth noting that a high level of DHEA-S can make laboratory tests for progesterone less accurate. The practical result is that progesterone levels may appear higher than they actually are.[39]

Action Steps

If you have been diagnosed with diminished ovarian reserve or have age-related infertility, an autoimmune condition, or a history of early miscarriage, it is helpful to get your DHEA-S and testosterone levels tested. If your levels are below the optimal range, talk to your doctor about taking a DHEA supplement to improve egg development.

Optimal DHEA-S:
95–270 mcg/dL, ideally closer to 180 mcg/dL

Optimal total testosterone:
8–60 ng/dL, ideally 25–45 ng/dL

Chapter 10

Supplements to Avoid

"We are drowning in informa-
tion but starved for knowledge."

— JOHN NAISBITT

MANY SUPPLEMENTS TOUTED as fertility boosters are supported by very little scientific evidence and may in fact worsen egg quality. The common theme among these supplements is that they sound good in theory because they have known antioxidant properties, but they are not a natural part of our cellular biology and have not been studied in women trying to conceive.

Supplements such as resveratrol are effective antioxidants, but they are not the antioxidants our ovarian cells are designed to use, unlike CoQ10, vitamin E, and melatonin. As a result, such supplements can have unpredictable and potentially undesirable effects on fertility.

This chapter describes some of the most popular supplements that should either be avoided completely or used carefully. They may be helpful in some limited circumstances, but there is no clear evidence of a benefit, and they may in fact be harmful. The supplements discussed are:

- resveratrol
- turmeric
- vitex
- maca
- pycnogenol
- royal jelly
- L-arginine

Resveratrol

Resveratrol is an antioxidant found in red wine and long hailed as promoting longevity and mitochondrial function. Based on these purported benefits, resveratrol has become a popular fertility supplement. There is some evidence that it can improve egg quality and mitochondrial function,[1] but this may come at a price.

Specifically, one study found that women who take resveratrol in the lead-up to embryo transfer are much less likely to get pregnant and more likely to miscarry.[2] The researchers who led that study suggested that resveratrol alters development of the uterine lining to make it less receptive to embryo implantation.

It is too early to draw any firm conclusions from this study because the women who chose to take resveratrol were significantly older and had a lower AMH than those not taking resveratrol. The lower implantation rate and higher miscarriage rate may simply reflect starting with lower egg quality in the resveratrol group, rather than a negative effect of the supplement. Nevertheless, the study provides reason to be cautious, and it fits with other research showing that resveratrol directly impacts endometrial cells.[3]

Two further human studies did not see negative effects of resveratrol on pregnancy or miscarriage rates but did not report much benefit either. In both studies, resveratrol was associated with a higher chance of eggs fertilizing and a greater proportion of good-quality blastocysts.[4] Overall, however, resveratrol had no impact on the chance of pregnancy or miscarriage. In one of these studies, resveratrol was compared to melatonin. Whereas resveratrol made little difference to overall outcomes, melatonin doubled the pregnancy rate and halved the miscarriage rate.[5] This suggests that even if resveratrol does have a benefit, it pales in comparison to melatonin.

In short, the limited research to date on resveratrol indicates that it may improve egg and embryo quality, but only to a limited extent. It may not increase overall success rates, perhaps because it interferes with development of the uterine lining. This may be less of an issue if you are trying to conceive through IVF and are planning on a frozen embryo transfer, because the effects of resveratrol on the endometrial lining are thought to be relatively short-lived.[6] Nevertheless, it may be wise to stop the supplement at least two weeks before egg retrieval, in case a fresh transfer is needed.

Turmeric/Curcumin

Turmeric and its active ingredient, curcumin, are widely used for their antioxidant and anti-inflammatory properties. In endometriosis, studies have found that turmeric can significantly reduce pain and other symptoms. But this is not necessarily good news for fertility, because turmeric may do so by reducing growth of endometrial cells that are needed for embryo implantation.

Preliminary research suggests that high doses of turmeric may in fact disrupt estrogen signaling and inhibit proper development of the uterine lining.[7] In 2021, doctors also described two cases of women preparing for frozen embryo transfer who initially achieved a good lining thickness, and then much of their lining suddenly disappeared, leading to cancellation of their embryo transfers.[8] In both cases, the women were taking high doses of turmeric. Animal studies suggest that curcumin may also interfere with egg and embryo development.[9] For all these reasons, high-dose turmeric supplements are generally best avoided when trying to conceive. Using turmeric as a spice in food is unlikely to be problematic.

Vitex

Vitex is a medicinal plant from the Mediterranean region that has been used for centuries to treat symptoms of PMS and menopause.[10] According to historical legend, this plant was also used by monks to suppress libido, giving rise to the names chasteberry and monk's pepper.[11]

There is very little evidence that vitex can improve fertility, and it has not been studied extensively in randomized trials. If vitex does have a benefit for women trying to conceive, it is likely by way of reducing prolactin and increasing progesterone.[12] Given that mechanism, vitex is likely only helpful if you have abnormal prolactin and progesterone levels. Even then, the evidence is not clear, and the potential benefit must be balanced against the lack of safety data. In one small animal study, the use of vitex before pregnancy was associated with a higher chance of miscarriage.[13]

If you have very low progesterone and are trying to conceive naturally, there are likely better avenues to pursue, including discussing progesterone treatment with a doctor who specializes in this issue. If that is not possible, even an over-the-counter progesterone oil or cream is likely a better option than vitex. The egg-quality supplements discussed in previous chapters are also likely to help by protecting the layer of cells in the ovarian follicle that are responsible for making progesterone.

Maca

Maca is a root traditionally grown in Peru and used as a food and herbal medicine by the Ancient Incas. In the same family as broccoli and radishes, it has been marketed as Peruvian ginseng and "nature's Viagra." Initial studies have suggested that maca may improve semen parameters,[14] but very little research has been done on the potential fertility benefits for women, other than a few studies suggesting that it may lower FSH in postmenopausal women.[15] Even on this point the evidence is inconsistent, with some studies finding that maca does not impact FSH or can even increase it.[16]

Apart from the lack of data, the primary concern with maca is the potential for contamination with heavy metals such as arsenic, lead, and cadmium. The two areas that produce most of the worldwide supply of maca, in Peru and China, are known for having soil contaminated with heavy metals as the result of local mining and industrial activity. As maca root grows, it can absorb these heavy metals from the soil. One study found that the amount of arsenic and cadmium in samples of maca from Peru was significantly above the safe limit.[17] Given the lack of evidence in favor of maca, it is not worth taking the risk with this supplement.

Pycnogenol

Pycnogenol is an extract from pine bark that has been shown to have antioxidant and anti-inflammatory properties. These properties led some IVF clinics to include pycnogenol on lists of supplements for egg quality, even though no evidence exists from any good-quality clinical trials.

From the clinical studies to date, all we can tell is that pycnogenol may reduce the pain of endometriosis. This may be due in part to its anti-inflammatory effects, but pycnogenol can also suppress growth factors involved in proliferation of endometrial cells. Although this may be helpful for symptomatic relief of endometriosis, it could be counterproductive for those trying to conceive because these growth factors are critical to development of the uterine lining.

Because pycnogenol is a mixture of compounds not naturally found in the body, it may have other unpredictable effects, and there is reason to be very cautious. At the time of writing, there have not been any good-quality clinical studies showing that pycnogenol can improve egg quality or fertility.

Given the lack of evidence, there is no reason to take pycnogenol when better antioxidant supplements are available, such as CoQ10 and melatonin. These antioxidants are naturally found inside ovarian follicles, and their supplement forms have been widely studied for safety and side effects in many large, double-blind, placebo-controlled clinical trials.

Royal Jelly

Royal jelly is a substance secreted by worker bees to provide food for the queen bee. This jelly is thought to contain hormones that make the queen bee extremely fertile and increase her lifespan. Based on this natural role, royal jelly has long been recommended as an alternative medicine in the fertility context. Just like pycnogenol, royal jelly is a mixture of compounds not naturally found in the human body.

At the time of writing, no good-quality clinical research supports the use of royal jelly in improving egg quality, and it has been found to occasionally cause life-threatening allergic reactions. These allergic reactions likely occur because royal jelly contains some of the same allergens found in bee venom.[18] In addition, because royal jelly contains a mixture of chemicals that act like hormones, it may have unpredictable effects and disrupt natural hormone balance.[19] Given the uncertain benefit and potential side effects, this is a supplement to avoid.

L-Arginine

L-arginine is an amino acid naturally found in ovarian follicles and one of the most widely recommended fertility supplements, but the evidence in its favor is inconsistent at best.

The theory behind using L-arginine to improve fertility is that it increases the production of nitric oxide, which dilates blood vessels and therefore increases blood flow to the ovaries and uterus, bringing with it hormones and nutrients that encourage follicles to grow.[20]

One of the earliest studies on L-arginine showed great promise, with high doses resulting in fewer cancelled IVF cycles and an increased number of eggs and embryos in women previously considered "poor responders."[21] Yet follow-up research in women with tubal infertility rather than poor ovarian function suggested that high doses of L-arginine can actually reduce the number and quality of eggs and embryos.[22] This fits with other research finding that women who naturally have very high L-arginine in ovarian follicles tend to have fewer eggs retrieved and fewer embryos in IVF.[23]

It may be that L-arginine is beneficial in certain amounts in women who have compromised ovarian function, but it becomes detrimental when the dose is too high or ovarian function is already good. In the two studies just mentioned, women were given 16 g of L-arginine per day. This is far more than the amount we normally get from food, which is around 4–6 g per day.

Although the research suggests it is best to avoid very high doses of L-arginine in the lead-up to egg retrieval or if trying to conceive naturally, there is likely no reason to be concerned about lower doses found in combination supplements, such as Serovital (which contains less than 1 g in four capsules and is discussed in chapter 16). At this low dose, L-arginine may even be beneficial, as found in a 2020 study that reported a slightly higher pregnancy rate in women taking 1 or 2 g of L-arginine per day before IVF.[24]

If you are preparing for embryo transfer, taking L-arginine

may have more value, as discussed in chapter 14. By boosting blood flow to the uterus, it may help to make the uterine lining more receptive to implantation.

Conclusion

Many commonly recommended fertility supplements are supported by little evidence of safety or efficacy, and they may in fact be counterproductive. The supplements to avoid or use with caution are:

- resveratrol
- turmeric
- vitex
- maca
- pycnogenol
- royal jelly
- high-dose L-arginine

Chapter 11

Your Complete Supplement Plan

"A good system shortens the road to the goal."
—Orison Swett Marden

THIS CHAPTER PROVIDES overall supplement plans for different scenarios, including the basic plan for those just getting started, versions of the intermediate plan for difficulty conceiving, PCOS, and egg freezing, and versions of the advanced plan for endometriosis, miscarriage, and IVF. Recommended supplement brands are listed at: **itstartswith-theegg.com/supplements**

Example Supplement Plans

The basic plan

If you have just started trying to get pregnant and have no reason to expect any difficulty, you are unlikely to need an extensive supplement regime. But a few basic supplements can likely shorten the time it takes to get pregnant while also reducing the risk of miscarriage and complications such as preterm birth and preeclampsia.

- Start taking a daily prenatal multivitamin as soon as possible, ideally one that includes at least 800 mcg of methylfolate.

- Consider a daily CoQ10 supplement. The most effective form is ubiquinol or high absorption ubiquinone, and the basic dose is 200 mg, preferably taken in the morning with food.

- Have your vitamin D level tested and consider supplementing with 4,000–5,000 IU of vitamin D3 per day if you are below the optimal target level (40 ng/ml or 100 nmol/L). If you have a significant deficiency, you can start with 10,000 IU per day for two weeks.

- If you do not eat fish regularly, consider adding an omega-3 fish oil supplement (500 mg), as will be discussed in chapter 12.

After a positive pregnancy test, you will generally stop CoQ10 and continue with your prenatal multivitamin and vitamin D, since both are important during pregnancy. Omega-3 fish oil and choline are also helpful during pregnancy, as discussed in my pregnancy book.

Intermediate plan: difficulty conceiving

If you are having trouble getting pregnant but have not yet moved on to treatments such as IUI or IVF, you can take a middle-ground approach: starting with the basic supplements and adding antioxidants. Women with unexplained infertility often have compromised antioxidant defenses in their ovarian follicles, and taking antioxidant supplements may reduce the time it takes to conceive. If you later progress to IVF, you can then move to the advanced plan, discussed later in this chapter.

- Consider adding the following supplements:
  › A prenatal multivitamin containing at least 800 mcg of methylfolate or natural food folate
  › Ubiquinol: 400 mg per day—one 200 mg capsule with breakfast and one with lunch
  › Additional vitamin C (500 mg) and vitamin E (200 IU). For a stronger antioxidant boost, you may also consider adding melatonin (such as a microdose of 300 mcg / 0.3 mg), alpha-lipoic acid, or N-acetylcysteine.
- If your vitamin D is below the optimal target level (40 ng/ml or 100 nmol/L), consider supplementing with 4,000–5,000 IU of vitamin D3 per day. If you have a significant deficiency, you can start with 10,000 IU per day for two weeks.

- If you have a B12 deficiency, consider supplementing with 1,000–2,000 mcg per day, preferably as hydroxylcobalamin and/or adenosylcobalamin. Methylcobalamin is also very effective but can sometimes cause side effects at higher doses.

- If you do not eat fish regularly, consider adding an omega-3 fish oil supplement (500 mg), as will be discussed in chapter 12.

After a positive pregnancy test, you will generally stop all supplements except your prenatal multivitamin and vitamin D, which are important during pregnancy. Omega-3 fish oil and choline are also helpful during pregnancy, as discussed in my pregnancy book.

Intermediate plan: polycystic ovary syndrome or irregular ovulation

PCOS is a common condition in which high insulin and high testosterone compromise egg quality and the hormones that control ovulation. To improve egg quality and rebalance hormones:

- consider taking the following supplements for two or three months before trying to conceive:
    › A prenatal containing 800 mcg of natural food folate or methylfolate
    › Myo-inositol: 4 g per day, divided into two doses—half in the morning and half at night
    › Ubiquinol: 400 mg per day—one 200 mg capsule with breakfast and one with lunch
    › R-alpha lipoic acid: 200 mg—preferably at least

30 minutes before a meal

> N-acetylcysteine: 600 mg—any time

> L-carnitine: 3 g per day—any time

> Melatonin: 1–3 mg—bedtime

- have your vitamin D level tested and consider supplementing with 4,000–5,000 IU of vitamin D3 per day if you are below the optimal target level (40 ng/ml or 100 nmol/L). If you have a significant deficiency, you can start with 10,000 IU per day for two weeks.

- if you have a B12 deficiency, supplement with 1,000–2,000 mcg per day, preferably as hydroxylcobalamin and/or adenosylcobalamin. Methylcobalamin is also very effective but can sometimes cause side effects at higher doses.

- If you do not eat fish regularly, consider adding an omega-3 fish oil supplement (500 mg), as will be discussed in chapter 12.

After a positive pregnancy test, you will generally stop all supplements except your prenatal multivitamin and vitamin D, which are important during pregnancy. Continuing with myo-inositol may be worthwhile since it can help to prevent gestational diabetes in women with PCOS. Omega-3 fish oil and choline are also helpful during pregnancy, as discussed in my pregnancy book.

Intermediate plan: egg freezing

When preparing to freeze your eggs, adding a few basic supplements and antioxidants may help you increase the number of good-quality eggs from a single retrieval and increase the chance of those eggs one day leading to a viable embryo.

- Consider adding the following supplements for three months before your egg retrieval:
  - › A prenatal multivitamin containing at least 800 mcg of methylfolate or natural food folate
  - › Ubiquinol: 400 mg per day—one 200 mg capsule with breakfast and one with lunch
  - › Additional vitamin C (500 mg) and vitamin E (200 IU).
  - › For a stronger antioxidant boost, you may also consider adding melatonin (such as 1mg), alpha-lipoic acid, or N-acetylcysteine.
- If your vitamin D is below the optimal target level (40 ng/ml or 100 nmol/L), consider supplementing with 4,000–5,000 IU of vitamin D3 per day. If you have a significant deficiency, you can start with 10,000 IU per day for two weeks.
- If you have a B12 deficiency, consider supplementing with 1,000–2,000 mcg per day, preferably as hydroxylcobalamin and/or adenosylcobalamin. Methylcobalamin is also very effective but can sometimes cause side effects at higher doses.
- If you do not eat fish regularly, consider adding an omega-3 fish oil supplement (500 mg), as will be discussed in chapter 12.

Advanced plan: endometriosis

Endometriosis impacts fertility in a variety of ways, but two major components are inflammation and oxidative damage to developing eggs. Research indicates it may be possible to counteract these problems to some extent with the right supplements.

- Consider taking the following supplements:
  › A prenatal with at least 800 mcg of natural food folate or methylfolate
  › CoQ10 (as ubiquinol or Bio-Quinon): 400 mg per day—one 200 mg capsule with breakfast and one with lunch. Some IVF clinics may recommend 600 mg per day for difficult cases.
  › R-alpha lipoic acid: 300 mg—preferably at least 30 minutes before a meal
  › N-acetylcysteine: 600 mg—any time
  › Vitamin C: 1000 mg—any time
  › Melatonin: 300 mcg–1 mg if trying to conceive naturally, 1–3 mg for IVF, taken at bedtime
- If you have had previous IVF cycles fail due to a low number of eggs retrieved, or if you have low AMH or a low follicle count, have your DHEA-S and testosterone levels tested. If your levels are low, talk to your doctor about taking a DHEA supplement. There has been very little research on the use of DHEA in women with endometriosis, but initial reports indicate that DHEA can help address the negative impact of endometriosis on ovarian reserve.

- Have your vitamin D level tested and consider supplementing with 4,000–5,000 IU of vitamin D3 per day if you are below the optimal target level (40 ng/ml or 100 nmol/L). Some believe aiming for an even higher target of 60 ng/ml may help reduce the inflammation associated with endometriosis. If you have a significant deficiency, you can start with 10,000 IU per day for two weeks.

- If you have a B12 deficiency, supplement with 1,000–2,000 mcg per day, preferably as hydroxylcobalamin and/or adenosylcobalamin. Methylcobalamin is also very effective but can sometimes cause side effects at higher doses.

- If you do not eat fish regularly, consider adding an omega-3 fish oil supplement (500 mg), as will be discussed in chapter 12.

After a positive pregnancy test, you will generally stop all supplements except your prenatal multivitamin and vitamin D, which are important during pregnancy. Omega-3 fish oil and choline are also helpful during pregnancy, as discussed in my pregnancy book.

Advanced plan: recurrent miscarriage

Although there are various medical causes of recurrent miscarriage, including blood clotting and immune disorders, nearly half of all early miscarriages are caused by chromosomal errors in the egg. By improving your egg quality, you may be able to reduce the chance of chromosomal errors occurring and thereby reduce your risk of miscarriage.

- Consider taking the following supplements for two or three months before trying to conceive:
    - › A prenatal with at least 800 mcg of methylfolate
    - › CoQ10 (as ubiquinol or Bio-Quinon): 400 mg per day—one 200 mg capsule with breakfast and one with lunch
    - › R-alpha lipoic acid: 200–300 mg—preferably at least 30 minutes before a meal
    - › Vitamin E: 200 IU—any time
    - › N-acetylcysteine: 600 mg—any time
    - › If you have insulin resistance, myo-inositol: 4 g per day, half in the morning and half at night
    - › Melatonin: 300 mcg–1 mg if trying naturally, 1–3 mg for IVF, taken at bedtime
- Have your vitamin D level tested and consider supplementing with 4,000–5,000 IU of vitamin D3 per day if you are below the optimal target level (at least 40 ng/ml or 100 nmol/L, although some believe a higher target is preferred to control inflammation). If you have a significant deficiency, you can start with 10,000 IU per day for two weeks.
- Consider having your DHEA-S and testosterone levels tested, particularly if age may be a factor or if you have low AMH or a low follicle count. Supplementing with DHEA may help increase the number of eggs that mature properly each month and potentially prevent some of the chromosomal errors that cause miscarriage, although there is little data on this.

- Make sure your male partner is also taking a daily multivitamin containing methylfolate, a CoQ10 supplement (at least 200 mg of ubiquinol or Bio-Quinon), and the advanced sperm quality supplements discussed in chapter 13.

- If you have a B12 deficiency, supplement with 1,000–2,000 mcg per day, preferably as hydroxylcobalamin and/or adenosylcobalamin. Methylcobalamin is also very effective but can sometimes cause side effects at higher doses.

- If you do not eat fish regularly, consider adding an omega-3 fish oil supplement (500 mg), as will be discussed in chapter 12.

After a positive pregnancy test, it is typical to stop all supplements except your prenatal multivitamin and vitamin D, which are important during pregnancy. Research suggests that continuing NAC and a lower dose of CoQ10 during the first trimester may also reduce the risk of miscarriage and preeclampsia, although neither supplement has been studied extensively in this context. Omega-3 fish oil and choline are important during pregnancy, as discussed in my pregnancy book.

Advanced plan: trying to conceive through IUI or IVF

If you have low ovarian reserve or age-related infertility, or you need to pursue IVF or IUI for some other reason, you have the most to gain from an aggressive plan to improve egg quality.

- Consider taking the following supplements for at least two or three months before your next IVF or IUI cycle:

  › A prenatal with at least 800 mcg of natural food folate or methylfolate

  › CoQ10 (as ubiquinol or Bio-Quinon): 400 mg per day—one 200 mg capsule with breakfast and one with lunch. Some clinics may recommend 600 mg per day for difficult cases.

  › R-alpha lipoic acid: 200–300 mg—preferably at least 30 minutes before a meal

  › N-acetylcysteine: 600 mg—any time

  › Vitamin E: 200 IU—any time. You may also decide to add vitamin C (500 mg) to boost antioxidant defenses even more.

  › Melatonin: 300 mcg–1 mg for IUI, 1–3 mg for IVF, taken at bedtime

- Have your DHEA-S and testosterone levels tested. If your levels are low, talk to your doctor about adding a supplement for at least three months before your next IUI or IVF cycle. The typical dose in studies is 25 mg three times per day, but 25 mg once per day may be a better starting point.

- Have your vitamin D level tested and consider supplementing with 4,000–5,000 IU of vitamin D3 per day if you are below the optimal target level (40 ng/ml or 100 nmol/L). If you have a significant deficiency, you can start with 10,000 IU per day for two weeks.

- If you have a B12 deficiency, supplement with 1,000–2,000 mcg per day, preferably as hydroxylcobalamin and/or adenosylcobalamin. Methylcobalamin is also very effective but can sometimes cause side effects at higher doses.

- If you do not eat fish regularly, consider adding an omega-3 fish oil supplement (500 mg), as will be discussed in chapter 12.

Different supplements are stopped at different times. It is typical to stop DHEA when you begin medication for IVF or IUI and to stop alpha-lipoic acid, vitamin C, and N-acetylcysteine the day before egg retrieval or insemination. CoQ10, melatonin, and vitamin E can be continued until embryo transfer since they may help promote the development of the uterine lining.

You can continue taking your prenatal multivitamin and vitamin D throughout your time trying to conceive and during pregnancy. Some may also choose to take NAC and a lower dose of CoQ10 during the first trimester to reduce the chance of miscarriage and preeclampsia, but there is little research on this point. Omega-3 fish oil and choline are important during pregnancy, as discussed in my pregnancy book.

PART 3

THE BIGGER
PICTURE

Chapter 12

The Egg-Quality Diet

*"We are indeed much more than what we
eat, but what we eat can nevertheless help us
to be much more than what we are."*

— ADELLE DAVIS

I T WILL COME as no surprise that diet can have a powerful influence on fertility, but much of the advice in this area is inconsistent and based on general ideas of a healthy diet, rather than solid scientific evidence. When we delve into the actual research on how diet impacts fertility, some surprising patterns emerge.

This chapter begins with the most powerful change you can make to your diet: balancing blood sugar.

Blood Sugar and Fertility

One of the key goals of a fertility diet is avoiding spikes in blood glucose because these spikes can disrupt hormones and compromise egg quality. To understand how to achieve steady blood sugar levels and why this is so important, we need to briefly delve into what happens when we eat carbohydrates.

After consuming carbohydrates such as bread or crackers, the starches are quickly broken down into individual glucose molecules and absorbed, triggering a rapid rise in blood glucose. This causes the pancreas to release insulin, which tells muscle cells to soak up glucose from the bloodstream. This system is important because if all the extra glucose stayed in the bloodstream, it would quickly cause damage.

Excess glucose damages cells in a variety of ways, triggering the production of free radicals and causing mitochondria to break apart or malfunction. To prevent this, the glucose needs to be safely stored away inside muscles or converted into fat. Insulin directs this process by telling muscle and fat cells to soak up glucose.

The higher the blood glucose level, the more insulin is released. Over time, if insulin is too high too often, the cells stop listening to insulin's message to soak up glucose, a condition called insulin resistance. Blood glucose levels remain high, the body compensates by making even more insulin, and chaos ensues.

All this sugar and insulin is a big problem for fertility. High glucose levels directly compromise egg quality, while high insulin disrupts the balance of other hormones that regulate the reproductive system.

Importantly, this is not a phenomenon limited to those with diabetes or true insulin resistance; the negative impact to fertility occurs when blood sugar and insulin levels are elevated but still within the normal range. That was demonstrated by a group of researchers in Denmark who found that women with blood sugar levels that were higher than average, but still within the normal range, were only half as likely to get pregnant over six months compared to women with lower glucose levels.[1]

One of the major factors that causes these higher-than-average blood sugar levels is the type of carbohydrates consumed. When you eat highly-processed carbohydrates made from refined flour, the starch molecules are easily accessible to digestive enzymes, so they can be broken down very quickly. This causes a massive spike in blood glucose levels.

By contrast, carbohydrate-rich foods that are closer to nature, such as nuts, seeds, or unrefined grains, take much longer to break down. That is because the starches are packed up tightly and are less accessible to digestive enzymes. As a result, glucose molecules are released gradually over time. The blood sugar response after eating whole, unrefined foods is therefore much slower and steadier. Instead of a sudden spike, there is a slow and steady climb, and glucose never reaches dangerous levels.

The Nurses' Health Study tracked tens of thousands of women over many years and found that women who followed a diet emphasizing these "slow" carbohydrates had a much lower rate of infertility due to ovulation problems.[2] This is likely because high insulin can disrupt hormones in the ovaries, which can interfere with ovulation.[3]

By modifying your diet to choose slow carbohydrates such as nuts, seeds, vegetables, beans, and lentils, instead of fast carbohydrates such as bread and cereal, you are more likely to maintain steady blood sugar and insulin levels. This in turn helps to maintain normal hormone levels in the ovaries. You can also avoid blood glucose spikes using other strategies discussed later in this chapter, such as eating high-carbohydrate foods only after foods containing fiber and protein, or going for a walk after meals.

These strategies are not only helpful for preserving the careful balance of hormones in the ovaries. They can also protect developing eggs from more direct impacts of high blood glucose.

Blood sugar, insulin, and egg quality

When blood sugar is very high, a chemical reaction occurs between glucose and either proteins or lipids within our cells. This reaction creates damaged proteins and lipids called "advanced glycosylation end products," or AGEs. These damaged molecules accumulate in the body over time as a result of high blood sugar levels.[4] AGEs are known to contribute to cosmetic aging by damaging collagen in the skin, as well as cardiovascular aging by causing cholesterol to clump together into plaques. Research shows they also contribute to ovarian aging.

Studies have found that women with higher levels of AGEs before starting IVF tend to have fewer eggs retrieved, fewer eggs fertilized, and fewer good-quality embryos. The pregnancy rate is also very different: 23% in women with normal levels, compared to just 3% in women with higher levels of glucose-induced damage.[5]

High blood glucose may also compromise egg quality by causing mitochondria to break into fragments or malfunction.[6] As explained in earlier chapters, mitochondria are the tiny power plants inside all our cells that produce the cellular energy needed for egg development. Any disruption in mitochondrial function compromises the ability to separate copies of chromosomes properly and can cause genetically abnormal eggs and embryos.

Research shows that high blood sugar levels impair mitochondrial function.[7] We would therefore expect an increase in the rate of chromosomal abnormalities, which is exactly what has been found in animal studies. Eggs from diabetic mice are much more likely to have an incorrect number of chromosomes.[8]

This could explain part of the link between insulin resistance and the risk of miscarriage. More than a decade ago, scientists revealed that in women with recurrent pregnancy loss, the rate of insulin resistance was nearly three times higher than normal.[9]

All this information suggests that we have a remarkable opportunity to prevent damage to developing eggs and potentially reduce chromosomal errors simply by getting blood sugar levels under control.

Mastering Your Blood Sugar

Achieving steady, even blood sugar levels does not require a strict low-carbohydrate diet. Instead, there are a variety of small shifts and strategies you can rely on to prevent blood sugar spikes, by focusing on either the amount, type, or timing of the carbohydrates you eat. You can choose which of these strategies to emphasize at different times, either alone or in combination.

Strategy 1: reduce the total amount of carbohydrates

The first strategy is to reduce your reliance on high-carbohydrate foods, while increasing fat, fiber, and protein. This appears to have a powerful impact on IVF success rates, even in women without noticeable insulin or blood sugar problems. In one study, researchers asked women with previous failed IVF cycles to eat fewer carbohydrates and more protein.[10] After two months, the women undertook another IVF cycle, with impressive results.

The greatest impact was on the percentage of eggs that made it to 5-day embryo stage. When the women followed their normal diet, 19% of eggs developed into blastocysts, but after two months of a lower carbohydrate and higher protein diet, 45% of eggs survived to the blastocyst stage. Ten out of the 12 women also became pregnant.

Importantly, this study indicates that you do not need to drastically cut carbohydrates to improve egg and embryo quality. A good ratio appears to be around 40% of calories from carbohydrates, 30% from protein, and 30% from fat.[11] This represents a healthy, balanced diet, and many people can easily reach these ratios by changing just one meal per day, such as having yogurt or eggs for breakfast rather than toast or cereal, or reducing a portion of rice or pasta at dinner while adding more protein or vegetables.

Strategy 2: choose "slow" carbohydrates

From a fertility standpoint, the best carbohydrates are those that are digested slowly, preventing sudden bursts of insulin. Good options include beans, lentils, nuts, seeds, most vegetables, and minimally processed whole grains such as quinoa, wild rice, brown rice, steel-cut oats, and buckwheat. You can also swap conventional bread and pasta for versions with more protein and fiber, such as chickpea or lentil pasta. Choosing more of these foods and minimizing foods made from highly processed or refined grains will help balance blood sugar and provide steady energy levels.

Choosing slow-release carbohydrates also means reducing sugar in all its forms. There is clear evidence that eating too much sugar compromises fertility.[12] Replacing standard sugar with natural forms such as maple syrup, dates, agave, or honey is likely no better. These sweeteners contain a combination of glucose, fructose, and sucrose—all of which cause similar rises in blood sugar and insulin.[13] For that reason, it makes sense to minimize all types of sweeteners.

Fruit also contains a significant amount of sugar, but it is likely fine to include in moderation. The sugar in whole fruit is packed together with fiber, which slows absorption and to some extent lessens the impact on blood sugar levels. Even so, it is better to have fruit after a meal that includes protein and vegetables to further slow the release of sugars.

If you find yourself needing a sweet treat, dark chocolate is a good choice. Also keep in mind that long-term daily habits matter most. The occasional indulgence is not worth feeling guilty about. You can also minimize the negative impact of refined carbohydrates and sugars with the next two strategies.

Strategy 3: fiber, protein, or vinegar before carbohydrates

Studies have found that you can significantly reduce blood sugar spikes by simply eating foods in the right order—specifically, by eating high-carbohydrate foods *after* vegetables or protein.[14] That could mean starting your meals with a salad and saving bread or pasta for the end of a meal. This is one of the key recommendations from Jessie Inchauspen, a bio-chemist and the author of *Glucose Revolution.*

A salad can lessen the impact on blood sugar even further if you add a vinegar-based dressing. That's because the acetic acid in vinegar not only inhibits the enzymes that break starch into sugar but also prompts cells to soak up and utilize glucose.[15] Studies have shown that one tablespoon of vinegar before a meal can reduce the glucose spike of that meal by up to 30%.[16]

In one study in Japan, adding a tablespoon of apple cider vinegar per day was found to improve hormone balance and restore ovulation in some women with PCOS.[17] Consuming vinegar before meals is another top recommendation from Inchauspen. She suggests diluting one tablespoon of vinegar in a glass of water or sparkling water, ideally ten minutes before a meal. It is best to drink through a straw to protect your teeth.

Strategy 4: exercise after meals

The final strategy you can rely on to lessen any blood sugar spikes is to add some physical activity after you eat. Whether going for a short walk or doing housework or light resistance exercises, even ten minutes of activity can significantly reduce spikes in blood sugar.[18] When your muscles are active, they soak up glucose from the bloodstream, preventing glucose and insulin spikes that can disrupt hormones and cause oxidative stress. Studies have found that exercising before a meal can also help prevent blood sugar spikes, but exercising after a meal has a greater impact.[19]

Few people have time to exercise after every meal, or even every day, but this is one more strategy you can turn to, especially when you want to indulge in a food that would otherwise have a significant impact on blood sugar.

Remember that all these strategies are merely tools at your disposal. You can choose which to rely on, either alone or in combination, in whatever way works best for you.

Is it necessary to eliminate gluten or dairy?

Gluten clearly contributes to infertility and miscarriage risk in those with celiac disease; that much is beyond doubt. The question is whether it is necessary for everyone else to avoid gluten and dairy while trying to conceive.

There is some concern that both gluten and dairy can contribute to autoimmunity and inflammation in those with a sensitivity, even in the absence of celiac disease. As will be discussed further toward the end of this chapter, for those with endometriosis, a history of recurrent miscarriage driven by immune factors, or a preexisting autoimmune disease such as a thyroid condition, it probably does make sense to avoid gluten. Dairy can also trigger inflammation and autoimmunity, but it less likely to be a problem than gluten.

The typical advice to avoid dairy while trying to conceive is often based on a concern that the hormones present in milk could compromise fertility. Yet the studies so far have not found a clear link. We know from the Nurses' Health Study that a higher intake of full-fat dairy was actually associated with a lower risk of ovulation disorder. In a more recent study of IVF outcomes, women with the highest dairy intake had the highest chance of live birth.[20]

You can, of course, choose to avoid gluten and dairy if you prefer a no-stone-unturned approach. There are numerous anecdotal reports of women battling infertility who were able to conceive after eliminating these foods. One option is to eliminate them for two weeks and see how you respond. If you feel better overall, that may indicate that you do indeed have a sensitivity and will benefit from avoiding gluten or dairy (or both) longer term.

Boosting Fertility with a Mediterranean Diet

If the first principle of a fertility-friendly diet is balancing blood sugar, the second is shifting towards a Mediterranean-style diet. This diet, based on the traditional eating patterns in Greece, Spain, and Southern Italy, emphasizes fish, olive oil, nuts, legumes, and antioxidant-rich vegetables. It has long been hailed as one of the healthiest dietary patterns, shown to increase life expectancy and lower the risk of heart disease, cancer, and diabetes.[21]

Most importantly for our purposes, the Mediterranean diet also lowers inflammation.[22] This matters because there is a growing body of evidence tying inflammation to infertility and miscarriage.[23] Researchers have also specifically found that eating this way can boost IVF success rates.

In 2018, researchers demonstrated that women who followed a Mediterranean-style diet for six months before IVF were much more likely to become pregnant.[24] The foods with the strongest links to improved success rates were vegetables, fruit, whole grains, legumes, fish, and olive oil.

This follows on from an earlier study on diet and IVF

success rates, which surveyed 161 couples at an IVF clinic in the Netherlands. The researchers found that women who more closely followed a Mediterranean diet before their IVF cycle had a 40% higher chance of becoming pregnant.[25] These women typically had a higher intake of vegetables, vegetable oil, fish, and legumes.

The researchers suggested two ways in which these foods could improve pregnancy rates so dramatically. The first is a higher level of specific vitamins, such as folate, B6, and B12, which are found in vegetables, fish, meat, dairy, and eggs. These vitamins can likely improve egg and embryo quality by lowering homocysteine.[26] Vitamin B6 alone could have a major impact on boosting fertility in women following a Mediterranean diet; one study found that supplementing with B6 can increase the chance of conception by 40% and decrease early miscarriage by 30%.[27] Fish is one the best sources of vitamin B6.

The second way in which the Mediterranean diet could improve fertility is by providing higher levels of important fatty acids.

Fertility-friendly fats and oils

One of the main features of the Mediterranean diet is its emphasis on anti-inflammatory fats and oils, particularly those found in fish, nuts, and olive oil.[28] In recent years, a wave of high-quality studies has demonstrated that these fats are beneficial for fertility. They improve egg and embryo quality in IVF and reduce the time it takes to get pregnant.[29]

In 2017, Harvard researchers found that women with above-average levels of omega-3 fats in their blood had a much higher chance of conceiving through IVF.[30] But only the specific omega-3s found in fish were linked to better odds of conceiving; the type found in plant sources (such as flaxseed oil) did not appear to have much impact.

Outside the context of IVF, a study of 2,000 women also reported that those with sufficient omega-3 intake conceived sooner than those with a low intake.[31] The researchers noted that this was likely because omega-3 fats reduce inflammation, support progesterone production, and increase uterine blood flow. These mechanisms may also be responsible for the link between higher omega-3 consumption and a lower risk of pregnancy loss.[32]

One interesting pattern to emerge in these recent studies is that above a certain level of omega-3 intake, consuming more does not confer any additional benefit. The threshold for improving fertility appears to be eating omega-3-rich fish approximately two times per week. The fish with the highest omega-3 levels and negligible mercury include salmon, sardines, and Atlantic mackerel. If these fish are a part of your regular diet, there is likely no benefit in supplementing with additional omega-3.

If you do not eat seafood regularly, or only eat types of fish with much lower omega-3 levels, it may make sense to add a low-dose fish oil supplement. A 2022 study found that women taking fish oil supplements and trying to conceive naturally have a significantly higher chance of getting pregnant each cycle.[33] In men, fish oil supplements have been shown to improve sperm quality.[34] A reasonable dose is approximately 500 milligrams per day of omega-3s. It is best to take omega-3 supplements with a meal containing some fat in order to allow for proper absorption.

Beyond the omega-3 fats found in fish, the Mediterranean diet may also improve fertility by virtue of its emphasis on olive oil.[35] Olive oil is not only rich in antioxidants but also contains a type of monounsaturated fat that is likely important for egg development, known as oleic acid.[36]

A 2017 study found that women with higher levels of oleic acid had more mature eggs retrieved before IVF.[37] Oleic acid accounts for around 70% of the total fat in olive oil and it is also the primary type of fat found in avocados and avocado oil.

Other fats found in olive oil, avocados, nuts, and seeds have also been linked to improved fertility.[38] In contrast, saturated fats, which are typically found in coconut oil, butter, and red meat, appear to negatively affect egg development and embryo quality.[39] This does not mean you need to avoid red meat, but it is worth choosing leaner cuts.

Taken as a whole, the research indicates that we can significantly improve fertility by aiming for a higher intake of fish, olive oil, nuts, and seeds, and a somewhat lower intake of saturated fat from coconut oil, butter, and red meat.

Rebalancing fat intake in this way may be particularly important for those with variants in folate metabolism genes, such as MTHFR, because a greater consumption of fish and a higher ratio of monounsaturated to saturated fat results in lower homocysteine levels.[40]

The Mediterranean diet and miscarriage

An anti-inflammatory Mediterranean diet could be particularly helpful for reducing the odds of pregnancy loss caused by inflammation or immune issues. Most of the strategies discussed in previous chapters have focused on preventing chromosome-related miscarriage, but there are also steps you can take to address other potential causes.

Some women show a pattern of repeated pregnancy losses even when testing shows no chromosomal abnormality. Clearly something else is going on in these cases and recent studies show that one likely culprit is inflammation.

As one example, researchers in Spain tested a dozen different blood markers in a group of women under 30 who had each experienced at least three miscarriages. The women showed two clear differences compared to women with no history of miscarriage: a higher level of inflammation (shown by a marker called C-reactive protein) and lower vitamin D levels.[41]

Vitamin D plays an important role in regulating the immune system, but we can also lower inflammation through diet. Numerous studies have found that following a Mediterranean diet can lower inflammation, and specifically lower C-reactive protein.[42] Shifting toward this type of diet may therefore reduce the risk of miscarriage driven by inflammation.

The term "inflammation" generally refers to nonspecific immune activity in which the immune system rages with no particular target. But in some cases, recurrent miscarriage can be caused by more direct immune activity, such as particular antibodies directed against the body's own proteins. This type of immune activity is referred to as "autoimmunity" and, in the miscarriage context, includes antiphospholipid antibody syndrome.

If you test positive for these or other antibodies, immune treatment may be helpful, but there are also dietary strategies to consider to help address the root causes.

A modified fertility diet for autoimmunity, endometriosis, and immune-mediated miscarriage

If you have fertility challenges involving the immune system, you may benefit by modifying your diet even further. This group includes those with:

- a preexisting autoimmune condition (such as thyroid disease, psoriasis, lupus, multiple sclerosis, Crohn's disease, or ulcerative colitis)
- endometriosis
- miscarriage with immune factors (such as antiphospholipid antibody syndrome).

In all these conditions, the immune system is reacting inappropriately to the body's own molecules and often triggering a very high level of inflammation. This inflammation can compromise egg quality and potentially contribute to miscarriage risk.

It is therefore worthwhile to place more emphasis on the dietary factors that influence general inflammation. This means an even greater focus on reducing sugar while emphasizing anti-inflammatory vegetables and healthy fats from fish and olive oil. But many women with immune system disruptions will benefit from going even further and eliminating foods that can sometimes trigger immune reactions in those with a sensitivity. Here, the two main culprits are gluten and dairy.

Gluten is the most important dietary trigger to avoid if you have immune issues. Even in the absence of any sensitivity to wheat or gluten, it appears that gluten can contribute to inflammation and autoimmunity. It likely does so by altering the gut microbiome and the permeability of the intestinal lining.[43] These changes allow microbial byproducts to cross through the gut barrier and activate the immune system.[44]

As a result, even the most conservative endocrinologists and rheumatologists often recommend eliminating gluten, especially when trying to conceive. Studies have also found that a gluten-free diet reduces pain in 75% of patients with endometriosis.[45]

A gluten-free diet may also be helpful for women with miscarriages driven by immune factors. We know that celiac disease is a common cause of recurrent miscarriage, but gluten could potentially contribute to pregnancy loss in the absence celiac disease, by impacting gut health and the immune system more generally. There is no definitive research on this point yet, but many reproductive immunologists recommend a gluten-free diet as a precaution. One such doctor was Jeffrey Braverman, a renowned reproductive immunologist who pioneered immune approaches to treating recurrent miscarriage. His advice was that "overall you can never go wrong with being off gluten."

Dairy is another food that is sometimes an issue, simply because it is one of the most common food allergens. It appears to be much less problematic than gluten, however. If you do not have a sensitivity to dairy, it may be fine to continue including it in your diet.

For those with more severe autoimmune diseases, there are of course further steps you can take if you choose. One common strategy is the autoimmune paleo diet, known as the AIP diet for short. This approach emphasizes animal proteins, fruits, vegetables, coconut oil, and animal fats, while excluding grains, legumes, and common allergens such as nuts, eggs, and dairy.

Some components of this diet, such as avoiding allergens, are likely to be helpful for many with autoimmune disease, but certain aspects of the AIP diet are counterproductive. Specifically, research shows that adding more coconut oil and other saturated fats can significantly increase inflammation. By contrast, the fats emphasized in the Mediterranean diet are much better at calming the immune system.

A better approach is likely starting with a Mediterranean-based diet and modifying it by eliminating the foods that can be problematic for those with autoimmunity, such as gluten, sugar, corn, and any foods that are flagged by food sensitivity testing.

For low-carbohydrate Mediterranean diet recipes that avoid common food allergens, see the *It Starts with the Egg Cookbook*. You can download a free PDF sample of recipes from the cookbook at **itstartswiththeegg.com/recipes**.

Alcohol and Fertility

The question of whether alcohol compromises fertility has been plaguing researchers for decades. In 1998, a small but highly publicized study reported that consuming just one to five alcoholic drinks per week could significantly reduce the odds of conceiving.[46] Yet this study involved just four hundred women. Much larger studies have now been done, and the results have been more reassuring.

A study of 40,000 women found an impact on fertility only with more than 14 alcoholic drinks per week.[47] The same result was evident in a 2016 study of 6,000 women, with researchers concluding that "consumption of less than 14 servings of alcohol per week seemed to have no discernible effect on fertility."[48]

It should be noted that these studies were performed in the context of women trying to conceive naturally, so the results do not necessarily extend to women with preexisting fertility problems who are trying to conceive through IVF.

In the context of IVF, moderate alcohol consumption may be slightly more problematic, but the effect still appears to be relatively small. In 2011, researchers at Harvard Medical School surveyed more than 2,000 couples undergoing IVF. They found that compared to women reporting fewer than four alcoholic drinks per week, women drinking more than this amount had a 16% lower chance of a live birth.[49] More recent studies found an impact on IVF success rates only when alcohol consumption exceeds six or seven drinks per week.[50]

Of course, it is still safer to err on the side of caution and keep alcohol intake to a minimum, but an occasional glass of wine when you know you are not pregnant is unlikely to have much impact.

Caffeine and Fertility

Another controversial issue is the amount of caffeine that is safe while trying to conceive. Here, the major concern is whether caffeine increases miscarriage risk.

It has been known for many years that consuming several cups of coffee per day *during* pregnancy can significantly increase the risk of miscarriage. Unfortunately, the same appears to be true for the time before pregnancy.

A 2018 study from more than 15,000 pregnancies found that compared to women who did not drink coffee, those who drank four or more cups per day before pregnancy had a 20% higher chance of miscarriage.[51]

The risk was not as pronounced for women drinking fewer coffees each day, but even a lower intake still raised the risk of miscarriage. That finding is consistent with prior studies, which reported that the miscarriage risk begins to rise at 50 to 150 mg of caffeine per day during pregnancy.[52] Translating that into real-world terms, the amount of caffeine in a single cup of coffee is typically around 100 to 200 mg. A cup of green tea typically contains around 25 mg of caffeine, whereas black tea often contains around 50 mg per cup. The studies therefore indicate that miscarriage risk begins to rise slightly with just one cup of tea or less than half a cup of coffee per day.

In addition, even though most studies have found no impact on fertility, some research does suggest that caffeine can make it more difficult to get pregnant. A Yale study revealed that women who used to drink tea or coffee in the past but stopped prior to fertility treatment had a higher pregnancy and live birth rate than current tea and coffee drinkers.[53] Another study also found a correlation between caffeine and a decrease in the number of good-quality embryos during IVF.[54]

So although it is probably not absolutely necessary to stop drinking tea and coffee altogether, there is reason to be cautious about how much caffeine you are consuming. One cup of tea or half a cup of coffee each day is likely fine, but gradually switching to decaffeinated tea and coffee is an even safer choice. When making decaf coffee at home, it might also be preferable to buy organic beans that have been decaffeinated by the Swiss Water Process rather than chemical solvents. For recommended brands, see www.itstartswiththeegg.com/coffee.

The Overall Fertility Diet

It is clear that spikes in blood sugar levels can cause major hormonal disruptions and reduce egg quality. Reducing overall carbohydrate intake, choosing more whole, natural foods in place of refined carbohydrates, and starting meals with vegetables and protein will help keep blood sugar levels steady. This in turn can balance a range of hormones and significantly improve egg quality.

Research has also revealed that the general pattern of the Mediterranean diet is associated with improved fertility, with significantly higher success rates in IVF. This is likely because the Mediterranean diet emphasizes vegetables, healthy fats, legumes, and seafood, all of which are higher in specific vitamins and fatty acids associated with lower inflammation and improved fertility.

Action Steps

To boost your fertility, choose a diet based on:

- slowly digested carbohydrates from unprocessed foods such as nuts, seeds, quinoa, wild rice, steel-cut oats, buckwheat, lentils, and other legumes
- leafy greens and other nonstarchy vegetables
- moderate amounts of fruit (up to two servings per day)
- lean, unprocessed protein such as fish, chicken, and beans
- healthy fats such as olive oil, avocado, nuts, and seeds
- You can further improve your egg quality and fertility by limiting:
  › refined carbohydrates such as white bread and highly processed breakfast cereals
  › added sugar and other sweeteners
  › caffeine and alcohol

It may also be worth eliminating gluten and possibly dairy if you have an inflammatory or autoimmune condition (including recurrent miscarriage, endometriosis, or thyroid antibodies).

Chapter 13

Improving Sperm Quality

"No individual can win a game by himself."
— PELE

FOR ANY COUPLE trying to conceive, sperm quality matters. It matters even more when the female partner has poor egg quality. That is because the DNA inside sperm will ordinarily accumulate some degree of damage by the time it reaches an egg. This includes physical breaks in the DNA strands and typos in the genetic code. Eggs have an extraordinary ability to correct this damage, with enzymes running along the sperm DNA shortly after fertilization and making repairs. Unfortunately, this machinery only functions well in good-quality eggs from younger women. As egg quality declines, damage to sperm DNA goes unchecked. This can cause an embryo to stop growing or fail to implant. It can also result in pregnancy loss.

The best solution to this problem is to focus on preventing damage in the first place, by addressing the underlying causes and supporting the natural defense systems that protect sperm DNA from harm. But first, we need to dispel some of the pervasive myths surrounding male fertility.

Myth no. 1: If semen analysis is normal, there is no need to focus on sperm quality

Male infertility contributes to nearly 50% of cases in which a couple has difficulty conceiving, but the male side of the equation is rarely given the attention it deserves.[1] All too often, poor sperm quality goes unrecognized because a clinic will perform a conventional semen analysis and stop there if the result is normal.

A conventional semen analysis focuses on three superficial measures: the number of sperm, how well they move, and their overall shape. A semen analysis can come back perfectly normal on these measures even when there is damage at a molecular level that could be standing in the way of conception. This damage includes oxidation and DNA fragmentation.

Sperm is basically a delivery vehicle for DNA; its entire job is to deliver a parcel of DNA to the egg. This DNA is wrapped up inside a protective layer, but it is still relatively exposed and vulnerable to damage. One of the most common types of damage that can occur is fragmentation, where physical breaks occur in the long DNA chains. This is often triggered by oxidation, a chemical reaction in which free radicals steal electrons. Free radicals are constantly produced as part of our normal metabolism, but a high level of oxidation can occur as a result of age, lifestyle factors, or medical issues, as discussed in this chapter. This oxidative damage in sperm is thought to be a contributing factor in up to 80% of all cases of male infertility.[2]

Although the data is somewhat inconsistent, many studies have reported that sperm with a high level of oxidative damage or DNA fragmentation is less likely to fertilize an egg.[3] Even if fertilization does occur, a resulting pregnancy is more likely to end in a miscarriage.[4] One recent study found the average level of DNA damage in sperm was twice as high in couples with a history of recurrent miscarriage.[5]

If you have a low sperm count, low morphology, or low motility, it is very likely you also have an unusually high level of oxidative damage, DNA fragmentation, or both. But a normal semen analysis does not rule out these issues. It is possible to have damage at the molecular level even if your semen analysis is normal.[6]

That is why it is worth understanding some of the hidden causes of damage to sperm—and the potential solutions. Even if your semen analysis is normal, there may be more subtle issues under the surface that you can address.

To get a sense of how much work you may need to do to optimize your sperm quality, it can be helpful to pursue further testing beyond the basic semen analysis. One of the options is DNA fragmentation testing. There is some controversy over the value of this testing, but it is likely worthwhile for couples with unexplained infertility, poor fertilization, or poor survival of embryos in IVF, a history of unexplained pregnancy loss, or another factor pointing to high level of DNA fragmentation, such as abnormal semen parameters.

According to Dr. Jonathan Ramsey, a British urologist who

has specialized in treating male fertility issues for decades, "Often this test can pick up abnormalities missed in a semen analysis as sperm may appear normal but contain high levels of genetic abnormalities resulting in male fertility problems." Dr. Ramsey advises that DNA fragmentation testing "can be useful for patients who have been trying to conceive for one year, are considering IVF treatment, have been unsuccessful with IVF treatment or have suffered a miscarriage."

Whether or not you opt for fragmentation testing, it is important to learn about the causes of sperm damage and what you can do to prevent it. This is particularly critical if the female partner is over 35 or she has poor egg quality. Although healthy eggs from younger women can effectively repair DNA damage in sperm, this ability declines with age and becomes compromised if the egg itself is damaged.[7]

Studies show that when it comes to the odds of getting pregnant and preventing miscarriage, one of the key issues is the balance between the extent of DNA damage in sperm and the egg's capacity to repair that damage.[8] If your partner is facing her own egg-quality challenges, you need to do everything you can to prevent sperm DNA damage because her eggs may be unable to do the necessary repair work.

Myth no. 2: Healthy men usually have good sperm quality

It is easy to assume that poor sperm quality only impacts men with obvious predisposing factors, such as being a smoker or heavy drinker, being overweight, or having a medical condition, erectile dysfunction, or low semen volume. Although all of these factors are indeed red flags for male fertility, there are many other hidden causes that you may not be aware of.

The first surprising cause of poor sperm quality is the presence of inflammatory bacteria. Recent advances in DNA sequencing technology have revealed that communities of microbes occur in almost every part of the body, including the pathway of glands and structures involved in sperm production, such as the prostate. Some types of microbes along this pathway may be harmless, whereas others can severely compromise male fertility.

Two common bacteria that are clearly detrimental to sperm quality are *Ureaplasma* and *Mycoplasma*. These bacteria are found in 20–30% of men, often without causing any symptoms.[9] Infections with *Ureaplasma* and *Mycoplasma* cause inflammation and an increase in free radicals, which results in DNA fragmentation.[10] For that reason, high DNA fragmentation is a strong sign that a low-level infection may be present.

Sometimes even a basic semen analysis will provide data points suggesting a possible infection. Clues include a low sperm concentration, abnormal morphology, or a high level of immune cells known as leukocytes. But not all infections impact semen parameters in this way.[11] For a more definitive answer, specific testing for infections is worthwhile, particularly in cases of unexplained infertility or poor fertilization in IVF, or if testing shows high DNA fragmentation. Testing options include a standard urine and semen culture or a microbiome test for bacterial DNA using a home collection kit, such as that developed by Fertilysis.

If harmful bacteria are found, antibiotic treatment can significantly improve sperm quality.[12] Ampicillin and doxycycline are among the most effective antibiotics for this purpose;

ciprofloxacin and related "floxacin" antibiotics should be avoided because they can damage sperm DNA and mitochondria.[13] If you are preparing for IVF, keep in mind that it may take more than a month for sperm quality to improve following antibiotic treatment.[14]

Another common cause of poor sperm quality in healthy men is a varicocele. This is an enlarged vein in the scrotum, similar to a varicose vein. It occurs when a valve in the blood vessel is absent or malfunctions, causing the vein to widen. The additional blood pooling in the vein can cause sperm damage in a variety of ways, including an increase in temperature, lack of blood flow where it is needed, and the accumulation of toxic metabolites. All these factors cause oxidative damage, resulting in DNA fragmentation. About 10% of men have varicoceles, but this rises to 30% of men in couples facing fertility problems, and up to 80% of men with secondary infertility—that is, difficulty conceiving after previously fathering a child.[15]

Dr. Ramsey explains that varicoceles often present as secondary infertility because "previously younger eggs were able to compensate for the less good-quality sperm... The reason for the subsequent secondary infertility is only because the passage of time has meant that his partner's eggs have become older and are unable to compensate for the inadequacies of his sperm."

Sometimes varicoceles can be seen with the naked eye or felt by a self-exam, but they are usually detected during a routine exam with a urologist. Correcting a varicocele with a quick medical procedure can significantly improve sperm quality, but studies have found it can take three to six months after the procedure to see the full benefit.[16] Protecting against further oxidative damage during this time using the supplements and strategies discussed later in this chapter can also make a big difference.

An additional factor that can contribute to poor sperm quality is age. It is commonly believed that men retain their fertility into their sixties, but the reality is that a typical 45-year-old man is significantly less fertile than a man 10 years younger, with sperm quality beginning to decline as early as age 35.[17] A large part of the reason for this decline is that sperm from older men have more DNA breakage, DNA mutations, and other chromosomal abnormalities.[18] In fact, DNA fragmentation in sperm doubles from ages 30 to 45.[19] This significantly increases the risk of miscarriage.[20]

It is not just the DNA inside sperm that suffers with increasing age. Sperm motility starts to decline at age 35, and age also negatively impacts sperm count and morphology.[21]

But it's not all bad news. Research shows that some of this decline can be prevented and reversed, with several studies finding that older men following a healthy diet and taking the right supplements have sperm quality similar to younger men. This brings us to the most significant myth of all.

Myth no. 3: Nothing can be done to improve sperm quality

Decades of scientific research contradicts this widely held belief and shows that it is possible to improve sperm quality and even improve the quality of the DNA within the sperm. Doing so can increase the chance of conceiving while reducing the risk of miscarriage and birth defects.

To understand what you can do to improve sperm quality, it helps to first understand a little more about how sperm become damaged in the first place.

The cycle of producing each sperm takes a little over two months.[22] During this time, many different environmental and lifestyle factors can impact the process. By far the most important factor impacting sperm quality during this time is oxidation.

As sperm are produced, a normal, healthy level of oxidation takes place as a result of biological processes, while an army of defenders stops this oxidation getting out of control. The defense system includes antioxidants such as vitamins C and E (semen contains a particularly high concentration of vitamin C), along with special enzymes that exist solely to protect sperm against oxidative damage. These enzymes are heavily dependent on zinc and selenium, which is why these minerals are so critical to male fertility.

When antioxidant defenses are compromised or overwhelmed by too many free radicals this causes damage to sperm DNA.[23] Research at the Cleveland Clinic has confirmed that men with high levels of oxidation in semen have more extensive DNA fragmentation and fewer normally functioning sperm.[24]

As mentioned earlier, medical issues such as infections and enlarged veins (varicoceles) can cause particularly high levels of oxidation.[25] If you are affected by one of these conditions, treating the underlying problem is critical to stopping the damage and improving your sperm quality. But even if you do not have one of these conditions, basic lifestyle factors can have a significant impact on the degree of oxidative damage in sperm, for better or worse.

Factors such as exposure to common toxins, smoking, alcohol consumption, and a diet high in refined carbohydrates and saturated fat can compromise sperm quality at a molecular level. Reducing exposure to those chemicals, shifting toward a healthier diet, and increasing intake of antioxidants through food and supplements can protect developing sperm, potentially allowing you to conceive sooner and reducing the odds of miscarriage.

How to Improve Your Sperm Quality

Take a daily multivitamin supplement

One of the simplest and most effective ways to improve sperm quality is by taking a daily multivitamin supplement that contains antioxidants such as vitamin E, vitamin C, selenium, and zinc. Dozens of studies have established that these and other antioxidants can improve sperm quality and increase the chance of conceiving.[26] This is true for couples trying to conceive naturally as well as those undergoing fertility treatment.

In 2022, a group of 30 leading urologists from around the world undertook a systematic review of all the randomized, placebo-controlled studies in this area and concluded that "the odds for a spontaneous clinical pregnancy are almost double … in infertile men after treatment with [antioxidants]."[27] Based on this evidence, the urologists affirmatively recommended that men having difficulty conceiving should supplement with antioxidants in order to improve sperm parameters, reduce oxidative stress, and increase the chance of pregnancy.

Research suggests that antioxidants may be particularly powerful when infertility is caused by DNA damage within sperm. In one study, men with elevated DNA fragmentation were given vitamins C and E daily for two months following a failed attempt to achieve fertilization by ICSI. ICSI is an approach similar to IVF, where sperm are injected directly into the eggs.[28] The researchers found an extraordinary improvement in the next attempt, with the clinical pregnancy rate jumping from 7% to 48%.

Different studies use different combinations of antioxidants, but the ones that have been studied the most in this context are vitamin C, vitamin E, zinc, folate, and selenium.[29] Vitamins C and E act directly as antioxidants, whereas zinc, folate, and selenium prevent oxidation in more complex ways, such as by assisting antioxidant enzymes. A deficiency in zinc or folate can also directly cause increased DNA damage.[30]

Although many studies have tried to find out which of these vitamins (or which combination) help the most, you can cover all bases and probably get the most benefit by simply taking a daily multivitamin. A multivitamin designed specifically for men is a good option because it will probably contain more zinc and selenium.

It is also helpful to choose a multivitamin that contains methylfolate rather than synthetic folic acid. That is because folate plays a critical role in protecting sperm DNA.[31] Common genetic variants can compromise the ability to convert synthetic folic acid to the active methylfolate form, resulting a deficiency of active folate. This appears to play a role in some cases of recurrent miscarriage. [32] We can likely circumvent the problem of poor folate metabolism by choosing a multivitamin that already contains methylfolate. For recommended multivitamins for men, see **itstartswiththeegg.com/male-supplements**

Ideally, you will start taking a multivitamin two or three months before trying to conceive, but boosting your vitamin and antioxidant levels for any time period before conception is helpful.

Add a Coenzyme Q10 supplement

Combining a multivitamin with additional antioxidants can provide even greater protection of sperm quality. The most useful additional supplement is probably CoQ10—a vital antioxidant molecule found in just about every cell in the body. It is particularly beneficial for sperm quality because it plays a critical role in cellular energy production.

Researchers have known for many years that there is a link between sperm quality and the level of CoQ10 naturally present in semen. Men with lower CoQ10 levels tend to have a lower sperm count and poor motility.[33]

More recently, several randomized, double-blind, placebo-controlled studies have reported that supplementing with CoQ10 improves sperm concentration, motility, and morphology.[34] It also significantly reduces DNA damage.[35] One way in which CoQ10 is thought to achieve these benefits is by increasing the activity of antioxidant enzymes, which prevent oxidative damage to sperm DNA.[36]

In addition to protecting sperm quality, supplementing with CoQ10 has many other benefits for general health, including reducing LDL cholesterol, inflammation, and heart disease.[37] A placebo-controlled study in Sweden found that taking CoQ10 significantly reduces heart disease deaths, with improved survival evident even 12 years later.[38]

When choosing a brand of CoQ10, a good form to take is known as ubiquinol (as explained in chapter 6), and the usual recommended dose is 200 mg per day.[39] For couples with particularly severe fertility issues, a dose of 400 mg may be more effective.

Protect sperm with Omega-3s

All men trying to conceive need adequate omega-3 fatty acids oil to prevent DNA damage in sperm. Unless you eat salmon or sardines regularly, it is likely you are not getting enough. Adding a daily omega-3 fish oil supplement will not only support your cognitive function and heart health, but also your sperm quality.

Double-blind, placebo-controlled trials have found that fish oil supplements improve sperm quality, with a particular improvement in DNA damage.[40] In a 2016 study, when men took a fish oil supplement for three months, the average percentage of sperm with DNA damage dropped from 22% to 9%.[41] The dose used in this study was 1,500 mg of fish oil containing 990 mg of DHA and 135 mg of EPA per day. For a similar dose, take two capsules of Nordic Naturals DHA Xtra.

Advanced sperm-quality supplements

In cases where sperm quality is known to be an issue or there is a history of failed IVF cycles or recurrent miscarriage, it is likely helpful to go further and add several additional supplements that have been found to improve sperm quality. The most effective supplements are:

- Alpha-lipoic acid
- L-carnitine
- N-acetylcysteine

Alpha-lipoic acid is a fatty acid found naturally in every cell of the body. It not only serves as an antioxidant but also plays a critical role in cellular energy production. Numerous studies have reported that supplementing with alpha-lipoic acid can significantly improve sperm quality.[42] As just one example, a randomized, double-blind, placebo-controlled study found that when men took alpha-lipoic acid every day for 12 weeks, there was a significant improvement in the total sperm count, sperm concentration, and motility.[43]

The recommended dose is 600 mg per day for a standard alpha-lipoic acid supplement. If your supplement is in the form of R-alpha lipoic acid, it is likely sufficient to take 200–300 mg per day. Note that alpha-lipoic acid is not recommended for those with underactive thyroid since it may interfere with conversion of Synthroid to active thyroid hormones.

Where testing shows that sperm motility is a concern, another useful supplement is L-carnitine. Randomized studies have found that on average, L-carnitine can improve motility by 8% and morphology by 5%.[44] Yet in men with a significant degree of oxidative damage to sperm, carnitine has a much greater impact. In those cases, it can increase the total number of motile sperm by more than twofold.[45] As a result, carnitine appears to be especially effective in men with poor sperm quality caused by varicoceles.[46] The usual dose is 1000 mg per day. (At higher doses it may reduce thyroid activity).

There is an alternative form of carnitine available in supplement form, called acetyl-l-carnitine. The body naturally maintains an equilibrium between the two forms, and studies have found that taking either can improve sperm quality.[47] L-carnitine may be preferred simply because it has been studied more extensively.

If your primary concern is DNA fragmentation or varicoceles, another supplement that may be particularly helpful is N-acetylcysteine (NAC). This amino acid derivative increases the natural production of glutathione—the master antioxidant that plays a key role in protecting sperm against oxidative damage. Studies have found that supplementing with NAC for several months can improve testosterone levels and semen parameters while reducing DNA damage.[48] In one study, men who supplemented with 600 mg of NAC per day for three months saw DNA fragmentation drop from 20% to 15%.[49] NAC may also help sperm quality recover sooner following varicocele repair.[50]

It is not necessary to take all of these supplements, but a combination does seem to have greater impact than any one supplement taken alone. In a double-blind, placebo-controlled study published in 2020, researchers investigated the combination of L-carnitine, CoQ10, B vitamins, zinc, and selenium in men with unexplained infertility.[51] After four months, 69% of men in the supplement group had a normal semen analysis, compared to just 22% in the placebo group. The chance of conceiving was also very different: 24% in the supplement group, compared to just 5% in the placebo group. This is a dramatic difference resulting from relatively little effort. You can get all of the components of the supplement combination used in that study with just a daily multivitamin plus L-carnitine and CoQ10. Where DNA fragmentation is a concern, you will likely see even greater benefit from adding omega-3 fish oil and NAC.

As a side note, maintaining an adequate vitamin D level may also be important for sperm quality because vitamin D plays a key role in fighting infection, reducing inflammation, and producing reproductive hormones.[52] Little research has been done on vitamin D and male fertility, but preliminary studies have found that men with higher vitamin D levels have higher sperm concentration, better morphology and motility, and higher levels of testosterone.[53] One study found a significant increase in sperm concentration and motility in vitamin D–deficient men after six months of supplementation.[54]

Herbal and plant-based fertility supplements such as maca and vitex are not recommended because they can have unpredictable effects on hormones and may be contaminated with heavy metals, as discussed in chapter 10. In addition, if you have low testosterone, this should be addressed by a urologist with an understanding of fertility issues. Supplementing with testosterone directly can halt sperm production for many months by suppressing other critical hormones.[55]

Boost your antioxidant levels through diet

Diet is another key strategy for improving sperm quality, with years of scientific research finding that men with a diet higher in antioxidants from fruit and vegetables are more likely to have good semen parameters and less sperm DNA damage.[56]

As just one example, a recent study in California revealed that men with the highest intake of vitamin C, vitamin E, zinc, and folate had much less sperm DNA damage.[57] In fact, the men with the highest intake of these antioxidants had sperm quality on par with much younger men. This extraordinary finding suggests that we may be able to prevent a large part of the decline in male fertility and increase in the risk of miscarriage that occurs with age, simply by placing greater emphasis on fruit, vegetables, nuts, and olive oil.

These foods are so beneficial because they provide a broader array of antioxidants than found in supplements. One example is lycopene, an antioxidant found in tomatoes that appears to be particularly helpful for sperm quality.[58]

Other powerful antioxidants include anthocyanins, which give berries their dark purple color, and beta-carotene, found in sweet potatoes and carrots. Additional well-known sources of antioxidants are green tea and dark chocolate, although little is known about how these antioxidants relate to sperm quality. Until we know more about which antioxidants are most beneficial, the best approach is to eat a wide variety of fruits and vegetables, especially the brightly colored varieties, which are typically higher in antioxidants.

It is also worth choosing fruits and vegetables that are naturally lower in pesticides. These include papaya, pineapple, mango, honeydew melon, avocado, cabbage, onion, and peas. In a recent study by researchers at the Harvard School of Public Health, men who ate more of these low-pesticide fruits and vegetables had a 169% higher total sperm count and a 173% higher sperm concentration.[59]

Lean in to a Mediterranean diet

Beyond antioxidants, a persuasive body of research indicates that you can dramatically improve sperm quality by shifting toward a Mediterranean diet.[60] In particular, the studies show that the best diet for male fertility is low in sugar, refined carbohydrates, processed meat, and saturated fat, and emphasizes fish, chicken, vegetables, beans, nuts, low-fat dairy, and unrefined whole grains.[61]

Even simply cutting back on sugar can make a difference. Numerous studies have found that sugar has a major impact on sperm quality.[62] Men who drink one or two sugary drinks per day have lower sperm concentration.[63] Studies have also found that higher sugar intake by men increases a couple's time to pregnancy.[64]

On the other hand, increasing consumption of healthier foods, such as nuts, can quickly improve sperm quality. A randomized, controlled trial found that eating a small handful of nuts each day increases sperm quality by reducing DNA fragmentation.[65] Another similar study reported that regularly eating walnuts can improve sperm motility and morphology.[66]

Cut back on alcohol

There is no doubt that heavy alcohol intake is associated with poor sperm quality,[67] but it appears that even moderate intake can compromise male fertility, particularly for couples trying to conceive through IVF.

In one study at the University of California, researchers found the risk of a failed IVF cycle more than doubled for men who drank one additional drink per day.[68] This was due in part to a higher miscarriage rate when men drank alcohol in the month before IVF.

Other studies have found that alcohol consumption decreases sperm count, sperm motility, and the chance of fertilization in IVF.[69] Alcohol intake is also known to increase oxidative stress and likely causes DNA damage in sperm.[70] The impact of alcohol on sperm DNA may explain a curious pattern observed in several studies: a higher rate of heart defects in babies whose fathers drank more alcohol before conception.[71]

Although the occasional drink may have little effect, beyond this amount it is worth exercising caution, particularly if you face an uphill battle trying to conceive.

If you are a smoker, it is also important to quit smoking as soon as you start trying to conceive. Data shows that paternal smoking before conception not only makes it more difficult to conceive but may also increase the risk of birth defects and childhood cancer.[72]

Reduce your exposure to environmental toxins

For many years, public health researchers have been sounding the alarm about consistently declining sperm counts. One of those researchers is Shanna Swan, a professor of environmental medicine and public health at the Icahn School of Medicine at Mount Sinai. Swan has studied the impact of the environment on health and fertility for more than two decades. In 2017, one of her studies revealed the true scope of the problem: from 1973 to 2011, the total sperm count of men in the developed world dropped by 59%.[73] The quality also declined, with a greater proportion of abnormal morphology, lower motility, and more DNA damage. Since that study was published, it has become clear the trend has continued and is even accelerating.[74]

Although some of the global decline in sperm count and sperm quality may be due to lifestyle factors or men having children later in life, according to Dr. Swan, the evidence is clear that "chemicals play a major causal role."

Everyday environmental toxins not only disrupt the activity of hormones that control sperm production, they are also a major contributor to the oxidative stress that is seen in up to 80% of infertile men. Toxins often cause increased oxidation by compromising the activity of antioxidant enzymes, along with causing a host of other harmful effects on sperm quality.

Over 80,000 chemicals are registered for use in the United States, yet only a small percentage have ever been analyzed for safety and even fewer for reproductive harm. Within the soup of chemicals we are exposed to on a daily basis, the toxins with the clearest evidence of harm to sperm quality are the same ones shown to harm developing eggs: phthalates and bisphenols. They are both ubiquitous chemical families that have long been known to disrupt hormone activity (so-called "endocrine disruptors").

Phthalates

Phthalates are a group of chemicals called "plasticizers" that are used in everything from cologne to laundry detergent to soft PVC plastic. As explained in more detail in chapter 2, these chemicals are banned in children's toys, and some phthalates are banned in personal care products in Europe, but very little has been done to curb the quantity of phthalates we are exposed to on a daily basis. This is despite the fact that scientists have known for more than 20 years that these chemicals are absorbed into the body and interfere with critical hormones.

By acting as endocrine disruptors, phthalates cause a range of harmful effects, including genital malformations in baby boys exposed in utero.[75] After many years of heated controversy, it now appears to be well established that phthalates also damage sperm in adult men.[76]

The concentration of phthalates that men are commonly exposed to has been shown to cause DNA damage in sperm while also reducing sperm quality by traditional measures. The damage may occur in a variety of ways, including altering hormone levels and causing oxidative stress. Specifically, higher phthalate levels have been linked to lower levels of testosterone and other hormones involved in male fertility.[77] A large study involving more than 10,000 people also revealed a link between higher levels of phthalates and more extensive oxidative stress throughout the body.[78]

Ultimately, even a small decline in sperm quality caused by phthalates may translate into a significant reduction in fertility. At the 2013 meeting of the American Society of Reproductive Medicine, researchers presented the results of a study investigating the relationship between phthalate levels and odds of conceiving in 500 couples. The researchers found that couples in which men had the highest levels of phthalates were 20% less likely to conceive over the course of a year.[79]

The single most important step to reducing phthalate exposure is avoiding highly processed food. Food processing results in a high degree of phthalate contamination because the processing equipment is often made from soft, flexible plastic. Studies have found that when individuals emphasize foods prepared in the home from natural ingredients, phthalate levels drop quicky and dramatically.[80]

The second major culprit is fragrance. Men can significantly reduce their exposure to phthalates simply by avoiding unnecessary fragrance such as cologne and fragranced laundry detergent and switching to shampoo, shaving cream, and deodorant labeled as "phthalate-free" (such as those made by Every Man Jack, Burt's Bees, and Caswell-Massey).

Bisphenols

Bisphenol A, or BPA for short, is another toxin that can disrupt hormones and therefore compromise male fertility. This chemical, and its closely related cousins, are commonly found in processed food and reusable plastic food and drink containers. Researchers have long been suspicious of BPA because it is an endocrine disruptor known to mimic the effects of estrogen.

In one of the earliest studies on the question of BPA and sperm quality, researchers at the University of Michigan found that higher urinary BPA levels were linked to lower sperm count, motility, and morphology, and a greater percentage of sperm DNA damage.[81] Other studies have reported similar patterns.[82]

Even though some controversy still remains over the impact of BPA on sperm quality, there is now more than enough evidence to warrant caution. The most important practical steps are to avoid canned and highly processed foods and replace plastic kitchenware with glass or stainless steel, as discussed in more detail in chapter 2. "BPA-free" plastic is not necessarily a safe option because many companies simply replace BPA with closely related compounds that are likely no better.

Chemicals in lubricants

Studies show that most lubricant brands significantly decrease sperm motility and increase DNA fragmentation.[83] In a 2014 study that compared 11 different lubricants, the brand with the least impact on sperm function was Pre-Seed.[84] A 2022 study reached the same conclusion, finding that Pre-Seed reduced motility to some extent but less than other purportedly sperm-friendly brands tested.[85] One newer brand that appears to have little impact on sperm is BabyDance.[86] The advantage of BabyDance over Pre-Seed is that it does not contain parabens, which are thought to act as hormone disruptors.

Fresher sperm is better

After tackling diet and toxins, there are a few other steps that can provide further improvement to sperm quality. One of those steps is making sure sperm has not accumulated for too long before ovulation or IVF.

For many years, fertility clinics have advised men to abstain from ejaculation for several days before an IVF or IUI procedure to ensure a higher sperm count. The most recent data suggests that might be counterproductive.[87] Although it is true that a higher sperm count will be obtained after a break of several days, the quality of sperm declines significantly. In particular, the longer sperm accumulates, the more DNA fragmentation occurs.[88]

Given a choice between higher sperm count or higher quality, the data indicates that fresher sperm with less DNA damage win. Although some researchers have reported similar outcomes either way, most studies have found that with fewer days' abstinence before ejaculation, there is a significantly higher chance of pregnancy.[89] There may also be a lower chance of miscarriage.[90] In other words, quality trumps quantity.

From a practical standpoint, if you are trying to conceive naturally, it likely makes sense to try every day starting at least four days before ovulation. If you are trying to conceive through IVF or IUI and your fertility clinic gives broad guidance on how long to abstain from ejaculation before giving your sample, such as one to three days, it is likely better to err on the shorter end of that time frame. It may also be worth questioning your doctor about their standard recommended time frame if you have very high DNA fragmentation. Some clinics now address high fragmentation by using a sample given just three hours after a previous ejaculation, with good results.[91]

Stay cool

Researchers have known for more than 40 years that elevated temperatures impair sperm quality. The impact of heat on sperm quality is readily apparent from the effect of a fever, which causes a drop in sperm count and motility.[92] The longer the fever, the worse the impact on sperm quality.

Other factors also increase temperature where it matters: sitting all day, taking hot baths or showers, and wearing tight-fitting underwear.[93] In one six-month study, researchers witnessed a 50% decrease in sperm parameters in men wearing tight-fitting underwear. Sperm parameters improved after subjects switched to loose-fitting boxers.[94] Cycling may also compromise sperm quality, with studies finding that regular cyclists have a lower concentration of sperm and lower percentage of sperm with normal morphology.[95]

Many fertility clinics advise men to avoid hot baths and showers in the week before sample collection, but that is likely not long enough. The full process of sperm production takes over two months, and it is likely that early stages of sperm production are just as vulnerable to heat. The longer you can keep things cool, the better.

Action Plan for Sperm Quality

- Optimizing sperm quality is important whenever egg quality is an issue, since a lower quality egg cannot perform the usual processes to repair DNA damage in sperm.

- If you have unexplained infertility, abnormal semen parameters, a history of IVF cycles in which few eggs fertilized or few embryos survived, or a history of unexplained miscarriage, it may be worth pursuing additional testing for DNA fragmentation and possible infections. It is also worth seeing a urologist for a routine exam to rule out varicoceles, particularly if you have high DNA fragmentation or secondary infertility.

- Even if you have no reason to be concerned about sperm quality, take a daily multivitamin, ideally starting several months before trying to conceive. It is best to choose a brand that contains methylfolate rather than synthetic folic acid.

- It is worth adding the following supplements to reduce DNA damage in sperm:
  - › CoQ10 (as ubiquinol or Bio-Quinon): 200 mg per day with breakfast. For couples with serious difficulties, consider increasing to 400 mg per day.
  - › Fish oil: two capsules of Nordic Naturals DHA Xtra or an equivalent to provide at least 900 mg of DHA

- If you have known sperm-quality issues, consider adding one or more of the following antioxidant supplements:

> › R-alpha lipoic acid: 200–300 mg per day, preferably on an empty stomach, but can be taken with breakfast if more convenient (particularly helpful for improving sperm count and concentration)

> › L-carnitine: 1,000 mg, with or without food (particularly helpful for improving motility and addressing damage caused by varicoceles)

> › N-acetylcysteine: 600 mg, with or without food (particularly helpful for addressing DNA damage, low testosterone, and damage caused by varicoceles)

- It may be worth getting your vitamin D level tested and supplementing if you are deficient.

- Further boost your vitamin and antioxidant levels with a diet rich in brightly colored fruits and vegetables.

- Limit sugar and red meat intake while shifting toward a Mediterranean diet that emphasizes fish, nuts, olive oil, and legumes.

- Reduce alcohol consumption, particularly in the lead-up to IVF.

- Take steps to reduce your exposure to toxins known to damage sperm, especially those found in highly processed food and fragrances.

- Keep in mind that fresher sperm is usually better, with less accumulated DNA damage.

- Stay cool where it counts with loose boxers and breaks from sitting.

Chapter 14

Preparing for Embryo Transfer

"Waiting makes me restless. When I'm ready, I'm ready."
— REBA MCENTIRE

AFTER DEVOTING MONTHS to improving egg quality, going through the arduous IVF process, and finally ending up with embryos ready to transfer, the focus shifts to helping those embryos implant. But the reality is, you are already more prepared than you think.

The single most significant factor that determines whether an embryo will implant is its quality—in particular, whether it is genetically normal. By focusing on improving egg quality (or making the difficult decision to use donor eggs or embryos), you have already taken the most important steps. There are still supplements that can help and decisions to be made, such as deciding between a fresh or frozen transfer and whether to opt for genetic testing, but these factors are less important than whether you start out with a good-quality embryo.

This chapter briefly discusses supplements that may help improve your uterine lining by encouraging blood flow and increasing thickness, but this is not an elaborate supplement regime that can make a dramatic difference. Supplements and lifestyle do not have as much impact when preparing for embryo transfer because once you have a good embryo, whether it implants comes down to luck and having a good endometrial lining.

Typically, the uterine lining does not need much support beyond the estrogen and progesterone given as part of a standard transfer protocol. When a genetically normal embryo fails to implant, it is generally either a matter of bad luck or an issue that cannot be addressed through supplements or lifestyle. These issues include hidden infections, autoimmunity, endometriosis, and scar tissue—all of which can cause so-called "implantation dysfunction." This condition requires more advanced testing to uncover and typically requires medical treatment to address. Because this issue can impact natural conception too, not just embryo transfer, it is covered in detail in chapter 15.

Most often, clinics recommend going ahead with at least one transfer and only pursuing additional testing later if failed transfers suggest there may be a problem. If you have very few embryos or a history of autoimmunity or infections, it might be reasonable to request some of the advanced testing for implantation issues discussed in chapter 15 before your first transfer, although your clinic may resist and advise that it is unnecessary.

For now, we will focus on the other decisions to be made in

the lead-up to transfer, as well as other measures that may aid in preparing your lining, such as supplements and acupuncture. These factors may help shift the odds in your favor, but at the end of the day, you have already done the hard work to improve your embryo quality, and that is likely what matters most.

Fresh or Frozen Transfer

In recent years, there has been a trend away from transferring fresh embryos shortly after egg retrieval, with many clinics instead preferring to freeze all embryos and wait a month to perform the first transfer. This approach is backed up by several large studies finding higher pregnancy rates after frozen embryo transfers.[1]

As one example, a study of almost 3,000 IVF cycles at some of the top clinics in the United States found the pregnancy rate for freeze-all cycles was 52%, compared to 45% for cycles with a fresh transfer.[2] A similar pattern was seen in a randomized trial of 1,600 women in China, published in the prestigious medical journal *The Lancet*.[3]

Not all studies have found higher success with frozen transfers, however.[4] It is possible that some clinics may simply be more skilled with fresh than frozen transfers. When a series of studies on this question were pooled and considered together, researchers concluded that "one strategy is probably not superior to the other."[5]

The best approach may depend more on your IVF clinic's strengths and weaknesses and your own unique circumstances. For example, if you have a thin endometrial lining after egg retrieval, that may weigh in favor of a frozen transfer at a later date. Another consideration is whether your embryos are strong enough to survive freezing and thawing. If you have very few embryos and they do not appear to be developing well, a fresh transfer will likely give you the best chance. On the other hand, if you decide to have your embryos genetically tested, that typically requires a frozen transfer.

In the end, it usually makes sense to trust your clinic's recommendation as to whether a fresh or frozen embryo transfer is the best approach for your particular circumstances.

Embryo Testing

The technology used to analyze embryos has advanced significantly in the past decade, identifying more and more abnormalities that previously would have gone undetected. Unfortunately, those advances in testing have not translated into higher success rates, perhaps because some of the embryos now being labeled as abnormal actually have the potential to develop into a healthy baby.

Genetic testing of embryos can no doubt provide useful information for many couples, helping increase the odds of implantation and reduce the odds of miscarriage. But getting that information sometimes comes at the cost of losing embryos in the process. Like so many other choices, deciding whether to test your embryos and whether to transfer an embryo reported as abnormal involves weighing the pros and cons in relation to your unique circumstances and priorities.

Types of embryo tests

The most common form of embryo testing looks for errors that have occurred spontaneously during egg or embryo development, such as an extra copy of a chromosome. This is called "preimplantation genetic testing for aneuploidy," abbreviated as PGT-A. It involves removing approximately five cells from the outer layer of a 5-day-old embryo and sending those cells to a lab for analysis.

The lab will determine whether any chromosomes are missing or duplicated, or whether a small piece of a chromosome has been gained or lost in any of the cells sampled from the embryo. The goal is to identify the embryos without any errors, known as "euploid" embryos, which have the greatest potential to successfully implant. Embryos with an abnormality (termed "aneuploid") are often discarded.

Another form of embryo testing, referred to as PGT-M, is used when a parent has a genetic disease and they wish to screen embryos to avoid passing down that particular gene. For couples affected by a serious genetic disease, it is often a relatively easy decision to pursue PGT-M.

This chapter focuses on PGT-A and the more difficult question of whether to opt for PGT-A testing in order to increase the chance of an embryo successfully implanting and reduce the chance of miscarriage. (PGT-A will be referred to as PGT for short in the remainder of this chapter.) This chapter will also discuss the types of abnormal embryos that may be worth transferring.

How does testing impact IVF success rates?

For women over 35, the evidence is fairly strong that a PGT-tested embryo will have a higher chance of implanting and a lower chance of miscarriage than an untested embryo.[6] In other words, there is a higher chance of pregnancy *per transfer*. That does not necessarily mean there is a higher chance of pregnancy *per egg retrieval*.

If you have one normal embryo and three abnormal embryos that are not viable, you still have the same overall chance of pregnancy from those four embryos, whether or not you opt for testing. Testing does not change the embryos you have, it just provides information about which embryos to transfer first, so you can reach the same outcome with fewer transfers.[7]

This ability to prioritize embryos is most useful for women over 35. In younger women, there is already a high chance that the best-looking embryo will be chromosomally normal. That was shown in a recent randomized study that compared the success rates when embryos were chosen on the basis of appearance alone or PGT testing. The study found that for women under 35, three-quarters of embryos with the best appearance were chromosomally normal. [8] The study also found the same chance of success whether transferring either a tested embryo or the single best-looking embryo.

For women starting out with a higher percentage of abnormal embryos, PGT is more useful because it can help avoid the time, cost, and heartache of failed embryo transfers and possibly miscarriage.

Opting to perform PGT testing is not without downsides, however. The numbers show that although testing increases the pregnancy rate per embryo transfer, some healthy embryos are also lost in the process.

Part of the explanation for this is that growing embryos to day 5 in order to perform a biopsy and then freezing the embryos, instead of performing a fresh transfer at day 3, can occasionally result in the loss of a viable embryo. For those with many embryos to choose from, this is not a major problem because it serves as a selection method for the best embryos. The situation is different for couples starting with only a few embryos, particularly if those embryos are viable but lower quality.

If your clinic tries to grow lower-quality embryos to day 5 in order to do PGT testing, the embryos may not make it. One study found that for women who had only a single viable embryo on day 3, doing an immediate fresh transfer rather than trying to grow the embryo to day 5 doubled the pregnancy rate.[9]

The potential for discarding viable embryos

There is also a growing concern that PGT testing can result in discarding supposedly abnormal embryos that have the potential to lead to a healthy baby. This issue was first raised in 2015 with a report published in the *New England Journal of Medicine* describing healthy babies born after transferring chromosomally abnormal embryos.[10]

The authors gave 18 women without any normal embryos the opportunity to transfer an embryo with a certain kind of abnormality (that is, a mosaic embryo). From those 18 transfers, six babies were born and all were found to have normal chromosomes. Several other studies have now reported the same astonishing outcome—healthy babies born from abnormal embryos.

This has led some to question whether PGT has any value at all. If embryos reported as abnormal can lead to perfectly healthy babies, what is the point of testing? However, the research shows that PGT results are still very informative and that only certain types of abnormal embryos have a good chance of becoming a healthy baby.

To understand why, it is helpful to know more about how PGT testing is performed. A 5-day embryo has an outer layer of cells, called the trophectoderm, and an inner ball of cells, called the inner cell mass. The trophectoderm eventually becomes the placenta, while the inner cell mass becomes the baby. To perform PGT, a sample of around five cells is taken from the trophectoderm.

If an embryo is reported as aneuploid, that typically means all cells tested had the same abnormality, such as an extra copy of a chromosome. In such a case, the abnormality can likely be traced all the way back to the original egg cell, which means the abnormality would impact the entire embryo. Some refer to these embryos as "uniform aneuploid." It is extremely rare for such embryos to implant and become a healthy baby. Most often, they fail to implant. If they do implant, they almost always lead to a first-trimester miscarriage.

In one study describing 100 transfers of embryos with uniform aneuploidies, there were only seven pregnancies. Out of those seven pregnancies, six resulted in miscarriage, leaving just one live birth.[11]

On the other hand, if only some of the sampled cells have an abnormality and others do not, this will be reported as "mosaic" or "intermediate copy number." Often these embryos are reported as abnormal and not considered suitable for transfer, but studies suggest they should be given a chance. That is because for mosaic embryos, there are two ways a PGT report may not truly reflect the state of the embryo.

First, the biopsied cells taken from the outer layer of the embryo may not accurately reflect the inner part of the embryo. If only some of the cells in the outer layer have a chromosomal abnormality, that means the error occurred later in development and may not be present in the part of the embryo that would become the baby.

Second, in mosaic embryos it is possible for the abnormal cells to be eliminated in a process of self-correction. The idea that embryos can correct genetic errors seems improbable, but there is a growing consensus among scientists that it does occur. If the inner cell mass contains a combination of normal and abnormal cells, the abnormal cells are more likely to stop growing and die off, while the normal cells can continue replicating and go on to form a healthy baby.[12] In other words, as development progresses, mosaic embryos have a mechanism to selectively eliminate cells with chromosomal abnormalities.

There is some controversy over this point, but research suggests that mosaic embryos with an abnormality impacting just one chromosome may have a similar chance of successfully implanting as normal embryos.[13] The chance of miscarriage with a mosaic embryo may be higher than with a normal embryo, but it is likely below 25%.[14]

Nevertheless, many doctors are reluctant to transfer mosaic embryos out of concern that a child may be born with a genetic abnormality. That concern appears to be largely unfounded. To date, almost all babies born from mosaic embryos have been genetically normal. There have been isolated cases of babies born with a chromosomal abnormality but without serious health consequences.[15] It is also possible to screen for genetic issues in pregnancy with noninvasive prenatal testing. Even so, many clinics refuse to transfer mosaic embryos, which is one factor to keep in mind when you are deciding whether to opt for PGT testing.

How to decide whether to test your embryos

Ultimately, whether to test your embryos can be a difficult decision that involves weighing your age, how many embryos you have, and your own priorities and concerns.

Selecting the best embryos makes more of a difference as you get older and likely have a higher percentage of abnormal embryos. In women over 40, the major advantage of testing is that it can help address the higher risk of miscarriage and chromosomal conditions such as Down syndrome. Given these concerns, some couples weigh the risks and benefits and decide that the need to avoid a miscarriage or genetic condition outweighs the risk of losing viable embryos by doing PGT.

Time can also be a consideration. Testing may show that all embryos are abnormal and that another egg retrieval is the best option. Without testing, many months could have been wasted on embryo transfers or potential pregnancy losses. With testing, it is possible to move on to another retrieval without delay.

Although testing has more value for women over 35, and particularly over age 40, it also carries more downsides. That is because PGT poses a small risk of losing viable embryos. Embryos may be lost as a result of trying to grow them to day 5 in the lab, damage from biopsy, or inaccurate results. Few embryos are lost in this way, but if your egg retrieval only produces one or two embryos, those embryos will have the best chance if they are transferred on day 3, without any testing.

A good compromise may be a fresh transfer with at least one embryo on day 3, and then testing any remaining embryos that survive to day 5.

If you do decide to test your embryos, it is worth asking your clinic for a copy of the PGT report and an explanation of the results so you can find out whether any of the embryos reported as abnormal are mosaic embryos that may be worth transferring. If your clinic refuses to transfer mosaics, you may be able to move the embryos to another clinic.

Supplements to Prepare for Transfer

In the lead-up to embryo transfer, which egg-quality supplements are worth continuing, and are there any additional supplements that can improve your uterine lining?

As a starting point, it is worth continuing your prenatal multivitamin, vitamin D, and, if you are deficient, vitamin B12. Having adequate levels of these vitamins in the months before pregnancy is incredibly important for protecting your future baby's health—reducing the odds of pregnancy loss, neural tube defects, and complications such as preeclampsia and preterm birth.

When it comes to adding further supplements to improve the uterine lining for embryo transfer, there is relatively little research on this point, but the two supplements with the most promise are vitamin E and L-arginine.

In 2019, a randomized, placebo-controlled study of women with repeated implantation failure found that supplementing with vitamin E significantly improved lining thickness.[16] An earlier study involving 60 patients with a thin lining also found that supplementing with either vitamin E or L-arginine improved endometrial thickness in about half of patients.[17] In that study, the doses used were 600 mg per day for vitamin E and 6 g per day for L-arginine. Although the women were assigned to receive either vitamin E or L-arginine to compare their effects, it may be even more effective to combine both supplements because they work in slightly different ways.

Vitamin E appears to boosts cell numbers in the uterine lining and promote the development of new blood vessels. L-arginine likely works by dilating blood vessels and thereby improving blood flow.

Beyond vitamin E and L-arginine, there is little evidence for further supplements. It is possible that CoQ10 can improve the uterine lining, based on one study reporting an increase in endometrial thickness in women taking CoQ10.[18] If CoQ10 does have this effect, it is likely by supporting energy production in the cells lining the uterus.

Another supplement that could potentially help improve the uterine lining is L-carnitine. In a randomized, double-blind study in Egypt, women with a previous failed embryo transfer took 3 g of L-carnitine per day before transfer. This was found to increase lining thickness and increase the pregnancy rate. L-carnitine has also been reported to improve endometrial thickness in women with PCOS.[19] This research is promising, but L-carnitine does not have a long history of use for female fertility and is not recommended if you are hypothyroid.

Recommended supplements to prepare for embryo transfer

- Prenatal multivitamin
- Vitamin D
- Vitamin B12 (if deficient)
- Vitamin E (200–400 IU per day)

Optional additional supplements

- L-arginine (6 g per day, starting after egg retrieval)
- CoQ10 (200–400 mg per day)
- L-carnitine (3 g per day)

Medications for Lining Preparation

In addition to the standard estrogen and progesterone treatments, some further medications are sometimes prescribed to improve endometrial lining in challenging cases. One of the most common add-ons is aspirin, which is thought to improve blood flow in the uterine lining. When used in the general population of IVF patients, there is little evidence that aspirin makes much of a difference,[20] but it may be helpful in specific situations.

In particular, low-dose aspirin may improve implantation rates in those with genetic blood-clotting disorders, a thin endometrial lining, or autoimmune conditions that can reduce blood flow or impact the uterine lining, such as antinuclear antibodies or antiphospholipid antibodies.[21]

For those with very thin endometrial lining, some doctors may prescribe Viagra suppositories. This relatively new treatment is backed by several studies and is thought to work by boosting blood flow.[22] Another treatment occasionally used for thin lining is Neupogen, also known as G-CSF. This is a growth factor normally given to cancer patients to promote the regeneration of immune cells. In theory it may also promote regeneration of the endometrial lining, but studies have produced inconsistent results.[23] Some researchers have found that although G-CSF may increase the thickness of the uterine lining, it may not have a significant impact on pregnancy rates.[24]

A more promising treatment for those with very thin lining, particularly due to either chronic infections or Asherman's syndrome, is platelet-rich plasma (PRP). This involves taking a vial of blood, concentrating the fraction containing growth factors and other components that promote healing, then reinjecting this fraction into the uterine lining. This is thought to promote healing in damaged tissues. Initial studies indicate higher pregnancy rates after PRP treatment in women with very thin lining.[25]

The Evidence for Acupuncture

Acupuncture has long been used as a treatment for infertility, but researchers are still trying to determine whether it actually improves IVF success rates. Many IVF clinics began recommending or offering acupuncture treatments in the early 2000s following the publication of a high-profile study led by Dr. Wolfgang Paulus in Germany.[26] Dr. Paulus showed that women who received acupuncture 25 minutes before and after embryo transfer had a 43% success rate, compared to a 26% success rate for those who did not get acupuncture. Many other groups have since tried to replicate these findings, often with disappointing results.

Now, almost 20 years later, when all the studies are pooled together, it appears there is little to no impact on the chance of pregnancy from just one or two acupuncture treatments around the time of embryo transfer.[27] Yet even just this isolated treatment may still have other benefits, with many physicians recommending acupuncture to IVF patients purely because it reduces stress and anxiety. It is not clear that stress actually impacts fertility as much as some may think, but relieving stress is a worthy goal in and of itself.

It is also clear that if stress relief is the goal, acupuncture works. Research has consistently found that in women undergoing IVF, acupuncture reduces the level of the stress hormone cortisol.[28] In 2009, Dr. Alice Domar, the Director of Mind/Body Services at Boston IVF, and a well-known expert on natural approaches to improving fertility, performed a study using the same acupuncture protocol as Dr. Paulus.[29] Patients were randomized to either lie quietly or receive an acupuncture treatment for 25 minutes before and after transfer. The study found no impact on pregnancy rates but concluded that "acupuncture patients reported significantly less anxiety post-transfer and reported feeling more optimistic about their cycle."

It is possible that this stress-relieving benefit may only be seen when acupuncture is available onsite at the IVF clinic. One study found that when women need to travel from the IVF clinic to a new location for their first acupuncture on the day of embryo transfer, the benefits seem to disappear.[30]

Rather than isolated acupuncture treatment on the day of

embryo transfer, there may be more value in receiving regular treatments several times per week during the IVF cycle itself and in the month before a frozen embryo transfer.

Although the evidence on that point is far from conclusive, there is some initial research suggesting that a series of acupuncture treatments may improve the odds in IVF cycles.[31] In one successful trial, patients received acupuncture twice per week for four weeks before egg retrieval, with additional treatments the day before and shortly after embryo transfer.[32] The pregnancy rate was significantly higher in the acupuncture group (53%) compared to the control group (41%).

If indeed acupuncture can improve the odds of success in IVF, there are several possible explanations. One is that acupuncture may promote blood flow to the ovaries and uterus, encouraging follicle growth and the development of the uterine lining. It has also been suggested that acupuncture may improve fertility by triggering the release of beneficial endorphins and reducing stress hormones. Regardless of the precise way in which acupuncture brings benefits for those trying to conceive, it does appear that a series of regular treatments is needed, not just isolated sessions immediately before or after embryo transfer.

At the end of the day, acupuncture is one approach to try if your budget permits and if you find it relaxing. If, however, finding the time and money for acupuncture is going to be an added burden and one more source of stress, it may not be right for you. There are a variety of other ways to reduce stress involved in the IVF process, such as walking in nature and meditation.

Bed Rest After Transfer

One of the most common questions that arises after an embryo transfer is whether there is any advantage to bed rest. It intuitively makes sense that resting may be helpful to allow the embryo to implant without disruption. Yet the data shows that bed rest immediately after embryo transfer has no real advantage and might even lower the chance of pregnancy, perhaps by reducing circulation.[33] Instead, the recommendation is to resume most activities but avoid strenuous exercise, saunas, heat packs, sexual activity, swimming, and baths for at least two weeks after transfer.

Pregnancy Testing and the Two-Week Wait

After embryo transfer, most doctors advise against using home pregnancy tests and encourage you to wait for the official blood test, usually 9–12 days after transfer. One reason for this advice is that if you are doing a fresh transfer, the hCG in your system from the trigger shot before retrieval can cause a false positive, and testing too early or with an unreliable brand can cause a false negative. Many doctors are concerned that a false negative may cause women to stop their medication prematurely. To avoid the emotional rollercoaster and potential for confusion, the standard advice is to wait until the blood test.

Often, this is the right approach. Yet in some cases, the wait after an embryo transfer is agonizing. It is perfectly reasonable to decide for yourself which will be better for your mental health—whether waiting for the official result and avoiding any false results or ambiguity, or testing at home to potentially get an answer sooner and have some control over when and where you find out.

Guidance for testing at home

If you decide to test at home, keep in mind that the sensitivity of home tests varies significantly between brands. This means that some brands are much better than others at detecting hCG at lower concentrations. One of the most sensitive and reliable brands is First Response Early Result.

With a fresh embryo transfer, the hCG from the trigger shot before egg retrieval can stay in your system for a while. As a result, a pregnancy test can give a false positive for around five days after a fresh transfer with a 5-day embryo. One way around this is to "test out" the trigger by starting to test around day 3 or 4 after transfer. You can start testing for pregnancy after you get negative tests that show the trigger is out of your system.

After a transfer with a fresh or frozen 5-day embryo and using a high-sensitivity test, most women get their first positive result between five to seven days after transfer. If tests are negative at eight days post-transfer, it is still possible that you are pregnant with a late-implanting embryo, but this is uncommon. Regardless of the result of home tests, you should always continue taking medication until a definitive result from your blood test.

The Beta-HCG blood test

Most doctors recommend performing the first hCG blood test at 9–12 days after transfer. Many pregnancies will test positive earlier, but this timing is intended to detect even late-implanting pregnancies. The precise level of hCG at this point can also offer clues as to the viability of the pregnancy.

If hCG is measured on day 12 after embryo transfer and it is over 100 mIU/ml by that point, there is a very high chance that the pregnancy is viable. There is still reason to be optimistic if hCG is over 60 mIU/ml, whereas a value below 40 mIU/ml on day 12 may indicate that the pregnancy is unlikely to continue.[34] If you start with a low value but another test several days later shows that hCG is rising normally, that is a very encouraging sign—the low initial value may just reflect a late implantation.

The rate at which hCG rises is an especially useful marker for predicting whether a pregnancy is viable. The typical rule is that hCG should double every two to three days during the earliest weeks. In 2022, researchers at Northwestern found that if hCG is over 100 mIU/ml by 10 days after transfer *and* hCG also doubles within 48 hours, there is an 85% chance of a live birth.[35] If only one of these milestones is met, the chance is much lower (at 34–55%), and if neither is met, there is just a 9% chance of a live birth. Although it can be heartbreaking to see a very low or slow-rising beta number, and these statistics can help you mentally prepare for possible outcomes, remember that even a low chance is still a chance and your embryo may defy the odds.

Action Steps

The two major decisions you will face in the lead-up to embryo transfer are whether to opt for a fresh or frozen transfer and whether to test your embryos. Frozen transfers may have a slight edge, although a fresh transfer may be the best approach if you have very few embryos and they may not survive freezing.

Deciding on embryo testing is a very personal decision that depends on your age, how many embryos you have, and how important it is to you to either prevent miscarriage or give every embryo the best possible chance. It is most helpful for women over 35 with many embryos to choose from, whereas it may not be worth the risk if you only have one or two embryos.

When preparing for a frozen embryo transfer, supplements and lifestyle play only minor roles because the most important factors that determine whether an embryo will implant are (i) whether it is a good-quality embryo, (ii) whether luck is on your side, and (iii) whether you have any health conditions that can impact your endometrial lining, such as a uterine infection, scarring, or autoimmune condition, as will be discussed in chapter 15. Nevertheless, supplements can help get your body ready for a healthy pregnancy and may support development of a healthy endometrial lining.

Recommended supplements to prepare for embryo transfer include:

- Prenatal
- Vitamin D
- Vitamin B12 (if deficient)
- Vitamin E (200–400 IU per day)

Optional additional supplements:

- L-arginine (6 g per day, starting after egg retrieval)
- CoQ10 (200–400 mg per day)
- L-carnitine (3 g per day)

PART 4

TROUBLESHOOTING STRATEGIES

Chapter 15

Immune and Implantation Factors

"Fall down seven times. Stand up eight."
— Japanese Proverb

SOMETIMES IMPROVING EGG and sperm quality is not enough. Even with the healthiest possible embryo, conditions involving the immune system and the uterus can sometimes prevent implantation or cause pregnancy loss. These conditions, which include silent infections, chronic endometritis, endometriosis, autoimmune antibodies, and scar tissue, often cause no symptoms and go undetected for years.

Many women only find out they have a problem with implantation after a long struggle with unexplained infertility, many failed embryo transfers, or repeated pregnancy losses. This chapter aims to prevent those years of heartbreak and make you aware of some of the underlying problems that are often missed, so you can request testing and treatment.

What Is Implantation Dysfunction?

As discussed in earlier chapters, a significant number of failed implantations and early pregnancy losses are due to chromosomal errors in the embryo, which the strategies discussed so far are designed to prevent. But even genetically normal embryos sometimes fail to implant or else implant and then result in miscarriage.

Newly developed tests have made it clear that behind many cases of implantation failure and unexplained infertility are issues related to the immune system and inflammation in the uterus. If certain immune cells in the lining of the uterus are in overdrive, whether because of a silent infection, autoimmunity, or other causes, an embryo will have difficulty implanting.

The same factors that can stop an embryo from implanting can also contribute to recurrent pregnancy loss. Rather than preventing implantation altogether, immune factors triggered by autoimmune antibodies or infection may cause the implantation to occur in a dysfunctional way.

The immune system plays a surprisingly important role in the development of the placenta and the connection of the mother and baby's blood supply. As one example, immune cells such as natural killer cells send messages that either increase or decrease development of blood vessels in the placenta. If this delicate process is disrupted, the detailed structure of blood vessels may not form correctly, raising the odds of miscarriage and pregnancy complications such as preeclampsia.[1]

In short, a range of issues with the uterine lining and immune system can contribute to failed embryo transfers, unexplained infertility, and recurrent pregnancy loss. If you are facing one of these challenges, this chapter will explain the testing options that can help you uncover the most common problems.

The testing discussed in this chapter may also be useful if you have an autoimmune condition, which can predispose you to other immune problems; a history of gynecological infections, which can put you at risk for endometritis; or chronic pelvic pain, which can indicate potential endometriosis.

In addition, you may consider requesting some of the tests in this chapter simply because you have very few embryos. In such cases, it might be reasonable to invest in testing to rule out some of the more common problems with implantation before an embryo transfer.

What to Test For

Six general categories of issues can cause implantation failure or recurrent pregnancy loss with a genetically normal embryo:

1. Hidden infections and chronic endometritis

2. Endometriosis

3. Immune factors, such as antiphospholipid antibodies and natural killer cells

4. Hormone imbalances and genetic blood-clotting disorders

5. Structural problems in the uterus, such as Asherman's syndrome

6. Parental genetic issues, such as translocations

It can be challenging to find a doctor willing to investigate these issues. Often, doctors prefer to wait until after three miscarriages to investigate potential causes, while fertility clinics often respond to failed embryo transfers by advising patients to keep trying and repeating the expensive and arduous process of IVF, without making any changes. Sometimes doctors will test for one or two problems they are most familiar with, such as genetic testing for translocations. These may be useful tests, but they are not the highest priority. Instead, testing should focus on the issues that are most common and the most treatable, such as silent infections in the uterine lining, endometriosis, and certain immune issues.

In recent years there have been huge advances in the ability to identify these common problems. New tests can now detect hidden infections and markers of endometriosis with a simple biopsy procedure. But these tests are not being offered to everyone who could benefit, likely because of the long lag time between medical discovery and updated medical practice. That is why it is so important to be aware of the testing options available so you can advocate for yourself and request the tests most likely to uncover a treatable problem. This chapter will discuss the main testing options, in order from the most common to least common causes of implantation dysfunction. You may not need to test for everything covered in this chapter and can start with the most likely culprits: endometritis, endometriosis, and antiphospholipid antibodies.

Hidden Infections and Chronic Endometritis

For decades, it was assumed that the uterus is a relatively sterile place, free of bacteria. Research has now shown that is not correct; the uterus is typically colonized by a small population of bacteria that have migrated through the cervix and formed a unique ecosystem. The presence of bacteria in the uterus is not a problem in itself, but the type of bacteria is hugely important.

Some species, such as *Lactobacilli*, are helpful for regulating the immune system, reducing inflammation, and creating a slightly acidic environment in the uterus. As a result, studies have found that women with a higher percentage of *Lactobacilli* in the uterus have a higher chance of getting pregnant after embryo transfer and a lower chance of miscarriage.[2]

Other types of bacteria, such as *Gardnerella* and *Ureaplasma*, have the opposite effect. They trigger an inflammatory response that makes it difficult for an embryo to implant and increases the chance of pregnancy loss and stillbirth.[3]

Although infections in other parts of the body are often cleared quickly, harmful bacteria can persist in the uterus for a long period of time, causing an inflammatory condition known as chronic endometritis.[4] (Although this sounds similar to endometriosis, they are separate conditions.) Studies have found chronic endometritis in up to 30% of women with repeated implantation failure or recurrent pregnancy loss.[5]

For many years, the infections that cause inflammation in the uterus were difficult to detect. Endometritis was diagnosed based on the presence of certain immune cells in an endometrial biopsy, but this could miss early-stage infections. Now, tests that use DNA-sequencing technology can determine the proportion of healthy bacteria present and identify whether you may have an overgrowth of the pathogenic bacteria that cause endometritis, providing much more granular information.

One of these tests is the EMMA/ALICE test, which involves a doctor performing an endometrial biopsy to take a small sample of uterine tissue, which is then sent for testing to assess the bacteria present. Another option is the Fertilysis micro-biome test, which can be ordered without a doctor. This test involves collecting a few drops of menstrual blood using a kit sent to your home. The sample is then sent to the laboratory for analysis, and a report is provided a few weeks later, along with treatment recommendations.

If you are not sure whether to invest in uterine microbiome testing, your insurance may cover the older method of testing for endometritis, which involves an endometrial biopsy to look for certain immune cells. Another option is a conven-tional vaginal swab test for bacterial vaginosis (BV). This swab test cannot directly determine whether harmful bacteria are present in the uterine lining, but up to 50% of women with BV are found to have endometritis, and a positive vaginal swab test for species such as *Gardnerella* or *Ureaplasma* provides reason enough to treat with antibiotics.[6]

If you do have harmful bacteria in the uterus, antibiotic treat-ment can be extremely helpful. Studies indicate that antibiotics can resolve endometritis about three-quarters of the time, dra-matically increasing the chance of getting pregnant and car-rying to term.[7] One study reported that the chance of live birth per pregnancy was just 7% with chronic endometritis, but this increased to 56% after treatment.[8] More difficult cases may require multiple rounds of antibiotics or advanced treatments, such as a uterine wash procedure with antibiotics and steroids, oral steroids, or treatment with platelet-rich plasma (PRP).[9]

Because the presence of beneficial bacteria such as *Lactobacilli* appears to be so important to fertility, you might wonder whether antibiotics may be counterproductive, by reducing the population of beneficial species and potentially causing even more disruption to the natural balance of the microbiome. Fortunately, one of the most common antibiotics for treating uterine infections, metronidazole, can kill many harmful species without impacting *Lactobacilli*. It can therefore shift the uterine microbiome to a healthier balance, with a greater proportion of beneficial species.[10]

While you are being treated with antibiotics, some doctors recommend antibiotic treatment for your partner, too, to make sure the infection will not be passed back and forth and recur.

Studies also suggest that combining antibiotics with probiotics may achieve better results.[11] The most helpful strains include *Lactobacillus rhamnosus* GR-1 and *Lactobacillus reuteri* RC-14. These two strains have been studied extensively for their ability to survive in the reproductive tract and combat harmful yeast and bacteria, including *Gardnerella*.[12] They form the basis of many women's health probiotics, including Jarrow FemDophilus and Rephresh ProB. They are also recommended during pregnancy to prevent group B strep colonization, as discussed in my pregnancy book.

Although these probiotic strains can eventually improve the reproductive microbiome if taken orally, studies have found that the most effective treatment regime is a combination of oral antibiotics and vaginal probiotic suppositories. That combination is much more likely to restore a healthy endometrial microbiome than antibiotics alone, probiotics alone, or antibiotics and oral probiotics.[13]

Endometriosis and the ReceptivaDX Test

For anyone trying to conceive, the most important thing to know about endometriosis is that it does not always cause symptoms. Endometriosis can contribute to implantation failure and unexplained infertility without causing pain or any other symptoms. As a result, most women with endometriosis who are going through fertility treatments do not even know they have it.[14] Even for women with severe pain from endometriosis, it takes an average of ten years to get diagnosed.

You might expect that the increasing public awareness of endometriosis in recent years would have improved the situation and that more women seeking fertility treatment would be getting diagnosed sooner. In fact, the opposite appears to be happening. More and more women with endometriosis are simply told they have unexplained infertility and are encouraged to pursue IVF without investigating potential causes.[15]

Researchers have found that silent endometriosis is one of the most common causes of unexplained infertility.[16] Many doctors are still not aware of this and only recommend investigating endometriosis when someone has chronic abdominal pain. Fortunately, newer testing options may change the equation and make it easier to find out if endometriosis may be present.

One promising test is ReceptivaDX, which can be performed in your doctor's office with a simple biopsy. It is worth asking for this testing if you have long-standing unexplained infertility or failed embryo transfers. It may also be worth considering if you have experienced multiple pregnancy losses, although it is a lower priority because endometriosis has a clearer link to infertility than to miscarriage.

How does endometriosis affect implantation?

Endometriosis is an inflammatory condition characterized by tissue similar to the lining of the uterus forming in other locations, often on the outside of the uterus, in the abdominal cavity, or on the ovaries. This tissue not only causes structural problems but also produces its own hormones and inflammatory mediators. The resulting hormonal disruptions and inflammation can make even the normal tissue in the uterine lining function differently. The uterine lining can become resistant to progesterone, which in turn makes it more difficult for embryos to implant, leading to unexplained infertility and failed embryo transfers. Endometriosis may also increase the chance of miscarriage, although the data on this point is inconsistent and the impact may be relatively small.[17]

Diagnosing endometriosis

The most accurate way to diagnose endometriosis is a procedure called a laparoscopy. This involves a surgeon making a small incision in the abdomen and then inserting a camera to look for any visible lesions. The surgeon may also remove lesions during this initial exploratory surgery.

Because a laparoscopy is a relatively expensive and invasive procedure, it is typically only performed when there are obvious symptoms, such as chronic pelvic pain. Sometimes, endometriosis can be seen on ultrasound or by MRI, so these screening options may be a worthwhile starting point, although they cannot rule out endometriosis and it will often be missed.

A newer testing option is the ReceptivaDX test, which looks for a marker called BCL6. This marker indicates a type of inflammation of the uterine lining that is most often caused by endometriosis. BCL6 seems to be specifically related to progesterone resistance in the endometrial lining, meaning that it can not only help identify when endometriosis is present but can also specifically indicate that endometriosis is likely making the uterine lining less receptive to implantation.[18]

The ReceptivaDX test is performed by your doctor collecting a sample by endometrial biopsy. The biopsy needs to be performed during the stage of the menstrual cycle when an embryo would normally implant, around a week after ovulation. The sample is then sent for analysis.

If the test shows elevated BCL6, that is a strong sign that endometriosis is present and impacting your fertility. Studies have found that 94% of women with unexplained infertility and elevated BCL6 have endometriosis.[19] The remaining 6% typically have inflammation caused by either a blocked fallopian tube or an infection.[20]

Although BCL6 testing is clearly a significant advance in the diagnosis of endometriosis, it is not perfect and can sometimes fail to identify even severe cases. There are reports of some women having a negative ReceptivaDX test and then discovering extensive endometriosis once they have a laparoscopy for other reasons. A negative result should not be considered conclusive and should not stop you from seeking further testing if you have chronic pelvic pain or some other clue that endometriosis may be an issue, such as grainy or pigmented eggs in IVF.

In addition, BCL6 testing is not yet recommended for women with an identified cause of infertility. When it is offered across the board to women undergoing IVF for other reasons, it does not appear to increase success rates. The main value of this testing is in those with unexplained infertility or failed embryo transfers.

If testing shows you have elevated BCL6, the chance of success with the next embryo transfer is 11% without treatment for endometriosis, but 50–60% with treatment.[21] That is why this testing is so incredibly useful: it not only identifies a problem that is extremely common, but one that can be treated.

Endometriosis treatment

The main treatment options are surgery to remove endometriosis lesions, or hormone-suppressing medications. There is controversy over which is the better approach, and the answer likely depends on your age and the severity of endometriosis. In general, both have been found to give a similar chance of the next embryo implanting and leading to a successful pregnancy.[22]

For younger women who have a good chance of conceiving naturally, surgery is typically recommended because it can often solve the problem. More than half of women in this category will get pregnant naturally in the first couple of years after surgery.[23]

For women with low ovarian reserve or severe endometriosis, some doctors advise a short period of suppressive medication and then moving straight to IVF. That is because surgery to remove endometriosis may not increase IVF success rates in the short term and can sometimes reduce the number of eggs available for retrieval.[24]

One approach for the toughest cases is to opt for IVF first, in order to freeze several embryos, before undergoing surgery to create the best environment for embryos to implant.

If you are considering surgery, it is critical to see the right kind of surgeon: an endometriosis excision specialist. Many ob-gyns perform a type of endometriosis surgery called ablation, which burns off the surface of lesions but does not fully remove them. The endometriosis tissue can regrow, sometimes more aggressively than before surgery. By contrast, excision surgery aims to remove each patch of endometriosis down to the root, even where it may be invading other tissues and organs. This provides much better long-term results, with little chance of recurrence for many years after complete excision. Excision surgery requires much greater skill than ablation, so it is only performed by a small number of endometriosis specialists. To find a specialist, see **nancysnookendo.com**.

Reproductive Immunology Testing

Activation of the immune system can have an enormous impact on the ability of an embryo to implant and lead to a successful pregnancy. Nowhere is that more evident than in the context of uterine infections. As discussed earlier, low-level infections can cause immune activity that stops embryos implanting or increases the risk of miscarriage.

Sometimes, however, the immune system can go into high-alert mode on its own in the absence of infection. This can happen without any identified trigger or when the immune system wrongly recognizes some component of the body's own cells as a foreign invader, a situation known as autoimmunity.

A significant proportion of women who have experienced multiple miscarriages or failed transfers have abnormal immune activation.[25] This can show up as antibodies directed against normal cell components, overactive natural killer cells, or a lack of regulatory cells that are supposed to calm the immune system.

In-depth testing and treatment for these immune issues is usually handled by specialists known as reproductive immunologists. This testing can be very expensive and involve a long wait for an appointment, but it is often the turning point after nothing else works.

Although it can be difficult to know whether to invest in reproductive immunology testing, the general rule is that the more failed embryo transfers or miscarriages you have had, and the more testing you have done to rule out other causes, the more likely you are to benefit from in-depth immune testing.

Whether or not you decide to go down the path of consulting a reproductive immunologist, or even while you are waiting for an appointment, it may be worth asking your current doctor for blood tests for some of the immune issues that are the least controversial and easiest to diagnose, namely autoimmune antibodies.

Autoimmune antibodies

Antibodies are produced by cells of the immune system to tag molecules as foreign invaders that should be eliminated. Although it is relatively normal for the immune system to accidentally produce some antibodies that recognize the body's own proteins, it is not normal to produce a high level of antibodies against one specific protein in the body. These are known as autoimmune antibodies.

Up to one-third of women with a history of unexplained infertility, failed embryo transfers, or recurrent miscarriage will test positive for autoimmune antibodies.[26] It is not clear whether these antibodies directly compromise the viability of an embryo or whether people with autoimmune antibodies are more likely to have other immune issues that pose a problem for early pregnancy. Either way, when autoimmune antibodies are present, treatment to regulate the immune system may be worth trying.

Whereas many tests for reproductive immunology issues require specialized laboratories and expertise to interpret the results, antibody tests can be ordered by a conventional fertility doctor or ob-gyn, or you can order the tests online in many countries.

The four types of antibodies that are most useful to test are: [27]

- antiphospholipid antibodies
- antithyroid antibodies
- antinuclear antibodies
- celiac antibodies

Antiphospholipid antibodies

Antiphospholipid antibodies occur when your immune system starts making antibodies against the fatty components of your cell membranes, known as phospholipids. These antibodies exist in various forms, but it is most common to test for three specific types: [28]

- cardiolipin antibodies
- beta2-glycoprotein antibodies
- phosphatidylserine antibodies

These antibodies trigger inflammation and make the blood clot more easily. Both inflammation and blood clots can disrupt the formation of the placenta, reducing blood flow to an embryo and increasing the risk of pregnancy loss.[29]

This is one of the few immune issues that is widely accepted by conventional doctors, with official guidelines recognizing that antiphospholipid antibodies contribute to around 15% of cases of recurrent miscarriage.[30] These antibodies are also much more common in women with unexplained infertility or failed embryo transfers. [31]

If you test positive for antiphospholipid antibodies, treatment can improve the chance of getting pregnant and carrying to term.[32] The aim is to address both inflammation and blood clotting, which typically involves a combination of several of the following medications:

- aspirin
- heparin or Lovenox
- hydroxychloroquine (Plaquenil)
- steroids such as prednisone or dexamethasone
- Intralipid or IVIG

Many people with antiphospholipid antibodies will have other immune abnormalities, such as higher levels of immune cells and markers of inflammation.[33] Fortunately, the same immune treatments that are used for antiphospholipid antibodies can help address some of these other immune abnormalities.

Although the primary aim of immune treatment is to protect implantation and development of the placenta, studies have reported that in women with antiphospholipid antibodies, immune treatments such as prednisone may also improve egg quality and the number of viable embryos in IVF, if treatment is started at least a month before egg retrieval. [34]

There also appears to be a relationship between antiphospholipid antibodies and celiac disease, the autoimmune condition triggered by gluten. Anecdotal reports suggest that antiphospholipid antibodies decline dramatically after adopting a strict gluten-free diet.[35] This is exactly what happened to one 34-year-old woman with antiphospholipid syndrome who had suffered two miscarriages. Once diagnosed with celiac disease, she began a gluten-free diet, and within six months the previously elevated antibodies were undetectable.[36]

Antithyroid antibodies

Antithyroid antibodies are autoimmune antibodies that bind to one or more components in the thyroid. The most relevant antithyroid antibodies to test are:

- thyroid peroxidase antibodies
- thyrotropin receptor antibodies
- thyroglobulin antibodies

If you were not tested for these antibodies as part of your general thyroid testing, it is worth getting this testing done when exploring possible immune issues. There is a clear link between thyroid antibodies, infertility, and pregnancy loss, even in women with normal thyroid hormone levels.[37] In the IVF context, women with thyroid antibodies tend to have fewer eggs retrieved, a lower chance of eggs fertilizing, and a lower chance of embryos implanting.[38]

The reason for this link is not entirely clear, but the evidence is growing that thyroid antibodies can have impacts beyond the thyroid. Thyroid peroxidase antibodies have recently been found to bind to proteins in the ovaries, endometrial lining, and placenta.[39]

If thyroid antibodies are directly triggering an immune response in the ovaries and in the cells needed for an embryo to properly implant, this could help explain why these antibodies compromise ovarian function and increase the chance of recurrent pregnancy loss. [40]

In addition, women with thyroid antibodies are more likely to have other immune abnormalities, such as elevated natural killer cells.[41] The presence of thyroid antibodies therefore provides an important clue that the immune system may not be functioning as it should and that further immune testing could be helpful.

Treatment with immune-suppressing steroid medication, such as prednisone or prednisolone, has been found to significantly improve pregnancy rates in those with thyroid autoimmunity.[42] When given before IVF, steroids can potentially increase the number and quality of eggs and increase the chance of an embryo implanting.[43] Starting aspirin plus prednisone on the day of embryo transfer does not seem to help,[44] but that could be because more time is needed to calm the immune system before transfer.

It is not clear whether immune treatment can impact the chance of miscarriage in those with thyroid autoimmunity.[45] If thyroid autoimmunity is the only immune issue and your thyroid hormone levels are maintained in the optimal range, you have a very good chance of a pregnancy continuing, even without any immune treatment.[46] That said, if you continue to experience pregnancy losses, it may be worth consulting a reproductive immunologist for a more comprehensive approach.

Whether or not you decide to pursue immune treatment, there are other strategies you can adopt to help lower thyroid antibodies. This includes correcting deficiencies in DHEA and vitamins D and B12, all of which are linked to thyroid antibody levels.[47] Supplementing with selenium can also help to reduce antibody levels and increase immune-calming regulatory T cells.[48]

Dietary changes can also make a huge difference in thyroid autoimmunity. The one change with the clearest evidence is eliminating gluten.[49] If you choose to go further, studies have found that a paleo diet can also improve thyroid autoimmunity, particularly an allergy-eliminating version such as the autoimmune paleo (AIP) diet.[50]

Another option is to test for possible food sensitivities. There are questions about the accuracy of these tests, but one study found that performing a blood test for food sensitivities and eliminating items flagged in the test results can help reduce thyroid antibodies.[51] In that study, the most common sensitivities were to wheat, eggs, dairy, yeast, corn, and peanuts.[52]

The fact that these particular foods often trigger immune responses may partly explain why so many people see improvement when following the AIP diet, which temporarily eliminates grains, dairy, nuts, and other common food allergens.[53]

In addition, there is growing evidence that the community of microbes in the digestive system, known as the microbiome, can influence autoimmunity. Eliminating or reducing grains, processed food, and sugar is one of the most effective ways to rebalance this ecosystem, thereby rebalancing the immune system.

The topic of using diet to influence immune activity is covered further in chapter 16.

Antinuclear antibodies

As the name suggests, antinuclear antibodies bind to molecules found in the nucleus of cells. These antibodies are more likely to be found in women with infertility and recurrent pregnancy loss: up to a quarter of women who have had multiple miscarriages have elevated antinuclear antibodies, compared to less than 10% of the general population. But it is unclear whether their presence means that immune treatment is needed.[54]

There is conflicting data on whether antinuclear antibodies actually increase the risk of pregnancy loss and whether steroids may help prevent further miscarriages.[55] The evidence is clearer if the issue is getting pregnant, with studies finding that steroid treatment before IVF in women with antinuclear antibodies can improve the results of IVF cycles.[56]

Specifically, studies have found that in women with antinuclear antibodies, the combination of prednisone and aspirin for three months before IVF can increase the percentage of embryos that fertilize and successfully implant.[57] One study also found that the combination of prednisone and Plaquenil before frozen embryo transfer can significantly improve pregnancy rates.[58]

Treatment may be more likely to help when antibody levels are particularly high. A value over 1:40 is often considered elevated, but some researchers have argued that this level may not signify a problem and that a more meaningful cutoff should be antibodies over 1:80.[59]

Celiac antibodies

Celiac disease is an autoimmune condition in which the presence of gluten triggers an immune attack against the body's own tissues. There is some controversy over the extent to which celiac disease contributes to infertility, but the weight of the evidence indicates that at a minimum, it increases the risk of pregnancy loss.[60]

A number of different celiac antibodies can be tested, but the most informative seems to be tissue transglutaminase IgA. The official guidelines in Germany recommend checking for transglutaminase antibodies after recurrent pregnancy loss, but this is not yet standard practice in other countries.[61] It may also be worth testing for transglutaminase antibodies if you have unexplained infertility or failed embryo transfers, but celiac disease is less likely to be the culprit than some of the other issues discussed so far.

If you are found to have celiac antibodies, adopting a strict gluten-free diet will quickly stop the autoimmune activity and give you the best chance of a healthy pregnancy.

Cellular immune testing

Beyond autoimmune antibodies, the testing and treatment of immune issues becomes much more controversial and complicated. This is particularly true when it comes to testing for the number and activity of certain immune cells, such as natural killer cells. The following section will provide a brief overview of some of the most common issues a reproductive immunologist may look for and the potential treatments, but this is by no means exhaustive.

In-depth reproductive immunology testing is most often recommended for recurrent pregnancy loss and late-term pregnancy loss, but it may also be worth considering for unexplained infertility or implantation failure, or if you have autoimmune antibodies. The presence of these antibodies often goes hand in hand with other immune system imbalances.[62]

If you are not considering detailed reproductive immunology testing at this stage, you can skip to the next section, on hormone and clotting issues.

Natural killer cells are immune cells that play a variety of different roles, including killing cancer cells and virus-infected cells. In the uterus, a unique form of natural killer cell encourages proper development of the placenta and formation of new blood vessels.

Although not yet widely accepted, some research suggests that either a high or low number of NK cells can be associated with recurrent pregnancy loss or implantation dysfunction.[63]

Natural killer cell activity can be tested in various ways. Blood tests can measure the number of NK cells present and how active they are in killing cells. A reproductive immunologist may also perform a uterine biopsy to more directly investigate the number and activity of natural killer cells found in the uterus.

Helper T cells are immune cells that regulate the activity of other parts of the immune system, including natural killer cells. Some types of helper T cells are pro-inflammatory, producing molecules that shift the immune system into high-alert mode. This includes Th1 and Th17 cells. Other types, such as Th2 cells, are anti-inflammatory, producing molecules that signal the immune system to calm down. Studies have suggested that women with recurrent miscarriage or multiple failed embryo transfers often have a higher proportion of Th1 or Th17 cells, triggering inflammation and immune activity.[64]

Regulatory T cells are immune cells that help regulate the activity of other immune cells, effectively calming the immune system and reducing inflammation. If the number of regulatory T cells is too low, this may prevent the shift of the immune system toward a more tolerant state necessary to sustain early pregnancy.

Immune-signaling molecules, also known as cytokines, are part of the communication system of the immune system. Cytokines are produced by cells of the immune system in order to regulate other cells, either dialing up or down specific immune activity. Cytokines include tumor necrosis factor (TNF) and a class of molecules known as interleukins. Some reproductive immunologists perform blood tests to measure these and other immune-signaling molecules in order to assess the activity of the immune system.

If TNF is high, that indicates that the immune system is in a more aggressive, inflammatory state. Medications that block TNF (such as Enbrel and Humira) are a mainstay of treatment for autoimmune diseases such as rheumatoid arthritis, but it is unclear whether these medications are helpful in the fertility context. Some believe they may suppress the immune system too much for implantation to occur.

Interleukins are a broad class of immune-signaling molecules, with each interleukin having a number, such as IL-1, IL-2, and so on. Some interleukins promote inflammation, and others act to suppress it. For example, IL-10 acts to calm the immune system.

Because different immune-signaling molecules are produced by different types of immune cells, they can provide information on the balance between opposing arms of the immune system. The Th1/Th2 cytokine ratio reflects the balance between inflammatory Th1 cells (represented by the level of TNF and interferon) and anti-inflammatory Th2 cells (represented by the level of IL-10).

Reproductive immunology treatments

If testing shows you have immune abnormalities that are characteristic of recurrent pregnancy loss or repeated implantation failure, a reproductive immunologist will attempt to rein in the immune system with a combination of medications that act together in concert to rebalance immune activity. Similar combinations are often used whether someone has excessive natural killer cell activity or an imbalance in T cells. Similar combinations are also used for addressing both implantation failure and recurrent pregnancy loss. One of the most often-used regimens is:

- a steroid such as prednisone
- aspirin
- intralipid or intravenous immunoglobulin (IVIG)
- heparin or Lovenox (if blood-clotting issues are present)

For women with a history of multiple unsuccessful embryo transfers, intralipid alone may improve the chance of pregnancy and live birth.[65] Yet other studies have suggested that combinations of medications are more effective. As one example, a study by Dr. Joanne Kwak-Kim and a group of leading reproductive immunologists in Chicago found that in women with a history of multiple miscarriages and failed embryo transfers, the combination of IVIG with prednisone, aspirin, and heparin resulted in a live birth rate of 40%, compared to just 2% without treatment.[66]

Sometimes the standard immune-suppressing medications are not enough, however, and doctors turn to a range of more advanced options. Studies indicate that the most effective options include:[67]

- Intrauterine PBMC infusion,
- Intrauterine PRP, and
- Neupogen

Intrauterine PBMC infusion is a treatment that involves taking a sample of blood, isolating certain immune cells, and then infusing those cells into the uterus. It likely works by increasing the number of regulatory T cells and has shown positive results in cases of implantation failure and recurrent miscarriage.[68]

Intrauterine PRP is a treatment that involves concentrating the fraction of a patient's own blood that contains growth factors and other components that promote healing, and injecting that fraction into the uterus. It may be particularly helpful for those with implantation failure, chronic endometritis, Asherman's syndrome, or thin endometrial lining.[69] (Asherman's syndrome is discussed later in this chapter.)

Neupogen is a man-made version of a naturally occurring growth factor called G-CSF. It is typically used to help regenerate the immune system after chemotherapy, but it is also used off-label to treat implantation failure and recurrent miscarriage, where it likely works by improving development of the uterine lining and increasing the number of regulatory T cells.[70]

A note on Vitamin D and immunology

Another important step to take in the process of treating potential immune issues is checking your vitamin D level and adjusting your supplement dose if needed. Vitamin D plays a critical role in regulating the immune system, and it is essential to make sure you are getting enough.

More specifically, vitamin D can reduce the production of autoimmune antibodies and help restore the proper balance of immune cells, including natural killer cell activity and regulatory T cells.[71]

In a study of women with recurrent miscarriage, those with low vitamin D were almost twice as likely to have autoimmune antibodies, including antiphospholipid and antithyroid antibodies.[72] The same study found that low vitamin D was also associated with higher natural killer cell numbers and cell-killing activity. Other studies have found that overactive cell killing by natural killer cells can be reduced after just three weeks of supplementing with vitamin D.[73]

People with autoimmune or inflammatory conditions typically require a higher dose of vitamin D in order to regulate the immune system, typically at least 5,000 IU per day.

Hormone and Clotting Issues

Leaving the topic of immunology, the next general category of testing addresses hormone and blood-clotting issues. These issues can play a role in recurrent miscarriage and possibly infertility, but many doctors only recommend the appropriate testing after three or more miscarriages. It is reasonable to be more proactive and ask for testing after even a single pregnancy loss or if you have unexplained infertility. The only reasons to hold off are cost and inconvenience.

Some of the hormonal and clotting issues that increase the chance of miscarriage and compromise fertility were covered in chapters 3 and 4. This includes thyroid function, vitamin D, B12, and progesterone.

In addition to these basic tests, further blood tests may uncover hormone dysfunction or an increased tendency toward blood clotting. These additional tests include:

- Fasting insulin
- Factor V Leiden and prothrombin gene mutations
- MTHFR
- Prolactin

Fasting insulin

A link between glucose metabolism, insulin, and recurrent miscarriage has been suspected for decades. Women with a history of multiple miscarriages are more likely to have high fasting insulin and other signs of insulin resistance, which occurs when cells are not responding well to insulin's message to soak up glucose from the bloodstream.[74]

According to Dr. Zev Williams, Chief of Reproductive Endocrinology at Columbia University Medical Center, "We have known for a while that women with insulin resistance have much higher rates of pregnancy loss, but the reason was unknown."[75] Now, Dr. Williams's research has revealed one possible explanation, finding that insulin can directly damage the placenta.[76] "Placenta cells from early pregnancy are uniquely vulnerable to elevated levels of insulin," Dr. Williams says.

Previously, many doctors tested for fasting glucose in order to rule out diabetes in those with recurrent miscarriage, but if insulin itself is the problem, that suggests testing glucose is not enough. High insulin could be problematic even when blood glucose is normal.

If you are found to have high fasting insulin, a low-carbohydrate diet and the other nutritional strategies in chapter 13 will go a long way toward rebalancing glucose and insulin levels. Supplementing with myo-inositol can also significantly improve insulin sensitivity—that is the main reason for its use in women with PCOS and gestational diabetes. [77] Another option is the medication metformin, which is commonly used to treat PCOS, insulin resistance, and gestational diabetes. Dr. Williams's study found that metformin can protect placental cells from the damaging impact of insulin. A ketogenic diet and time-restricted eating can also significantly improve insulin sensitivity, although there are potential drawbacks, as discussed in chapter 16.

Inherited blood-clotting disorders

A number of different genes influence the tendency to form blood clots. Certain mutations in these genes, such as Factor V

Leiden and prothrombin gene mutations, increase blood clotting, which may reduce blood flow through the placenta and increase the risk of miscarriage.

The official guidance in most countries is that miscarriage alone is not a sufficient reason to test for genetic blood-clotting disorders.[78] But many reproductive immunologists disagree and argue that women who have had several miscarriages should be screened.

If testing shows you have an increased tendency to form blood clots, the typical treatment is a combination of low-dose aspirin and an anti-clotting medication, such as heparin or Lovenox. Studies have found that for women with an inherited blood-clotting disorder, this treatment can significantly increase the chance of carrying a pregnancy to term.[79]

MTHFR

The MTHFR enzyme plays an important role in processing folate into its active form, methylfolate. Although there is some controversy on this point, women with certain variations in the MTHFR gene appear to have a higher chance of miscarriage.[80] That is likely because a lack of methylfolate causes a buildup of homocysteine, which increases blood clotting and may therefore reduce blood flow through the placenta.[81] A lack of active folate may also cause DNA damage in eggs and sperm, so this issue is relevant to men too.[82]

There are several common versions of the MTHFR gene, with different levels of activity. The lowest-activity version is C677T and A1298C has an intermediate level of activity. Having two copies of C677T significantly compromises your ability to process folate, whereas having a single copy of A1298C may not have that much impact.

The problem of poor folate conversion can be largely circumvented by taking a multivitamin that contains methylfolate rather than synthetic folic acid. If you are already taking methylfolate, this testing is a lower priority. The main value in MTHFR testing is knowing whether it is worthwhile to take additional measures to lower homocysteine, such as adhering more closely to a Mediterranean diet and ensuring that you are getting sufficient vitamin B12. It has also been suggested that individuals with compromised folate metabolism should avoid synthetic folic acid added to processed foods, although there is little evidence that small amounts of folic acid pose a problem.

Prolactin

Prolactin is a hormone produced during pregnancy and breastfeeding to control various hormones and encourage milk production. It is normally low in women who are not pregnant or breastfeeding but can be elevated in those with certain medical conditions, such as underactive thyroid. If prolactin is elevated, it can disrupt development of the uterine lining, causing a short window of implantation and a higher chance of pregnancy loss.[83] When treated with medication to lower prolactin, the chance of miscarriage decreases.[84]

In the United States, prolactin is one of the few blood tests widely offered to women after pregnancy loss, but the guidance in other countries is to perform this test only in those with abnormal cycles or other hormonal abnormalities, because prolactin is rarely the cause of miscarriages or infertility when other hormones are normal.

Uterine Issues and Asherman's Syndrome

If you have unexplained infertility or recurrent pregnancy loss, one of the standard steps in the diagnostic workup is either a saline ultrasound or an X-ray with dye to check for physical issues with the uterus. These physical issues can include an abnormally shaped uterus and fibroids, both of which are usually easy to identify and can be corrected with surgery. A more difficult and troubling issue that can evade diagnosis is scar tissue in the uterus from Asherman's syndrome.

Asherman's syndrome usually occurs when a medical procedure damages the foundational layer of cells in the uterus, causing scar tissue to form. The scar tissue, also known as adhesions, can effectively fuse the front and back walls of the uterus together, preventing pregnancy or causing pregnancy loss.

Asherman's syndrome most often forms after a dilation and curettage ("D&C") procedure to remove tissue after a miscarriage or termination, or to remove retained placenta after delivery. The uterus is in a more delicate state during pregnancy, and the curettage procedure, which involves scraping tissue from the uterus, can sometimes damage the deeper layers of cells, triggering the formation of scar tissue. Asherman's can also occur after other events that cause trauma to the uterus, such as postpartum hemorrhage, infection, or surgery to remove fibroids.

Asherman's may be rare in general, but it is all too common in women with infertility or recurrent miscarriage. The risk is highest for those who have had multiple D&Cs, with studies finding Asherman's in over 30% of women who have had three or more of these procedures.[85] It is also found in 20% of women who have had a single postpartum curettage procedure.[86]

The main clues that Asherman's may be present are lighter or absent periods and a thin endometrial lining. If the deeper layer of cells in the uterus is damaged, these cells can no longer regenerate a normal lining each month, which can cause lighter or even absent periods. But this is not always the case, and more than half of women with Asherman's have normal cycles.[87]

Unfortunately, some doctors will only consider Asherman's if periods are absent, which causes many women to go through expensive and futile IVF procedures with undiagnosed uterine scarring. "It's just really frustrating," says Professor Vancaillie, an Asherman's specialist in Australia.[88]

If you have unexplained infertility or recurrent pregnancy loss and have had a D&C procedure, uterine surgery, or any postpartum complications, it may be worth investigating this issue, even if it requires some persistence to find a doctor willing to listen and willing to perform the necessary diagnostic procedure.

Asherman's can often be seen on a saline ultrasound or uterine X-ray with dye, but it is missed about a quarter of the time with these methods. The gold standard for diagnosis is a hysteroscopy—a procedure in which a doctor passes a thin tube with a camera through the cervix to see inside the uterus. If scar tissue is seen, it can be treated during the same procedure using small instruments to cut the adhesions. The goal is to remove as much scar tissue as possible, releasing the adhesions that glue the walls of the uterine cavity together.

Removing the adhesions is often enough to restore fertility and prevent further pregnancy losses, but in some cases other treatments are needed to help regenerate the uterine lining. This can include medications such as estrogen, or more experimental treatments such as stem cell injections, Neupogen, or platelet-rich plasma.[89]

A note on the endometrial receptivity assay (ERA)

The logic behind the ERA test is appealing. This test aims to determine the optimal time for embryo transfer for a particular individual by assessing when the endometrial lining is most receptive. It is done by taking progesterone for a set number of days as if preparing for an embryo transfer, then on the day that one would typically perform a transfer, a doctor performs an endometrial biopsy. The lab then assesses the stage of the endometrial lining on that particular day to determine whether it would have been ideal for an embryo transfer or whether a transfer should be performed earlier or later.

Unfortunately, the results of this testing have been disappointing. The most recent studies have consistently found that performing an ERA test and adjusting the timing of embryo transfer based on the result does not improve success rates.[90] Although it may be helpful in some cases, there is likely much more to gain from other forms of endometrial testing, including testing for potential infections or endometriosis.

Parental Genetic Testing

The final category of issues that can play a role in implantation dysfunction and recurrent miscarriage is genetic issues in the parents, such as translocations and HLA matching. In earlier chapters we saw that genetic abnormalities in embryos often cause failed implantation and miscarriages. Those genetic abnormalities are typically errors that occur spontaneously during egg or sperm development—they are not passed down from multiple generations and found in the parents' own cells. In rare cases, however, genetic issues passed down from one or both parents can compromise the viability of an embryo. For this reason, it can be helpful for both partners to undergo genetic testing for a few specific issues, such as chromosome translocations and HLA type.

Translocations

A translocation occurs when someone has a fault in the arrangement of DNA in their chromosomes. For example, a part of one chromosome may have broken off and attached to another chromosome during early development. Or parts of two chromosomes may have been swapped. These errors, known as balanced translocations, do not pose any issue to the individual because all the genetic information is present—some of it is just in a different location.

That different location becomes a problem when the two copies of that person's chromosomes are separated to form an egg or sperm. A sperm may have the copy of one chromosome that is missing a section, but may not get the copy of the other chromosome that has that section added on. The sperm will be missing genetic information, and an embryo formed from that sperm may not implant or will result in miscarriage.

Testing for this type of genetic issue is called "parental

karyotype testing." It is fairly routine for couples with unexplained infertility or recurrent miscarriage, even though translocations are rare. Researchers have found translocations in less than 5% of couples with implantation failure or miscarriage.[91]

If you are found to have a translocation, it is a matter of persistence and waiting until you are lucky enough to make an embryo that does not have the genetic error. Couples can try to conceive naturally, accepting the higher risk of miscarriage, or opt for IVF with a special type of PGT testing using a custom-made probe. This is known as PGT-SR and it allows embryos to be tested for the genetic error caused by the translocation. Between these two options, the decision often comes down to emotional and financial resources—balancing the physical and mental toll of enduring miscarriages against the expense of IVF.

HLA matching

Some experts believe that parental genetics may also influence an embryo's chance of implanting and leading to a viable pregnancy if there is too much similarity in certain genetic markers between the parents.

In organ transplantation, the goal is to find a donor with a tissue match, meaning certain molecules on the surface of cells are the same. The molecules being matched in that context are called human leukocyte antigen (HLA) molecules. These are proteins appearing on the surface of cells that the immune system uses to determine whether a cell is the body's own or something altered or foreign that should be destroyed. They can be thought of as cellular fingerprints, and an embryo will have a combination of HLA molecules from the mother and father displayed on the surface of its cells.

One might expect an embryo that is too different from the mother's HLA type to be rejected by the mother's immune system, like an organ from a mismatched donor. But the way a mother's immune system prepares and responds to pregnancy is much more sophisticated.

There is limited evidence and a great deal of controversy in this area, but according to one theory, when an embryo has a different HLA type from the mother, it is recognized as an embryo and the immune system switches to a more tolerant state. If the embryo is too similar to the mother's own cells, the immune system may not recognize it as an embryo but instead view the embryo as the mother's own cells that have become cancerous or infected by a virus and need to be destroyed.

According to this theory, parents with closely matching HLA types may have more difficulty conceiving and be more likely to miscarry because the embryo will match the mother too closely.[92] There is only limited evidence supporting this theory, however, and several studies have found no link.[93]

If you decide to have this testing done, it is likely worth consulting a reproductive immunologist because the interpretation of results can be complex. For example, some studies have suggested that even when there is not a match between parents, the presence of certain versions of some of the HLA molecules, such as DQ-alpha, can increase the risk of miscarriage.[94] This could be due to the role these genes play in autoimmunity, so some doctors may recommend immune treatment.

In the event of an HLA match, one of the treatment options is a controversial immune treatment called lymphocyte immunotherapy (LIT). This involves taking a sample of immune cells from the prospective father and injecting those cells under the prospective mother's skin to train her immune system to generate the protective immune response needed for pregnancy. So far, the studies on LIT have produced mixed results.[95] It is currently prohibited in the United States, but many couples choose to travel to other countries for this treatment after more conservative options have failed.

Action Plan

If you have unexplained infertility or a history of unsuccessful embryo transfers or miscarriages, there could be an underlying issue that goes beyond egg or sperm quality. Issues involving the uterine lining, immune system, hormones, blood clotting, and genetics can compromise the ability of an embryo to implant or increase the chance of pregnancy loss. Since many of these issues can be treated very effectively, testing is often worth the investment. Testing for these issues includes:

- an endometrial biopsy for chronic endometritis or a microbiome test for infections that cause endometritis (such as the EMMA/ALICE test)
- the ReceptivaDX test for endometriosis
- antiphospholipid, antinuclear, antithyroid, and celiac antibodies
- advanced immunology testing with a reproductive immunologist
- fasting insulin, blood-clotting disorders, MTHFR, and prolactin
- hysteroscopy for Asherman's, particularly if you have had a D&C
- parental genetic testing for translocations and HLA matching

Until medical practice catches up with the science, it may take some persistence to find a doctor who is familiar with testing and treating some of these issues. The tests that are a higher priority are those for chronic endometritis, endometriosis, antiphospholipid antibodies, and insulin resistance, since these are incredibly common and treatment can make a big difference.

Chapter 16

Troubleshooting Low Ovarian Reserve

"The trick in life is learning how to deal with it."
— Helen Mirren

ARLIER CHAPTERS DESCRIBED the strategies for improving ovarian function that are supported by the clearest evidence. In most cases, applying those strategies will be enough. But if you have extremely poor egg quality or very low ovarian reserve, you may need more help.

This chapter explains some of the options to consider if you are trying to conceive in your late thirties or early forties, have premature ovarian aging or extremely low AMH, or have had IVF cycles with very few or no eggs retrieved.

If you are facing even greater challenges, such as premature ovarian insufficiency or premature ovarian failure, some of the strategies in this chapter may improve your odds, but there will remain a very low chance of being able to conceive with your own eggs. The same is true if you are in your mid-forties or later; even with every tool available, the chance of success is low. That said, sometimes it is possible to overcome the odds, and this chapter is intended to give you all the options to consider.

This chapter focuses on addressing underlying causes of poor ovarian function, such as oxidative damage, inflammation, and autoimmunity, using strategies such as the ketogenic diet and intermittent fasting, platelet-rich plasma, red-light therapy, and additional supplements.

These approaches are somewhat speculative and not supported by the same degree of evidence as the topics covered in earlier chapters. Nevertheless, some may be worth considering if your odds of success are otherwise very low and you want to try everything possible before closing the door on trying to conceive with your own eggs.

Diminished, Not Depleted

In the past few years, there has been a flurry of research investigating novel strategies to boost ovarian reserve. Progress in this area has been met with great skepticism because if the problem is truly a finite supply of eggs, then it logically follows that nothing can be done to improve the situation.

Yet the reality is, if you have signs of low ovarian reserve, such as low AMH and few follicles visible on ultrasound, the problem is not necessarily the total number of eggs you have left. Even at menopause, women still have over 1,000 follicles remaining.

Instead, the problem may be the recruitment or survival of eggs in the early stages of the development process. In other words, you may have thousands of eggs left but may be lacking the hormones and growth factors that activate dormant follicles. Alternatively, you may be continuously recruiting a good number of follicles to leave the dormant stage and start developing into mature eggs, but they are dying off prematurely. They may be dying off because they have accumulated damage as a result of age, exposure to high blood sugar, autoimmunity, or other conditions that cause inflammation.

Eggs have elaborate mechanisms for detecting this damage. If an immature egg senses that it is defective, it will quickly self-destruct. The more difficult conditions are in ovarian follicles, the more eggs will self-destruct before they reach the stage of producing AMH or growing large enough to be visible on ultrasound. Importantly, your AMH and ovarian follicle count are not purely measures of how many eggs you have left. They also reflect how many follicles are surviving early development.

So how do we improve survival? The first part of the equation is giving the strategies discussed in previous chapters more time. Although most activity in egg development occurs during the final three to four months before an egg is ovulated, the initial development starts much earlier. The total time from when a dormant follicle is recruited from the long-term storage pool until it is mature and ready for ovulation is around 10 months.

If your ovarian follicles are accumulating more damage, perhaps because you are older or have more inflammation or insulin resistance, you may need the protective steps discussed in previous chapters throughout this full egg development timeline. When you consider that it can take weeks or months for dietary changes and supplements to have an impact at a cellular level, and that your eggs may need support during the entire 10-month development timeline, it becomes clear that it may take a year to see the full benefit of the strategies covered in previous chapters.

During this time, the most important supplements are likely CoQ10, folate, B12, antioxidants, DHEA, and melatonin. These supplements make the most difference to mitochondrial function, oxidative damage, inflammation, and, in the case of DHEA, to providing the raw materials needed to make hormones for early-stage egg development.

New research suggests that a very specific type of inflammation that naturally increases with age may also play a key role in ovarian aging. As cells throughout the body accumulate damaged molecules over the course of a lifetime, this activates a mechanism known as the inflammasome, which causes egg cells to die off.[1]

Supplementing with melatonin may be one of the best ways of inhibiting this specific kind of inflammation.[2] As a result, if you have very low ovarian reserve, it may be worth taking a low dose of melatonin longer term, even if trying to conceive naturally, as discussed in chapter 7. This differs from the traditional use of melatonin in the fertility context, which is typically a high dose for one month before IVF.

Following a low-carbohydrate Mediterranean diet throughout the egg development timeline can also reduce the inflammation and oxidative stress that causes early follicles to die off. A key component of this approach is minimizing the spikes in glucose and insulin that compromise egg quality over the long term.

Sometimes, however, the core strategies discussed in previous chapters are not enough. If you are in your forties or have another underlying cause of premature ovarian ageing, too much damage may be occurring, and you may continue to show signs of poor ovarian function. This chapter explains additional strategies you can choose from when more help is needed. The strategies include:

- tackling autoimmunity and inflammation
- a ketogenic diet and intermittent fasting
- ovarian platelet-rich-plasma injections
- red light therapy
- human growth hormone/Serovital
- PQQ
- acai
- resveratrol
- NAD precursors

Tackling Inflammation and Autoimmunity

If you have poor ovarian function for your age, one of the potential root causes is immune activity or inflammation. The most extreme version of this is premature ovarian insufficiency (POI). This condition can have a genetic component, but most women with POI have autoimmune antibodies against either the thyroid, adrenals, ovaries, or hormone receptors. If the immune system can be reined in, there is a possibility of improved ovarian function.

Less extreme forms of ovarian dysfunction are often driven by similar immune issues. For example, studies have found that women with antithyroid antibodies or other autoimmune antibodies are more likely to have diminished ovarian reserve and fewer eggs retrieved in IVF cycles. As explained in chapter 15, treatment with immune-suppressing steroids such as prednisone for several months before IVF may increase the number and quality of eggs. Supplementing with DHEA may also help if you are deficient.

There is also value in more holistic approaches to regulating the immune system, particularly if you have signs of systemic inflammation such as frequent headaches, skin issues, fatigue, or muscle and joint pain. One of the most effective ways to combat this is an anti-inflammatory diet that addresses gut health and rebalances the microbiome.

Many recent studies have demonstrated that the gut microbiome has a major impact on inflammation throughout the body, and this likely impacts ovarian function.[3] The gut microbiome is something we have the power to influence dramatically through diet, with steps such as avoiding sugar and refined starches and increasing vegetables, lean proteins, and anti-inflammatory fats. This dietary shift can quickly reduce inflammation throughout the body.[4] Probiotics may also help, along with an omega-3 supplement and higher-dose vitamin D. More advanced options include gut microbiome testing and addressing an overgrowth of pathogenic microbes, as covered in more detail in my book *The Keystone Approach*, which focuses on autoimmunity and the microbiome.

Finally, some experts have also suggested that mold exposure could be a factor driving immune-related poor ovarian function in younger women. There has been very little research on this point, but it is something to consider if you are concerned about mold in your home.

Intermittent fasting and the ketogenic diet

Although following a low-carbohydrate Mediterranean diet can go a long way toward improving ovarian function, some argue there may be greater benefit from reducing carbohydrate intake even further and following a ketogenic diet.

When carbohydrate intake is below 20–50 g per day, the body transitions from primarily burning glucose to primarily burning fat, a state known as ketosis. There are plausible mechanisms for how a ketogenic diet could improve ovarian function, including a reduction in inflammation, an improvement in mitochondrial function, and activation of longevity enzymes known as sirtuins.[5]

In the PCOS context, the most recent studies have found that following a ketogenic diet can significantly boost the chance of getting pregnant.[6] Yet there has been little research in women without PCOS. We must also balance the potential benefits against the potential downsides, such as hormone disruptions.

Dr. Robert Kiltz, the founder of CNY Fertility, is a firm proponent of the ketogenic diet for fertility, after seeing it work for so many of his patients. Dr Kiltz reports that "around ten years ago, I noticed something incredible happening at my fertility practice. I had patients who had been struggling to get pregnant for years, then on their own, they changed their diets by eliminating carbs and sugar, and suddenly they were pregnant."[7]

According to Dr. Kiltz, the most likely explanation for this phenomenon is a reduction in inflammation. "In the majority of cases I treat, infertility is an inflammatory disease," he says. Dr. Kiltz further explains that "my observations as a fertility doctor led me to believe that the constant sugar and fiber fermenting in our bowels spreads inflammation to tissue and organs throughout the entire lower abdominal region, including our tubes, ovaries [and] uterus..."[8] A ketogenic diet is intended to reduce this inflammation by removing the carbohydrates that are fermented by unfriendly gut microbes.

Dr. Kiltz also recommends intermittent fasting, such as eating just once per day. Intermittent fasting and the ketogenic diet often go hand in hand because it is easier to fast when you can efficiently burn fat for energy. Both approaches are also purported to have similar benefits for inflammation and mitochondrial function, so many people choose to adopt both strategies for maximum benefit.

Some argue that intermittent fasting has additional benefits because it allows the body to go into a healing and damage-cleanup mode called autophagy. In this mode, old damaged molecules are broken down, and stem cells are activated to produce new cells and new mitochondria. An animal study published in 2023 indicated that intermittent fasting may indeed improve egg quality and reduce chromosomal errors in eggs by increasing mitochondrial function.[9]

Yet there are potential downsides to both a ketogenic diet and intermittent fasting. Some people feel better than ever with these dietary approaches, but others experience problems such as hormone disruptions, lower thyroid function, and compromised sleep. Occasionally, women following a ketogenic diet may also stop ovulating, but this appears to be rare. A 2023 study reported minimal impacts on women's hormones after intermittent fasting with a four- to six-hour eating window. The only notable change was a small reduction in DHEA.[10]

In the end, whether the benefits outweigh these potential negative impacts may differ between individuals. Following a ketogenic diet is most likely to be helpful if your ovarian function is significantly compromised by autoimmunity, inflammation, or high insulin, or if you are overweight.

If you decide to experiment with a ketogenic diet, one option is to take a moderate approach in order to minimize the potential impact on hormones. This could mean aiming for around 4o g of carbohydrates per day, rather than the 10–20 g in stricter versions of the ketogenic diet.

In a similar vein, a gentle approach to intermittent fasting could mean limiting your eating hours to two meals per day, with a late brunch and early dinner.

To get the most benefit from a ketogenic diet or intermittent fasting, it is important to continue with the general anti-inflammatory diet principles shown to improve fertility: prioritizing nutrient density and emphasizing fats from fish, olive oil, and avocados, rather than sources such as coconut oil. If you would like to try this approach, you can download anti-inflammatory ketogenic meal plans, food lists, and recipes in my online program at **itstartswiththeegg.com/join**

Lowering inflammation with LDN

When conventional measures are not enough to tackle immune activity that may be compromising ovarian function, another option is the medication LDN, which stands for low-dose naltrexone. Although this is a prescription medication, it falls firmly in the camp of alternative medicine, and many doctors will not be familiar with LDN or comfortable prescribing it.

Naltrexone is approved to treat opioid addiction, where it works by temporarily blocking opioid receptors. In much lower doses, naltrexone causes an increase in natural endorphin production, which is thought to reduce inflammation. LDN may also reduce inflammation by stopping the immune system from overreacting to the gut microbiome. Initial studies in autoimmune diseases such as Crohn's disease show promise,[11] but it has not been studied in the fertility context.

Despite the lack of evidence, some alternative doctors are strong advocates for the use of LDN in women with poor ovarian function, particularly if they also have an autoimmune condition. One such doctor is Dr. Phil Boyle, director of the NaPro Fertility Care Clinic in Dublin.

Dr. Boyle has prescribed naltrexone to more than 2,500 of his fertility patients. He reports that "at this point, I find it is clinically appropriate to try LDN in up to 50% of my subfertile patients. Of those, about 80% experience a positive response to the LDN."[12]

This experience does not overcome the lack of scientific research, but overall, this medication is considered quite safe and low-risk. The main side effects are sleep disruptions such as vivid dreams, and headaches.

LDN is relatively inexpensive, typically costing less than $150, but because the dose used is much lower than the FDA-approved dose, it must be ordered from a specialist compounding pharmacy. At time of writing, most fertility doctors are not familiar with LDN, so it is typically necessary to consult a functional medicine or integrative doctor or use a telemedicine service that specializes in prescribing LDN. This may be changing, however, with some IVF clinics such as CNY now including LDN in their immune protocols for IVF.

Ovarian Rejuvenation with Platelet-Rich Plasma

One of the most promising strategies for restoring ovarian function in those with age-related infertility or premature ovarian insufficiency is PRP, which stands for platelet-rich plasma. Chapter 15 mentioned the potential value of PRP injections in the uterus to address implantation problems caused by Asherman's syndrome, endometritis, or a thin lining. Another use of PRP for fertility, explained in this section, is injecting the solution directly into the ovaries, with the goal of restoring ovarian function.

To perform this treatment, a vial of a patient's blood is processed to remove red blood cells, leaving behind a concentrated solution that contains a range of growth factors. These growth factors promote healing and cell regeneration, while reducing inflammation. PRP has been used for decades to treat joint injuries, particularly among professional athletes.

Using PRP to improve ovarian function is a relatively new technique offered by some IVF clinics, but the results so far have been encouraging, especially in women with a history of many unsuccessful IVF cycles or with premature ovarian insufficiency (POI).

Women with POI typically have irregular or absent cycles and an FSH over 30–40 mIU/L. The chance of getting pregnant is extremely low, but PRP may be able to improve the odds in some cases.

Published case reports include a 37-year-old woman with a high FSH value and an undetectable AMH. A month after PRP, her FSH dropped to the normal range, and her previously absent cycles resumed. After two IVF cycles, she was able to obtain three embryos and eventually gave birth to twins.[13]

In another similar case, a 40-year-old woman who had premature menopause with very high FSH and low AMH saw her cycles resume within two months of PRP treatment. Within four months, she conceived naturally.[14]

These extraordinary stories are not necessarily typical and most women with POI are still unable to conceive after PRP,[15] but they suggest that in rare cases this treatment could make a difference when the situation otherwise appears hopeless.

PRP may have even greater value for those with a milder form of ovarian dysfunction, falling into the category of age-related infertility or diminished ovarian reserve. Numerous controlled studies of ovarian PRP in this context have reported increases in AMH, decreases in FSH, many naturally conceived pregnancies, and improvements in IVF outcomes.[16] These improved IVF outcomes include a higher number of good-quality embryos and often a higher pregnancy rate.[17]

If you have age-related fertility challenges, the odds of success in IVF will still be low, even after PRP. Yet there have been some dramatic success stories, such as the published case of a 41-year-old woman with 12 failed IVF cycles. Six weeks after PRP treatment, her AMH doubled. She then conceived naturally and gave birth to a healthy baby.[18]

One of the most encouraging findings from the studies on PRP for diminished ovarian reserve is an apparent increase in egg and embryo quality. One study compared the proportion of genetically normal embryos from women before PRP and then three months after PRP. The average age of the women was 40, and just 8% of their embryos were normal in the cycle before PRP. After PRP, 39% of their embryos were normal, and a quarter got pregnant.[19]

It is unclear how exactly PRP can improve fertility, but it is likely related to the many growth factors found in platelets. These growth factors regulate inflammation, sensitize follicles to FSH, and may help recruit more dormant follicles to start actively growing. Perhaps those who see an improvement after PRP start out deficient in critical growth factors needed to support the survival or recruitment of ovarian follicles? Hopefully, future research will provide more understanding of the mechanisms underlying PRP, so clinics can better predict which patients will benefit from it.

On balance, PRP appears to be a promising option for restoring ovarian function, particularly in women with very high FSH and low AMH. Yet it does not help everyone and it is possible you may not see any improvement. As with any medical procedure, it carries theoretical risks, such as infection, but PRP has been used for a range of medical conditions for many years, and complications are extremely rare.

The most significant downside of PRP is the expense. Each treatment can cost thousands of dollars, and some clinics recommend multiple rounds of treatment. Because PRP seems to have a dramatic impact for some women and very little impact for others, this expense can be a significant gamble.

It often makes sense to combine PRP with IVF because there appears to be a short window of greatest effect from one to three months after treatment. Planning an egg retrieval for this time takes maximum advantage of this window.

Yet IVF is not always necessary, and if finances are limiting, one option is to combine PRP with trying to conceive naturally. Some of the studies have reported a higher rate of natural pregnancies within the three months after PRP than we would expect even from IVF. In a study of over 300 women with POI, 7% got pregnant naturally within one or two months after PRP.[20] That number is likely to be much higher for women with diminished ovarian reserve rather than POI. In addition, although ovarian function will likely start to wane several months after treatment, some of the improvement in FSH and AMH may remain for up to 12 months.[21]

Red Light Therapy

Red light therapy involves using a device that emits light at a specific wavelength within the red or infrared spectrum. The device is held close to the skin for several minutes, with the goal of the light energy reaching certain tissues and having a biological effect.

There is some evidence that red light therapy can promote localized tissue healing and reduce inflammation in the specific area treated. That has been observed in animal and human studies in a range of scenarios, particularly in joint and tendon injuries.[22] In addition, there is some evidence that at a biochemical level, specific wavelengths of red light can promote energy production by mitochondria.

What is less clear is whether these purported benefits translate into improved fertility. In theory, a reduction in inflammation or increase in mitochondrial function in the ovaries or uterine lining would be beneficial. The problem is that the light energy may not reach that far. Studies indicate that at common wavelengths used for red light therapy, more than 80% of the energy is absorbed or scattered within the first 3 millimeters, which is the very beginning of the fat layer beneath the skin.[23]

It is questionable whether red light therapy could have any impact on fertility if only a tiny percentage of light energy can reach the target tissues deep in the abdomen. In studies in mice, where this is less of an issue, researchers have found positive effects, with a greater proportion of actively developing follicles.[24]

So far, the studies in humans have been very limited. Many of the claims about the fertility benefits of red-light therapy are based on early studies in Japan that reported good pregnancy rates among older women with long-standing infertility.[25] In those studies, the red-light device was typically applied to the neck, based on the theory that this would impact the blood supply to the brain, which is the master regulator of hormones and fertility. It is often reported that another group in Denmark found that 65% of women with infertility became pregnant after red light therapy to the abdomen, but this report originated from a manufacturer of the devices and was not published in a reputable journal.[26]

Overall, the current evidence in favor of red-light therapy for female fertility is relatively weak, but there is little evidence of potential harm.

Further Supplements for Ovarian Reserve

Although some fertility supplements are easy to recommend because they have been studied extensively, and others are clearly worth avoiding, this section addresses the gray area—supplements that may be useful, but more research is needed. These are options to consider if you have severely compromised ovarian function and are interested in trying everything that could possibly help.

Serovital and growth hormone/ Omnitrope

Serovital is an amino acid–based supplement purported to have anti-aging effects by increasing the normal production of human growth hormone. Growth hormone is certainly important to fertility, because it plays a role in the development and survival of ovarian follicles. The natural decline in growth hormone that occurs with age may be one component of age-related infertility.

For that reason, growth hormone is often given to women with low ovarian reserve in preparation for IVF. It is a relatively expensive prescription injection sold under the brand name Omnitrope. The effectiveness of this medication is not yet clear and some studies have found little benefit.[27] Nevertheless, most studies to date have reported some improvement in the number or quality of eggs and embryos after growth hormone treatment.[28] It seems more likely to have a beneficial effect in those with age-related infertility or poor follicle growth in a prior IVF cycle.

Growth hormone may also be more effective in women who start with a low level of insulin-like growth factor 1, also known as IGF-1.[29] Doctors at the PIVET Medical Center in Australia suggest supplementing with growth hormone only if IGF-1 is below 20 nmol/L, which is equivalent to 153 ng/mL.[30] IGF-1 is a routine blood test that can be ordered from a standard testing laboratory.

The duration of treatment may also matter. Growth hormone likely has the greatest impact when taken for at least a month before IVF. During this time frame, it appears to increase the number of hormone receptors on ovarian cells, which makes the follicles respond better to FSH during the stimulation phase.[31] Growth hormone may have further benefits if taken for even longer, by increasing the survival of early-stage follicles that are two or three months away from maturity.[32]

The problem with using Omnitrope for several months is the cost, because each vial is quite expensive. That is where Serovital comes in, as a cheaper over-the-counter supplement that naturally increases growth hormone production. In addition to the benefit of lower cost, some IVF clinics are more comfortable recommending Serovital than prescribing Omnitrope, given that Omnitrope is only approved for growth hormone deficiency and must be prescribed off-label for fertility. Serovital does not require a prescription and it can be taken longer-term by those trying to conceive naturally, not just in preparation for IVF.

Serovital is a combination of five amino acids that together boost the natural production of growth hormone. It is marketed as an anti-aging supplement, based on the concept that growth hormone reduces wrinkles and body fat while increasing energy and improving sleep. Serovital is also used to treat fibromyalgia.[33] Studies have reported that Serovital does indeed increase growth hormone and IGF-1,[34] but it has not been specifically studied in the fertility context.

One of the amino acids in Serovital is L-arginine, which you may recall from chapter 10 has produced conflicting results when given to women preparing for IVF, with some reports of chaotic egg development. This is likely due to very high doses of L-arginine causing some follicles to develop rapidly and out of sync. At low doses, this does not seem to be a concern and L-arginine may be beneficial, as found in a 2020 study that reported a slightly higher pregnancy rate in women taking 1 or 2 g of L-arginine per day before IVF.[35] In Serovital, the amount of L-arginine is less than 1 g in the suggested dose of four capsules.

In the absence of clinical studies on Serovital in the fertility context, the best information we have to rely on is the real-world experience of people taking this supplement and the fertility clinics that recommend it. These reports are overwhelmingly positive, with many IVF clinics reporting improved results when their patients take Serovital for at least three months before IVF.

The usual dose is a packet of four capsules taken on an empty stomach at least two hours before breakfast or two hours after dinner. This timing is intended to optimize absorption of the amino acids and the production of growth hormone, which is increased by fasting. It may also be preferable to take Serovital at bedtime to mirror our natural circadian rhythms more closely. The natural production of growth hormone typically peaks between 2 a.m. and 4 a.m. Data shows it also peaks approximately two hours after taking Serovital.

PQQ

PQQ is a supplement gaining popularity based on its ability to improve mitochondrial function. For that reason, it is often included as a secondary ingredient in CoQ10 supplements. Studies indicate that PQQ not only acts as an efficient antioxidant but also increases the generation of new mitochondria and their ability to produce cellular energy.[36]

Human studies have found that in addition to boosting the number and activity of mitochondria, PQQ increases blood flow and energy metabolism in the brain and appears to reduce inflammation.[37]

Despite all these positive signs, little research has been done in the fertility context. A small number of animal studies have found that PQQ acts to protect ovarian cells from chemical damage and promotes their survival.[38] We do not yet know whether this protective effect or the ability of PQQ to promote mitochondrial activity translates into improved fertility in humans.

Acai

Acai is a fruit native to Central and South America that is particularly rich in antioxidants. The clear link between oxidative damage and ovarian aging led to the idea that supplementing with acai may improve IVF outcomes in women with low ovarian reserve.

One of the top fertility clinics in the United States, CCRM, is known for recommending acai supplements to patients preparing for IVF. Dr. Schoolcraft and his colleagues at CCRM have also published several studies in this area, with some positive results.

The clinic found that in aging mice, supplementing with acai led to a small improvement in the number of eggs and an even greater improvement in egg quality. Better egg quality was clear from a higher percentage of eggs that developed into blastocysts and a higher rate of embryo implantation.[39] Overall, the eggs from older mice treated with acai seemed to perform on par with eggs from younger mice.

This research was followed up with a preliminary human trial involving more than 100 patients at CCRM. Women in the study took 1800 mg of a freeze-dried acai supplement for around 10 weeks before IVF. This resulted in a small increase in the number of eggs but a significant increase in the number of embryos, particularly genetically normal embryos. On average, women in the acai group ended up with three normal embryos, compared to just one normal embryo in the control group.[40] A previous publication from CCRM also described a high implantation rate in women taking acai before IVF.[41]

Although these results are encouraging, the antioxidants found in acai are not part of our natural biology, and it is possible that acai may have unpredictable effects. In addition, there are many low-quality acai supplements on the market, and the form used in the CCRM study is only available to patients at that clinic. If you decide to add acai to your regime, freeze-dried acai powder or frozen acai berries may be a more reliable source than capsules.

Resveratrol

Resveratrol is another supplement widely used for age-related infertility and diminished ovarian reserve. The main rationale for taking resveratrol is that it is an antioxidant, but it may also activate sirtuin enzymes associated with longevity and anti-aging. At this stage there is very little evidence that resveratrol improves fertility, and there is reason for concern that it may disrupt implantation or harm developing embryos.[42]

As discussed in chapter 10, a randomized study of women preparing for embryo transfer found that supplementing with resveratrol significantly decreased the pregnancy rate and increased the miscarriage rate.[43] It is unclear whether that effect is real because it has not been observed in other studies, but animal studies also suggest that resveratrol may negatively impact implantation by altering the endometrial lining.

If you have severely diminished ovarian function and are preparing for IVF, you may decide it is worth temporarily sacrificing your endometrial lining for the potential benefits to egg quality. There is some logic to this, because you can stop resveratrol before egg retrieval and later do a frozen transfer. One major downside to be aware of is that you may be reducing the chance of conceiving naturally while preparing for IVF. In addition, women with very few eggs retrieved often have the best results with a fresh day 3 embryo transfer, so it is safest to stop resveratrol at least two weeks before egg retrieval.

NAD, TruNiagen, and NMN

NAD stands for nicotinamide adenine dinucleotide. NAD is found in every cell in the body, where it performs a vital role in energy production. We naturally produce NAD from niacin, also known as vitamin B3, but the efficiency of this process declines with age, resulting in a depletion of NAD and compromised cellular energy production.

The link between aging, lower NAD, and lower energy production has sparked interest in ways to boost levels of NAD to combat age-related diseases and infertility.

We cannot supplement with NAD directly, so the solution is to supplement with a precursor that can then be converted into NAD inside our cells. These precursors include niacin and intermediates along the pathway of conversion from niacin to NAD. There is a great deal of controversy over which precursor is the most effective, with ongoing battles between competing researchers and companies.

The form that has been studied most extensively is nicotinamide riboside, or NR for short. This is known by the brand names Niagen or TruNiagen. In the 2000s, researchers discovered that NR raises NAD levels more effectively than the standard form of niacin. As a result, it boosts cellular energy production. In aging mice, it also increases the number of ovarian follicles and decreases chromosomal abnormalities.[44]

Another NAD precursor is NMN, which stands for nicotinamide mononucleotide. This compound is almost identical to NR but with the addition of a single phosphate group. NMN has produced similar positive results in mouse studies, with an increase in the number and quality of eggs retrieved in

IVF.[45] One of the most interesting findings of this research was the observation that in mice supplemented with NMN, the cellular machinery that processes and separates chromosomes could function just like that of young mice, likely preventing chromosomal errors during egg development.[46]

This research has naturally generated a great deal of excitement, but at time of writing, there has been little research in humans to confirm the potential benefits of either NR or NMN for fertility. The mouse studies are very promising, but as noted by Leonard Guarente, the chief scientist at one of the major companies developing these supplements, "not everything that works in mice works in humans."[47] Even so, many fertility doctors have started recommending NR or NMN based on the promising animal studies.

One potential risk to be aware of is the possibility that NAD precursors could drive tumor growth. Tumors, like other cells, depend on NAD for energy production and it has been suggested that these supplements may help cancers spread.[48] There is very little evidence for this, but until more long-term studies are done, it is a personal decision whether these supplements are worth the risk.

If you do wish to take an NAD precursor, deciding which is the better form is no easy task. A heated controversy has erupted on this point, with contradictory claims driven by commercial interests.

On one side of the debate is the argument that NMN is more stable and more effective than NR, because it is further along the pathway of conversion to NAD. On the other side is the argument that NMN cannot enter cells directly and must be broken down to NR first. [49] In the end, both points may be moot because it has been suggested that both compounds may be broken down to niacin and other niacin derivatives in the gut and liver.[50]

If that is true, the most cost-effective way to increase NAD could be the niacin derivative niacinamide, also known as nicotinamide. This naturally occurring form of vitamin B3 is often used in multivitamins and has been shown to raise NAD more effectively than niacin.[51] It may not be quite as effective as NR or NMN, but animal studies have reported similar improvements in egg quality.[52] The advantage of niacinamide is that it is much less expensive, costing less than $10 for a three-month supply, compared to $100 or more for a similar supply of TruNiagen or NMN.

In contrast to the cloud of suspicion over whether these other NAD precursors increase cancer growth, niacinamide has been suggested to have the opposite effect, with a potential role in preventing and treating cancer.[53] This, too, is uncertain, with a clinical study published in the prestigious *New England Journal of Medicine* in 2023 finding no impact on the rate of developing skin cancer after 12 months of supplementing with niacinamide.[54]

Another question hanging over niacinamide is whether it may inhibit the longevity enzymes known as sirtuins, which are thought to play a role in fertility.[55] This appears to occur only at high doses, with one study finding that lower doses could actually increase sirtuin activity,[56] but again, more research is needed. One potential solution is to take 500 mg of niacinamide in a controlled-release form to maintain a low, steady dose.

The bottom line on NAD precursors is that animal studies are very promising, but we do not yet have clear evidence from human trials. There are more questions than answers in this area, particularly as to whether these supplements increase cancer growth and which form is preferable. Based on the information available to date, the benefits of NR or NMN may not justify their high cost, although this may change as further research comes to light.

Action Steps

If you have very low ovarian reserve, additional strategies may help improve the number and quality of eggs by reducing inflammation and promoting survival of early-stage follicles. In approximate order from the most to the least likely to make a difference, these strategies include

- ovarian PRP
- tackling autoimmunity and inflammation
- a ketogenic diet and intermittent fasting
- human growth hormone/ Serovital
- acai (for egg quality, not quantity)
- NAD precursors (for age-related infertility)
- PQQ
- resveratrol
- red light therapy

Epilogue

EGG QUALITY HAS such profound implications for fertility that all women who are trying to conceive deserve to know what they can do to protect their own egg quality. If you found this book useful, please help spread the word to others who are trying to conceive.

References

Introduction

1   Sugiura-Ogasawara M, Ozaki Y, Katano K, Suzumori N, Kitaori T, Mizutani E. Abnormal embryonic karyotype is the most frequent cause of recurrent miscarriage. Hum Reprod. 2012 Aug;27(8):2297-303 ("Suguira-Ogasawara 2012").

2   Macklon NS, Geraedts JP, Fauser BC. Conception to ongoing pregnancy: the 'black box' of early pregnancy loss. Hum Reprod Update. 2002 Jul-Aug;8(4):333-43 ("Macklon 2002").

Chapter 1: Understanding Egg Quality

1   Sugiura-Ogasawara M, Ozaki Y, Katano K, Suzumori N, Kitaori T, Mizutani E. Abnormal embryonic karyotype is the most frequent cause of recurrent miscarriage. Hum Reprod. 2012 Aug;27(8):2297-303; Macklon NS, Geraedts JP, Fauser BC. Conception to ongoing pregnancy: the 'black box' of early pregnancy loss. Hum Reprod Update. 2002 Jul-Aug;8(4):333-43

2   Macklon 2002.

3   Hassold T, Hall H, Hunt P. The origin of human aneuploidy: where we have been, where we are going. Hum Mol Genet. 2007;16(Spec No. 2):R203–R208. ("Hassold and Hunt 2007"); Macklon 2002; Sher G, Keskintepe L, Keskintepe M, Ginsburg M, Maassarani G, Yakut T, Baltaci V, Kotze D, Unsal E.Oocyte karyotyping by comparative genomic hybridization provides a highly reliable method for selecting "competent" embryos, markedly improving in vitro fertilization outcome: a multiphase study. Fertil Steril. 2007 May;87(5):1033-40.

4   Fragouli E, Alfarawati S, Goodall NN, Sánchez-García JF, Colls P, Wells D. The cytogenetics of polar bodies: insights into female meiosis and the diagnosis of aneuploidy. Mol Hum Reprod. 2011 May;17(5):286-95. ("Fragouli 2011").

5   van den Berg MM, van Maarle MC, van Wely M, Goddijn M. Genetics of early miscarriage. Biochim Biophys Acta. 2012 Dec;1822(12):1951-9; ("van den Berg 2012"). Macklon 2002

6   Macklon 2002.

7   Suguira-Ogasawara 2012.

8   Kushnir VA, Frattarelli JL. Aneuploidy in abortuses following IVF and ICSI. J Assist Reprod Genet. 2009 Mar;26(2-3):93-7;

Kim JW, Lee WS, Yoon TK, Seok HH, Cho JH, Kim YS, Lyu SW, Shim SH. Chromosomal abnormalities in spontaneous abortion after assisted reproductive treatment. BMC Med Genet. 2010 Nov 3;11:153; van den Berg 2012

9   Macklon 2002.

10 Allen EG, Freeman SB, Druschel C, Hobbs CA, O'Leary LA, Romitti PA, Royle MH, Torfs CP, Sherman SL. Maternal age and risk for trisomy 21 assessed by the origin of chromosome nondisjunction: a report from the Atlanta and National Down Syndrome Projects. Hum Genet. 2009 Feb;125(1):41-52.

11 Fragouli 2011; Macklon 2002.

12 Thomas, C., Cavazza, T., & Schuh, M. (2021). Aneuploidy in human eggs: contributions of the meiotic spindle. Biochemical Society Transactions, 49(1), 107-118.
    Kuliev A, Zlatopolsky Z, Kirillova I, Spivakova J, Cieslak Janzen J. Meiosis errors in over 20,000 oocytes studied in the practice of preimplantation aneuploidy testing. Reprod Biomed Online. 2011 Jan;22(1):2-8.; Fragouli 2011

13 Munné S, Held KR, Magli CM, Ata B, Wells D, Fragouli E, Baukloh V, Fischer R, Gianaroli L. Intra-age, intercenter, and intercycle differences in chromosome abnormalities in oocytes. Fertil Steril. 2012 Apr;97(4):935-42.

14 Id.

15 Hassold T, Hunt P. Maternal age and chromosomally abnormal pregnancies: what we know and what we wish we knew. Curr Opin Pediatr. 2009 Dec;21(6):703-8.

16 Nagaoka SI, Hassold TJ, Hunt PA. Human aneuploidy: mechanisms and new insights into an age-old problem. Nat Rev Genet. 2012 Jun 18;13(7):493-504; Fragouli 2011;

17 Bentov Y, Yavorska T, Esfandiari N, Jurisicova A, Casper RF. The contribution of mitochondrial function to reproductive aging. J Assist Reprod Genet. 2011 Sep;28(9):773-83.

18 Van Blerkom J. Mitochondrial function in the human oocyte and embryo and their role in developmental competence. Mitochondrion. 2011 Sep;11(5):797-813. ("Van Blerkom 2011").

19 Van Blerkom 2011.

20 Shigenaga MK, Hagen TM, Ames BN. Oxidative damage and mitochondrial decay in aging. Proc Natl Acad Sci USA. 1994 91:10771–8.

21 Eichenlaub-Ritter U, Wieczorek M, Lüke S, Seidel T. Age related changes in mitochondrial function and new approaches to study redox regulation in mammalian oocytes in response to age or maturation conditions. Mitochondrion. 2011 Sep;11(5):783-96; Van Blerkom 2011.

22 Interview with Dr. Robert Casper, published in The Spectator, 11/19/2011. http://www.spectator.co.uk/features/7396723/resetting-the-clock/

Chapter 2: Protecting Eggs from Toxins

1   Dr. Patricia Hunt, personal communication. 2/6/2014.

2   Hunt PA, Koehler KE, Susiarjo M, Hodges CA, Ilagan A, Voigt RC, Thomas S, Thomas BF, Hassold TJ. Bisphenol a exposure causes meiotic aneuploidy in the female mouse. Curr Biol. 2003 Apr 1;13(7):546-53. ("Hunt 2003").

3   Hunt 2003.

4   Kitamura S, Suzuki T, Sanoh S, Kohta R, Jinno N, Sugihara K, Yoshihara S, Fujimoto N, Watanabe H, Ohta S. Comparative study of the endocrine-disrupting activity of bisphenol A and 19 related compounds. Toxicol Sci. 2005 Apr;84(2):249-59;
    Welshons WV, Nagel SC, vom Saal FS. Large effects from small exposures. III. Endocrine mechanisms mediating effects of bisphenol A at levels of human exposure. Endocrinology. 2006 Jun;147(6 Suppl):S56-69. ("Welshons 2006").

5   Lamb, J. D., M. S. Bloom, F. S. Vom Saal, J. A. Taylor, J. R. Sandler, and V. Y. Fujimoto. "Serum Bisphenol A (BPA) and reproductive outcomes in couples undergoing IVF." Fertil Steril. 2008; 90: S186;
    Fujimoto VY, Kim D, vom Saal FS, Lamb JD, Taylor JA, Bloom MS. Serum unconjugated bisphenol A concentrations in women may adversely influence oocyte quality during in vitro fertilization. Fertil Steril. 2011 Apr;95(5):1816-9;
    Mok-Lin E, Ehrlich S, Williams PL, Petrozza J, Wright DL, Calafat AM, Ye X, Hauser R. Urinary bisphenol A concentrations and ovarian response among women undergoing IVF. Int J Androl. 2010 Apr;33(2):385-93. ("Mok-Lin 2010")
    Ehrlich S, Williams PL, Missmer SA, Flaws JA, Ye X, Calafat AM, Petrozza JC, Wright D, Hauser R. Urinary bisphenol A concentrations and early reproductive health outcomes among women undergoing IVF. Hum Reprod. 2012 Dec;27(12):3583-92
    Ehrlich S, Williams PL, Missmer SA, Flaws JA, Berry KF, Calafat AM, Ye X, Petrozza JC, Wright D, Hauser R. Urinary bisphenol A concentrations and implantation failure among women undergoing in vitro fertilization. Environ Health Perspect. 2012 Jul;120(7):978-83

6   Mínguez-Alarcón, L., Messerlian, C., Bellavia, A., Gaskins, A. J., Chiu, Y. H., Ford, J. B., ... & Earth Study Team. (2019). Urinary concentrations of bisphenol A, parabens and phthalate metabolite mixtures in relation to reproductive success among women undergoing in vitro fertilization. Environment international, 126, 355-362.

7   Id.

8   Mínguez-Alarcón, L., Gaskins, A. J., Chiu, Y. H., Souter, I., Williams, P. L., Calafat, A. M., ... & EARTH Study team. (2016). Dietary folate intake and modification of the association of urinary bisphenol A

concentrations with in vitro fertilization outcomes among women from a fertility clinic. Reproductive Toxicology, 65, 104-112

9   Ao, J., Huo, X., Zhang, J., Mao, Y., Li, G., Ye, J., ... & Zhang, J. (2022). Environmental exposure to bisphenol analogues and unexplained recurrent miscarriage: A case-control study. Environmental Research, 204, 112293.

Adu-Gyamfi, E. A., Rosenfeld, C. S., & Tuteja, G. (2022). The impact of bisphenol A on the placenta. Biology of Reproduction, 106(5), 826-834.

Lathi, R. B., Liebert, C. A., Brookfield, K. F., Taylor, J. A., Vom Saal, F. S., Fujimoto, V. Y., & Baker, V. L. (2014). Conjugated bisphenol A in maternal serum in relation to miscarriage risk. Fertility and sterility, 102(1), 123-128.

Butts, S., Holder, S., Mostisser, C., Mesaros, C., Imbalzano, M., Coutifaris, C., & Bartolomei, M. S. (2015). BPA levels at implantation are associated with elelvated miscarriage risk in IVF cycles. Fertility and Sterility, 104(3), e87.

10 R.B. Lathi et al, Maternal Serum Bisphenol-A (BPA) Level Is Positively Associated with Miscarriage Risk, O-6, 69th Annual Meeting of the American Society for Reproductive Medicine, October 14, 2013.

Sugiura-Ogasawara M, Ozaki Y, Sonta S, Makino T, Suzumori K. Exposure to bisphenol A is associated with recurrent miscarriage. Hum Reprod. 2005 Aug;20(8):2325-9

Shen, Y., Zheng, Y., Jiang, J., Liu, Y., Luo, X., Shen, Z., ... & Liang, H. (2015). Higher urinary bisphenol A concentration is associated with unexplained recurrent miscarriage risk: evidence from a case-control study in eastern China. PloS one, 10(5), e0127886.

11 Can A, Semiz O, Cinar O. Bisphenol-A induces cell cycle delay and alters centrosome and spindle microtubular organization in oocytes during meiosis. Mol Hum Reprod. 2005 Jun;11(6):389-96. ("Can 2005").

Lenie S, Cortvrindt R, Eichenlaub-Ritter U, Smitz J.Continuous exposure to bisphenol A during in vitro follicular development induces meiotic abnormalities. Mutat Res. 2008 Mar 12;651(1-2):71-81.

Xu J, Osuga Y, Yano T, Morita Y, Tang X, Fujiwara T, Takai Y, Matsumi H, Koga K, Taketani Y, Tsutsumi O. Bisphenol A induces apoptosis and G2-to-M arrest of ovarian granulosa cells. Biochem Biophys Res Commun. 2002 Mar 29;292(2):456-62.

Brieño-Enríquez MA, Robles P, Camats-Tarruella N, García-Cruz R, Roig I, Cabero L, Martínez F, Caldés MG. Human meiotic progression and recombination are affected by Bisphenol A exposure during in vitro human oocyte development. Hum Reprod. 2011 Oct;26(10):2807-18.

12 Li, Q., Davila, J., Kannan, A., Flaws, J. A., Bagchi, M. K., & Bagchi, I. C. (2016). Chronic exposure to Bisphenol A affects uterine function during early pregnancy in mice. Endocrinology, 157(5), 1764-1774.

See also: Aldad, T. S., Rahmani, N., Leranth, C., & Taylor, H. S. (2011). Bisphenol-A exposure alters endometrial progesterone receptor expression in the nonhuman primate. Fertility and sterility, 96(1), 175-179.

13 Adu-Gyamfi, E. A., Rosenfeld, C. S., & Tuteja, G. (2022). The impact of bisphenol A on the placenta. Biology of Reproduction, 106(5), 826-834.

14 Meeker JD, Sathyanarayana S, Swan SH.Phthalates and other additives in plastics: human exposure and associated health outcomes. Philos Trans R Soc Lond B Biol Sci.
2009 Jul 27;364(1526):2097-113.

15 Hauser R, Calafat AM. Phthalates and human health. Occup Environ Med. 2005 Nov;62(11):806-18.;

16 David Byrne, EU Commissioner for Consumer Protection and Health, November 10th, 1999. http://europa.eu/rapid/press-release_IP-99-829_en.htm?locale=FR

17 Ferguson, K. K., McElrath, T. F., & Meeker, J. D. (2014). Environmental phthalate exposure and preterm birth. JAMA pediatrics, 168(1), 61-67.
Minatoya, M., & Kishi, R. (2021). A review of recent studies on bisphenol A and phthalate exposures and child neurodevelopment. International Journal of Environmental Research and Public Health, 18(7), 3585.

18 Begum, T. F., Fujimoto, V. Y., Gerona, R., McGough, A., Lenhart, N., Wong, R., ... & Bloom, M. S. (2021). A pilot investigation of couple-level phthalates exposure and in vitro fertilization (IVF) outcomes. Reproductive Toxicology, 99, 56-64.
Mínguez-Alarcón, L., Bellavia, A., Gaskins, A. J., Chavarro, J. E., Ford, J. B., Souter, I., ... & EARTH Study Team. (2021). Paternal mixtures of urinary concentrations of phthalate metabolites, bisphenol A and parabens in relation to pregnancy outcomes among couples attending a fertility center. Environment international, 146, 106171.

19 Machtinger, R., Gaskins, A. J., Racowsky, C., Mansur, A., Adir, M., Baccarelli, A. A., ... & Hauser, R. (2018). Urinary concentrations of biomarkers of phthalates and phthalate alternatives and IVF outcomes. Environment international, 111, 23-31.

20 Hong YC, Park EY, Park MS, Ko JA, Oh SY, Kim H, Lee KH, Leem JH, Ha EH. Community level exposure to chemicals and oxidative stress in adult population. Toxicol. Lett. 2009;184(2):139–144;
Ferguson KK, Loch-Caruso R, Meeker JD.Urinary phthalate metabolites in relation to biomarkers of inflammation and oxidative stress: NHANES 1999-2006.Environ Res.
2011 Jul;111(5):718-26. ("Ferguson 2011").
Huang XF, Li Y, Gu YH, Liu M, Xu Y, Yuan Y, Sun F, Zhang HQ, Shi HJ. The effects of Di-(2-ethylhexyl)-phthalate exposure on fertilization and embryonic development in vitro and testicular genomic mutation in vivo. PLoS One. 2012;7(11):e50465

Duty S. M., Singh N. P., Silva M. J., Barr D. B., Brock J. W., Ryan L., Herrick R. F., Christiani D. C., Hauser R. 2003b. The relationship between environmental exposures to phthalates and DNA damage in human sperm using the neutral comet assay. Environ. Health Perspect. 111, 1164–1169. ("In conclusion, this study represents the first human data to demonstrate that urinary MEP, at environmental levels, is associated with increased DNA damage in sperm.")

21 Erkekoglu, P., Giray, B., Rachidi, W., Hininger-Favier, I., Roussel, A. M., Favier, A., & Hincal, F. (2014). Effects of di (2-ethylhexyl) phthalate on testicular oxidant/antioxidant status in selenium-deficient and selenium-supplemented rats. Environmental Toxicology, 29(1), 98-107.

22 Emojevwe, V., Nwangwa, E. K., Naiho, A. O., Oyovwi, M. O., & Ben-Azu, B. (2022). Toxicological outcome of phthalate exposure on male fertility: Ameliorative impacts of the co-administration of N-acetylcysteine and zinc sulfate in rats. Middle East Fertility Society Journal, 27(1), 1-15.
Ogli, S. A., & Odeh, S. O. (2020). Oral Ascorbic Acid And α-Tocopherol Protect On Di-(2-Ethyl Hexyl) Phthalate (DEHP) Induced Effects On Gonadotoxicity In The Adult Male Wistar Rats. European Journal of Medical and Health Sciences, 2(3).

23 Chang, W. H., Chou, W. C., Waits, A., Liao, K. W., Kuo, P. L., & Huang, P. C. (2021). Cumulative risk assessment of phthalates exposure for recurrent pregnancy loss in reproductive-aged women population using multiple hazard indices approaches. Environment international, 154, 106657.
Toft G, Jönsson BA, Lindh CH, Jensen TK, Hjollund NH, Vested A, Bonde JP. Association between pregnancy loss and urinary phthalate levels around the time of conception. Environ Health Perspect. 2012 Mar;120(3):458-63.
Mu, D., Gao, F., Fan, Z., Shen, H., Peng, H., & Hu, J. (2015). Levels of phthalate metabolites in urine of pregnant women and risk of clinical pregnancy loss. Environmental science & technology, 49(17), 10651-10657.
Messerlian, C., Wylie, B. J., Mínguez-Alarcón, L., Williams, P. L., Ford, J. B., Souter, I. C., ... & Earth Study Team. (2016). Urinary concentrations of phthalate metabolites in relation to pregnancy loss among women conceiving with medically assisted reproduction. Epidemiology (Cambridge, Mass.), 27(6), 879.

24 Adir, M., Combelles, C. M., Mansur, A., Ophir, L., Hourvitz, A., Orvieto, R., ... & Machtinger, R. (2017). Dibutyl phthalate impairs steroidogenesis and a subset of LH-dependent genes in cultured human mural granulosa cell in vitro. Reproductive toxicology, 69, 13-18.
Yi, H., Gu, H., Zhou, T., Chen, Y., Wang, G., Jin, Y., ... & Zhang, L. (2016). A pilot study on association between phthalate exposure and missed miscarriage. Eur Rev Med Pharmacol Sci, 20(9), 1894-1902.

25 Rudel RA, Gray JM, Engel CL, Rawsthorne TW, Dodson RE, Ackerman JM, Rizzo J, Nudelman JL, Brody JG. Food packaging and bisphenol A and bis(2-ethyhexyl) phthalate exposure: findings from a dietary intervention. Environ Health Perspect. 2011 Jul;119(7):914-20.

26 Buckley, J. P., Kim, H., Wong, E., & Rebholz, C. M. (2019). Ultra-processed food consumption and exposure to phthalates and bisphenols in the US National Health and Nutrition Examination Survey, 2013–2014. Environment international, 131, 105057
Zota, A. R., Phillips, C. A., & Mitro, S. D. (2016). Recent fast food consumption and bisphenol A and phthalates exposures among the US population in NHANES, 2003–2010. Environmental health perspectives, 124(10), 1521.

27 Buckley, J. P., Kim, H., Wong, E., & Rebholz, C. M. (2019). Ultra-processed food consumption and exposure to phthalates and bisphenols in the US National Health and Nutrition Examination Survey, 2013–2014. Environment international, 131, 105057
Zota, A. R., Phillips, C. A., & Mitro, S. D. (2016). Recent fast food consumption and bisphenol A and phthalates exposures among the US population in NHANES, 2003–2010. Environmental health perspectives, 124(10), 1521.
Rudel RA, Gray JM, Engel CL, Rawsthorne TW, Dodson RE, Ackerman JM, Rizzo J, Nudelman JL, Brody JG. Food packaging and bisphenol A and bis(2-ethyhexyl) phthalate exposure: findings from a dietary intervention. Environ Health Perspect. 2011 Jul;119(7):914-20.

28 Lakind JS, Naiman DQ. Daily intake of bisphenol A and potential sources of exposure: 2005-2006 National Health and Nutrition Examination Survey. J Expo Sci Environ Epidemiol. 2011 May-Jun;21(3):272-9.

29 Van Holderbeke, M., Geerts, L., Vanermen, G., Servaes, K., Sioen, I., De Henauw, S., & Fierens, T. (2014). Determination of contamination pathways of phthalates in food products sold on the Belgian market. Environmental research, 134, 345-352.

30 Bae B, Jeong JH, Lee SJ. The quantification and characterization of endocrine disruptor bisphenol-A leaching from epoxy resin. Water Sci Technol. 2002;46(11-12):381-7.

31 Tsalbouris, A., Kalogiouri, N. P., Kabir, A., Furton, K. G., & Samanidou, V. F. (2021). Bisphenol A migration to alcoholic and non-alcoholic beverages–An improved molecular imprinted solid phase extraction method prior to detection with HPLC-DAD. Microchemical Journal, 162, 105846.

32 Montuori P, Jover E, Morgantini M, Bayona JM, Triassi M. Assessing human exposure to phthalic acid and phthalate esters from mineral water stored in polyethylene terephthalate and glass bottles. Food Add Contamin. 2008;25(4):511–518;

Sax L. Polyethylene terephthalate may yield endocrine disruptors. Environ Health Perspect. 2010;118:445–8; Farhoodi M, Emam-Djomeh Z, Ehsani MR, Oromiehie A. Effect of environmental conditions on the migration of di(2-ethylhexyl)phthalate from PET bottles into yogurt drinks: influence of time, temperature, and food simulant. Arabian J Sci Eng. 2008;33(2):279–287.

33   Ehrlich, S., Calafat, A. M., Humblet, O., Smith, T., & Hauser, R. (2014). Handling of thermal receipts as a source of exposure to bisphenol A. Jama, 311(8), 859-860.

34   FDA's 2010 Survey of Cosmetics for Phthalate Content. Accessed at https://www.fda.gov/cosmetics/cosmetic-ingredients/phthalates-cosmetics

35   Al-Saleh, I., & Elkhatib, R. (2016). Screening of phthalate esters in 47 branded perfumes. Environmental Science and Pollution Research, 23, 455-468.

36   Caporossi, L., Alteri, A., Campo, G., Paci, E., Tranfo, G., Capanna, S., ... & Papaleo, B. (2020). Cross sectional study on exposure to BPA and phthalates and semen parameters in men attending a fertility center. International journal of environmental research and public health, 17(2), 489.

37   Hsieh, C. J., Chang, Y. H., Hu, A., Chen, M. L., Sun, C. W., Situmorang, R. F., ... & TMICS Study Group. (2019). Personal care products use and phthalate exposure levels among pregnant women. Science of the total environment, 648, 135-143.

38   Jurewicz, J., Radwan, M., Wielgomas, B., Karwacka, A., Klimowska, A., Kałużny, P., ... & Hanke, W. (2020). Parameters of ovarian reserve in relation to urinary concentrations of parabens. Environmental Health, 19, 1-8.

Smith, K. W., Dimitriadis, I., Ehrlich, S., Ford, J., Berry, K. F., & Souter, I. (2011). The association of urinary paraben concentrations with measures of ovarian reserve among patients from a fertility center. Fertility and Sterility, 96(3), S197.

Smith, K. W., Souter, I., Dimitriadis, I., Ehrlich, S., Williams, P. L., Calafat, A. M., & Hauser, R. (2013). Urinary paraben concentrations and ovarian aging among women from a fertility center. Environmental health perspectives, 121(11-12), 1299-1305.

39   Id.

40   Melin, V. E., Melin, T. E., Dessify, B. J., Nguyen, C. T., Shea, C. S., & Hrubec, T. C. (2016). Quaternary ammonium disinfectants cause subfertility in mice by targeting both male and female reproductive processes. Reproductive Toxicology, 59, 159-166.

41   Interview with EurActiv, 05/09/2012. http://www.euractiv.com/sustainability/us-scientist-routes-exposure-end-interview-512402

42   Bornehag, C. G., Lindh, C., Reichenberg, A., Wikström, S., Hallerback, M. U., Evans, S. F., ... & Swan, S. H. (2018). Association of prenatal

phthalate exposure with language development in early childhood. JAMA pediatrics, 172(12), 1169-1176.

Braun JM, Yolton K, Dietrich KN, Hornung R, Ye X, Calafat AM, Lanphear BP. Prenatal bisphenol A exposure and early childhood behavior. Environ Health Perspect. 2009 Dec;117(12):1945-52.

Cabaton, Nicolas J., Perinaaz R. Wadia, Beverly S. Rubin, Daniel Zalko, Cheryl M. Schaeberle, Michael H. Askenase, Jennifer L. Gadbois et al. "Perinatal exposure to environmentally relevant levels of bisphenol A decreases fertility and fecundity in CD-1 mice." Environmental health perspectives 119, no. 4 (2011): 547;

Tharp, Andrew P., Maricel V. Maffini, Patricia A. Hunt, Catherine A. VandeVoort, Carlos Sonnenschein, and Ana M. Soto. "Bisphenol A alters the development of the rhesus monkey mammary gland." *Proceedings of the National Academy of Sciences* 109, no. 21 (2012): 8190-8195; Tian, Yu-Hua, Joung-Hee Baek, Seok-Yong Lee, and Choon-Gon Jang. "Prenatal and postnatal exposure to bisphenol a induces anxiolytic behaviors and cognitive deficits in mice." *Synapse* 64, no. 6 (2010): 432-439;

Jang, Young Jung, Hee Ra Park, Tae Hyung Kim, Wook-Jin Yang, Jong-Joo Lee, Seon Young Choi, Shin Bi Oh et al. "High dose bisphenol A impairs hippocampal neurogenesis in female mice across generations." *Toxicology* (2012). Somm, Emmanuel, Valérie M. Schwitzgebel, Audrey Toulotte, Christopher R. Cederroth, Christophe Combescure, Serge Nef, Michel L. Aubert, and Petra S. Hüppi. "Perinatal exposure to bisphenol a alters early adipogenesis in the rat." *Environmental Health Perspectives* 117, no. 10 (2009): 1549.

Braun, Joe M., Amy E. Kalkbrenner, Antonia M. Calafat, Kimberly Yolton, Xiaoyun Ye, Kim N. Dietrich, and Bruce P. Lanphear. "Impact of early-life bisphenol A exposure on behavior and executive function in children." *Pediatrics* 128, no. 5 (2011): 873-882.

43 Latini G, et al. In utero exposure to di-(2-ethylhexyl)phthalate and duration of human pregnancy. Environmental Health Perspectives. 2003;111:1783–1785.

Meeker JD, Hu H, Cantonwine DE, Lamadrid-Figueroa H, Calafat AM, Ettinger AS, Hernandez-Avila M, Loch-Caruso R, Téllez-Rojo MM. Urinary phthalate metabolites in relation to preterm birth in Mexico city. Environ. Health Perspect. 2009;117(10):1587–1592.

Whyatt RM, Adibi JJ, Calafat AM, Camann DE, Rauh V, Bhat HK, Perera FP, Andrews H, Just AC, Hoepner L, Tang D, Hauser R. Prenatal di(2-ethylhexyl) phthalate exposure and length of gestation among an inner-city cohort. Pediatrics. 2009;124(6):e1213–e1220.

Swan SH, Main KM, Liu F, Stewart SL, Kruse RL, Calafat AM, Mao CS, Redmon JB, Ternand CL, Sullivan S, Teague JL; Study for Future Families Research Team. Decrease in anogenital distance among male infants with prenatal phthalateexposure. Environ Health Perspect.

2005 Aug;113(8):1056-61. Erratum in: Environ Health Perspect. 2005 Sep;113(9):A583. ("Swan 2005").

Swan SH. Environmental phthalate exposure in relation to reproductive outcomes and other health endpoints in humans. Environ Res. 2008 Oct; 108(2):177-84

Chapter 3: Unexpected Obstacles to Fertility

1   Stabler, S.P. Vitamin B12 deficiency. N. Engl. J. Med. 2013, 368, 2041–2042.

Klee, G.G. Cobalamin and folate evaluation: Measurement of methylmalonic acid and homocysteine vs. vitamin B and folate. Clin. Chem. 2000, 46, 1277–1283.

Scarpa, E.; Candiotto, L.; Sartori, R.; Radossi, P.; Maschio, N.; Tagariello, G. Undetected vitamin B12 deficiency due to false normal assay results. Blood Transfus. Trasfus. Sangue 2013, 11, 627–629.

Olson, S.R.; Deloughery, T.G.; Taylor, J.A. Time to abandon the serum cobalamin level for diagnosing vitamin B12 deficiency. Blood 2016, 128, 2447

2   Gaskins, A. J., Chiu, Y. H., Williams, P. L., Ford, J. B., Toth, T. L., Hauser, R., ... & EARTH Study Team. (2015). Association between serum folate and vitamin B-12 and outcomes of assisted reproductive technologies. The American journal of clinical nutrition, 102(4), 943-950.

3   Cirillo, M., Fucci, R., Rubini, S., Coccia, M. E., & Fatini, C. (2021). 5-methyltetrahydrofolate and vitamin B12 supplementation is associated with clinical pregnancy and live birth in women undergoing assisted reproductive technology. International Journal of Environmental Research and Public Health, 18(23), 12280.

4   Bala, R., Verma, R., Verma, P., Singh, V., Yadav, N., Rajender, S., ... & Singh, K. (2021). Hyperhomocysteinemia and low vitamin B12 are associated with the risk of early pregnancy loss: A clinical study and meta-analyses. Nutrition Research, 91, 57-66.

Cavallé-Busquets, P., Inglès-Puig, M., Fernandez-Ballart, J. D., Haro-Barceló, J., Rojas-Gómez, A., Ramos-Rodriguez, C., ... & Murphy, M. M. (2020). Moderately elevated first trimester fasting plasma total homocysteine is associated with increased probability of miscarriage. The Reus-Tarragona Birth Cohort Study. Biochimie, 173, 62-67.

Mishra, J., Tomar, A., Puri, M., Jain, A., & Saraswathy, K. N. (2020). Trends of folate, vitamin B12, and homocysteine levels in different trimesters of pregnancy and pregnancy outcomes. American Journal of Human Biology, 32(5), e23388.

5   Zittan, E., Preis, M., Asmir, I., Cassel, A., Lindenfeld, N., Alroy, S., ... & Flugelman, M. Y. (2007). High frequency of vitamin B12 deficiency in asymptomatic individuals homozygous to MTHFR C677T mutation is associated with endothelial dysfunction and homocysteinemia. American Journal of Physiology-Heart and Circulatory Physiology, 293(1), H860-H865.

6   Schijns, W., Homan, J., van der Meer, L., Janssen, I. M., van Laarhoven,
    C. J., Berends, F. J., & Aarts, E. O. (2018). Efficacy of oral compared with
    intramuscular vitamin B-12 supplementation after Roux-en-Y gastric
    bypass: a randomized controlled trial. The American Journal of Clinical
    Nutrition, 108(1), 6-12.

    Yazaki, Y., Chow, G., & Mattie, M. (2006). A single-center, double-
    blinded, randomized controlled study to evaluate the relative efficacy of
    sublingual and oral vitamin B-complex administration in reducing total
    serum homocysteine levels. Journal of Alternative & Complementary
    Medicine, 12(9), 881-885.

    Strong, A. P., Haeusler, S., Weatherall, M., & Krebs, J. (2016). Sublingual
    vitamin B12 compared to intramuscular injection in patients with type
    2 diabetes treated with metformin: a randomised trial. The New Zealand
    Medical Journal (Online), 129(1436), 67.

    Bensky, M. J., Ayalon-Dangur, I., Ayalon-Dangur, R., Naamany, E.,
    Gafter-Gvili, A., Koren, G., & Shiber, S. (2019). Comparison of sublingual
    vs. intramuscular administration of vitamin B12 for the treatment of
    patients with vitamin B12 deficiency. Drug delivery and translational
    research, 9, 625-630.

    Wang, H., Li, L., Qin, L. L., Song, Y., Vidal-Aaball, J., & Liu, T. H.
    (2018). Oral vitamin B 12 versus intramuscular vitamin B 12 for vitamin
    B 12 deficiency. Cochrane Database of Systematic Reviews, (3).

    Butler, C. C., Vidal-Aaball, J., Cannings-John, R., McCaddon, A., Hood,
    K., Papaioannou, A., … & Goringe, A. (2006). Oral vitamin B12 versus
    intramuscular vitamin B12 for vitamin B12 deficiency: a systematic
    review of randomized controlled trials. Family practice, 23(3), 279-285.

    Sharabi, A., Cohen, E., Sulkes, J., & Garty, M. (2003). Replacement
    therapy for vitamin B12 deficiency: comparison between the sublingual
    and oral route. British journal of clinical pharmacology, 56(6), 635-638.

7   Schijns, W., Homan, J., van der Meer, L., Janssen, I. M., van Laarhoven,
    C. J., Berends, F. J., & Aarts, E. O. (2018). Efficacy of oral compared with
    intramuscular vitamin B-12 supplementation after Roux-en-Y gastric
    bypass: a randomized controlled trial. The American Journal of Clinical
    Nutrition, 108(1), 6-12.

    Yazaki, Y., Chow, G., & Mattie, M. (2006). A single-center, double-
    blinded, randomized controlled study to evaluate the relative efficacy of
    sublingual and oral vitamin B-complex administration in reducing total
    serum homocysteine levels. Journal of Alternative & Complementary
    Medicine, 12(9), 881-885.

    Strong, A. P., Haeusler, S., Weatherall, M., & Krebs, J. (2016). Sublingual
    vitamin B12 compared to intramuscular injection in patients with type
    2 diabetes treated with metformin: a randomised trial. The New Zealand
    Medical Journal (Online), 129(1436), 67.

Bensky, M. J., Ayalon-Dangur, I., Ayalon-Dangur, R., Naamany, E., Gafter-Gvili, A., Koren, G., & Shiber, S. (2019). Comparison of sublingual vs. intramuscular administration of vitamin B12 for the treatment of patients with vitamin B12 deficiency. Drug delivery and translational research, 9, 625-630.

Wang, H., Li, L., Qin, L. L., Song, Y., Vidal-Alaball, J., & Liu, T. H. (2018). Oral vitamin B 12 versus intramuscular vitamin B 12 for vitamin B 12 deficiency. Cochrane Database of Systematic Reviews, (3).

Butler, C. C., Vidal-Alaball, J., Cannings-John, R., McCaddon, A., Hood, K., Papaioannou, A., ... & Goringe, A. (2006). Oral vitamin B12 versus intramuscular vitamin B12 for vitamin B12 deficiency: a systematic review of randomized controlled trials. Family practice, 23(3), 279-285.

Sharabi, A., Cohen, E., Sulkes, J., & Garty, M. (2003). Replacement therapy for vitamin B12 deficiency: comparison between the sublingual and oral route. British journal of clinical pharmacology, 56(6), 635-638.

8 Paul, C., & Brady, D. M. (2017). Comparative bioavailability and utilization of particular forms of B12 supplements with potential to mitigate B12-related genetic polymorphisms. Integrative Medicine: A Clinician's Journal, 16(1), 42.

9 Id.

10 Eussen, S. J., de Groot, L. C., Clarke, R., Schneede, J., Ueland, P. M., Hoefnagels, W. H., & van Staveren, W. A. (2005). Oral cyanocobalamin supplementation in older people with vitamin B12 deficiency: a dose-finding trial. Archives of internal medicine, 165(10), 1167-1172.

11 Wang, H., Li, L., Qin, L. L., Song, Y., Vidal-Alaball, J., & Liu, T. H. (2018). Oral vitamin B 12 versus intramuscular vitamin B 12 for vitamin B 12 deficiency. Cochrane Database of Systematic Reviews, (3).

Oh, R. C., & Brown, D. L. (2003). Vitamin B12 deficiency. American family physician, 67(5), 979-986.

Lane, L. A., & Rojas-Fernandez, C. (2002). Treatment of vitamin B12–deficiency anemia: oral versus parenteral therapy. Annals of Pharmacotherapy, 36(7-8), 1268-1272.

12 Schijns, W., Homan, J., van der Meer, L., Janssen, I. M., van Laarhoven, C. J., Berends, F. J., & Aarts, E. O. (2018). Efficacy of oral compared with intramuscular vitamin B-12 supplementation after Roux-en-Y gastric bypass: a randomized controlled trial. The American Journal of Clinical Nutrition, 108(1), 6-12.

13 Sourander, A., Silwal, S., Surcel, H. M., Hinkka-Yli-Salomäki, S., Upadhyaya, S., McKeague, I. W., ... & Brown, A. S. (2023). Maternal Serum Vitamin B12 during Pregnancy and Offspring Autism Spectrum Disorder. Nutrients, 15(8), 2009.

14 Garland, C. F., Gorham, E. D., Mohr, S. B., Grant, W. B., Giovannucci, E. L., Lipkin, M., ... & Garland, F. C. (2007). Vitamin D and prevention of

breast cancer: pooled analysis. The Journal of steroid biochemistry and molecular biology, 103(3-5), 708-711.

Murdaca, G., Tonacci, A., Negrini, S., Greco, M., Borro, M., Puppo, F., & Gangemi, S. (2019). Emerging role of vitamin D in autoimmune diseases: An update on evidence and therapeutic implications. Autoimmunity reviews, 18(9), 102350.

15 Argano, C., Mallaci Bocchio, R., Natoli, G., Scibetta, S., Lo Monaco, M., & Corrao, S. (2023). Protective Effect of Vitamin D Supplementation on COVID-19-Related Intensive Care Hospitalization and Mortality: Definitive Evidence from Meta-Analysis and Trial Sequential Analysis. Pharmaceuticals, 16(1), 130.

Durmuş, M. E., Kara, Ö., Kara, M., Kaya, T. C., Şener, F. E., Durmuş, M., ... & Özçakar, L. (2023). The relationship between vitamin D deficiency and mortality in older adults before and during COVID-19 pandemic. Heart & Lung, 57, 117-123.

Petrelli, F., Oldani, S., Borgonovo, K., Cabiddu, M., Dognini, G., Ghilardi, M., ... & Ghidini, A. (2023). Vitamin D3 and COVID-19 outcomes: an umbrella review of systematic reviews and meta-analyses. Antioxidants, 12(2), 247.

16 Iliuta, F., Pijoan, J. I., Lainz, L., Exposito, A., & Matorras, R. (2022). Women's vitamin D levels and IVF results: a systematic review of the literature and meta-analysis, considering three categories of vitamin status (replete, insufficient and deficient). Human Fertility, 25(2), 228-246.

Aleyasin A, Hosseini MA, Mahdavi A, Safdarian L, Fallahi P, Mohajeri MR, Abbasi M, Esfahani F.Predictive value of the level of vitamin D in follicular fluid on the outcome of assisted reproductive technology.Eur J Obstet Gynecol Reprod Biol. 2011 Nov;159(1):132-7.

Anifandis GM, Dafopoulos K, Messini CI, Chalvatzas N, Liakos N, Pournaras S, Messinis IE. Prognostic value of follicular fluid 25-OH vitamin D and glucose levels in the IVF outcome. Reprod Biol Endocrinol. 2010 Jul 28;8:91.

Aleyasin A, Hosseini MA, Mahdavi A, Safdarian L, Fallahi P, Mohajeri MR, Abbasi M, Esfahani F.Predictive value of the level of vitamin D in follicular fluid on the outcome of assisted reproductive technology.Eur J Obstet Gynecol Reprod Biol. 2011 Nov;159(1):132-7.

Anifandis GM, Dafopoulos K, Messini CI, Chalvatzas N, Liakos N, Pournaras S, Messinis IE. Prognostic value of follicular fluid 25-OH vitamin D and glucose levels in the IVF outcome. Reprod Biol Endocrinol. 2010 Jul 28;8:91.

17 Rudick B, Ingles S, Chung K, Stanczyk F, Paulson R, Bendikson K. Characterizing the influence of vitamin D levels on IVF outcomes. Hum Reprod. 2012 Nov;27(11):3321-7. ("Rudick 2012").

18 Ozkan S, Jindal S, Greenseid K, Shu J, Zeitlian G, Hickmon C, Pal L. Replete vitamin D stores predict reproductive success following in vitro fertilization. Fertil Steril. 2010 Sep;94(4):1314-9.

19 Firouzabadi RD, Rahmani E, Rahsepar M, Firouzabadi MM. Value of follicular fluid vitamin D in predicting the pregnancy rate in an IVF program. Arch Gynecol Obstet. 2014 Jan;289(1):201-6

20 Meng, X., Zhang, J., Wan, Q., Huang, J., Han, T., Qu, T., & Yu, L. L. (2023). Influence of Vitamin D supplementation on reproductive outcomes of infertile patients: a systematic review and meta-analysis. Reproductive Biology and Endocrinology, 21(1), 17.

Walz, N. L., Hinchliffe, P. M., Soares, M. J., Dhaliwal, S. S., Newsholme, P., Yovich, J. L., & Keane, K. N. (2020). Serum Vitamin D status is associated with increased blastocyst development rate in women undergoing IVF. Reproductive BioMedicine Online, 41(6), 1101-1111.

Doryanizadeh, L., Morshed-Behbahani, B., Parsanezhad, M. E., Dabbaghmanesh, M. H., & Jokar, A. (2021). Calcitriol effect on outcomes of in vitro fertilization in infertile women with vitamin D deficiency: a double-blind randomized clinical trial. Zeitschrift für Geburtshilfe und Neonatologie, 225(03), 226-231.

Abedi, S., Taebi, M., & Esfahani, M. H. N. (2019). Effect of vitamin D supplementation on intracytoplasmic sperm injection outcomes: a randomized double-blind placebo-controlled trial. International Journal of Fertility & Sterility, 13(1), 18.

Hasan, H. A., Barber, T. M., Cheaib, S., & Coussa, A. (2023). Preconception vitamin D level and In Vitro Fertilization-pregnancy outcome. Endocrine Practice.

Rudick B, Ingles S, Chung K, Stanczyk F, Paulson R, Bendikson K. Characterizing the influence of vitamin D levels on IVF outcomes. Hum Reprod. 2012 Nov;27(11):3321-7. ("Rudick 2012").

Ozkan S, Jindal S, Greenseid K, Shu J, Zeitlian G, Hickmon C, Pal L. Replete vitamin D stores predict reproductive success following in vitro fertilization. Fertil Steril. 2010 Sep;94(4):1314-9

Firouzabadi RD, Rahmani E, Rahsepar M, Firouzabadi MM. Value of follicular fluid vitamin D in predicting the pregnancy rate in an IVF program. Arch Gynecol Obstet. 2014 Jan;289(1):201-6

21 Ruddick 2012). Rudick B, Ingles S, Chung K, Stanczyk F, Paulson R, Bendikson K. Characterizing the influence of vitamin D levels on IVF outcomes. Hum Reprod. 2012 Nov;27(11):3321-7.

22 Luk J, Torrealday S, Neal Perry G, Pal L. Relevance of vitamin D in reproduction. Hum Reprod. 2012 Oct;27(10):3015-27 ("Luk 2012").

23 Aramesh, S., Alifarja, T., Jannesar, R., Ghaffari, P., Vanda, R., & Bazarganipour, F. (2021). Does vitamin D supplementation improve ovarian reserve in women with diminished ovarian reserve and vitamin

D deficiency: a before-and-after intervention study. BMC Endocrine Disorders, 21(1), 1-5.

Bacanakgil, B. H., İlhan, G., & Ohanoğlu, K. (2022). Effects of vitamin D supplementation on ovarian reserve markers in infertile women with diminished ovarian reserve. Medicine, 101(6).

24 Masbou, A. K., Kramer, Y., Taveras, D., McCulloh, D. H., & Grifo, J. A. (2018). Vitamin D deficiency at time of frozen embryo transfer is associated with increased miscarriage rate but does not impact folliculogenesis. Fertility and Sterility, 109(3), e37-e38.

Mumford, S. L., Garbose, R. A., Kim, K., Kissell, K., Kuhr, D. L., Omosigho, U. R., ... & Plowden, T. C. (2018). Association of preconception serum 25-hydroxyvitamin D concentrations with livebirth and pregnancy loss: a prospective cohort study. The Lancet Diabetes & Endocrinology.

25 Masbou, A. K., Kramer, Y., Taveras, D., McCulloh, D. H., & Grifo, J. A. (2018). Vitamin D deficiency at time of frozen embryo transfer is associated with increased miscarriage rate but does not impact folliculogenesis. Fertility and Sterility, 109(3), e37-e38.

26 Ota, K., Dambaeva, S., Han, A. R., Beaman, K., Gilman-Sachs, A., & Kwak-Kim, J. (2013). Vitamin D deficiency may be a risk factor for recurrent pregnancy losses by increasing cellular immunity and autoimmunity. Human reproduction, 29(2), 208-219.

Chen, X., Yin, B., Lian, R. C., Zhang, T., Zhang, H. Z., Diao, L. H., ... & Zeng, Y. (2016). Modulatory effects of vitamin D on peripheral cellular immunity in patients with recurrent miscarriage. American Journal of Reproductive Immunology, 76(6), 432-438.

27 Hollis, B. W., & Wagner, C. L. (2022). Substantial vitamin D supplementation is required during the prenatal period to improve birth outcomes. Nutrients, 14(4), 899.

28 Wagner, C. L., Baggerly, C., McDonnell, S. L., Baggerly, L., Hamilton, S. A., Winkler, J., ... & Hollis, B. W. (2015). Post-hoc comparison of vitamin D status at three timepoints during pregnancy demonstrates lower risk of preterm birth with higher vitamin D closer to delivery. The Journal of steroid biochemistry and molecular biology, 148, 256-260.

Tamblyn, J. A., Pilarski, N. S., Markland, A. D., Marson, E. J., Devall, A., Hewison, M., ... & Coomarasamy, A. (2022). Vitamin D and miscarriage: a systematic review and meta-analysis. Fertility and sterility.

Hollis, B. W., & Wagner, C. L. (2017). New insights into the vitamin D requirements during pregnancy. Bone research, 5, 17030.

29 Hollis, B. W., & Wagner, C. L. (2011). Vitamin D requirements and supplementation during pregnancy. Current opinion in endocrinology, diabetes, and obesity, 18(6), 371.

30 Hollis, B. W., Johnson, D., Hulsey, T. C., Ebeling, M., & Wagner, C. L. (2011). Vitamin D supplementation during pregnancy: Double-blind,

randomized clinical trial of safety and effectiveness. Journal of bone and mineral research, 26(10), 2341-2357.

31 Grossmann RE, Tangpricha V. Evaluation of vehicle substances on vitamin D bioavailability: a systematic review. Mol Nutr Food Res. 2010 Aug;54(8):1055-61;
Raimundo FV, Faulhaber GA, Menegatti PK, Marques Lda S, Furlanetto TW. Effect of High- versus Low-Fat Meal on Serum 25-Hydroxyvitamin D Levels after a Single Oral Dose of Vitamin D: A Single-Blind, Parallel, Randomized Trial. Int J Endocrinol. 2011;2011:809069.

32 Rao, M., Zeng, Z., Zhou, F., Wang, H., Liu, J., Wang, R., ... & Tang, L. (2019). Effect of levothyroxine supplementation on pregnancy loss and preterm birth in women with subclinical hypothyroidism and thyroid autoimmunity: a systematic review and meta-analysis. Human Reproduction Update, 25(3), 344-361.
Yoshioka, W., Amino, N., Ide, A., Kang, S., Kudo, T., Nishihara, E., ... & Miyauchi, A. (2015). Thyroxine treatment may be useful for subclinical hypothyroidism in patients with female infertility. Endocrine journal, 62(1), 87-92.
Alexander Erik, K., Pearce Elizabeth, N., Brent Gregory, A., Brown Rosalind, S., Grobman William, A., Lazarus John, H., ... & Peeters Robin, P. (2017). 2017 Guidelines of the American Thyroid Association for the diagnosis and management of thyroid disease during pregnancy and the postpartum. Thyroid.
Maraka, S., Mwangi, R., McCoy, R. G., Yao, X., Sangaralingham, L. R., Ospina, N. M. S., ... & Montori, V. M. (2017). Thyroid hormone treatment among pregnant women with subclinical hypothyroidism: US national assessment. Bmj, 356

33 Abalovich, M., Alcaraz, G., Kleiman-Rubinsztein, J., Pavlove, M. M., Cornelio, C., Levalle, O., & Gutierrez, S. (2010). The relationship of preconception thyrotropin levels to requirements for increasing the levothyroxine dose during pregnancy in women with primary hypothyroidism. Thyroid, 20(10), 1175-1178.
Alexander Erik, K., Pearce Elizabeth, N., Brent Gregory, A., Brown Rosalind, S., Grobman William, A., Lazarus John, H., ... & Peeters Robin, P. (2017). 2017 Guidelines of the American Thyroid Association for the diagnosis and management of thyroid disease during pregnancy and the postpartum. Thyroid.

34 Rao, M., Zeng, Z., Zhou, F., Wang, H., Liu, J., Wang, R., ... & Tang, L. (2019). Effect of levothyroxine supplementation on pregnancy loss and preterm birth in women with subclinical hypothyroidism and thyroid autoimmunity: a systematic review and meta-analysis. Human Reproduction Update, 25(3), 344-361.
Yoshioka, W., Amino, N., Ide, A., Kang, S., Kudo, T., Nishihara, E., ... & Miyauchi, A. (2015). Thyroxine treatment may be useful for subclinical

hypothyroidism in patients with female infertility. Endocrine journal, 62(1), 87-92.

35 Leng, T., Li, X., & Zhang, H. (2022). Levothyroxine treatment for subclinical hypothyroidism improves the rate of live births in pregnant women with recurrent pregnancy loss: a randomized clinical trial. Gynecological Endocrinology, 38(6), 488-494.

Rao, M., Zeng, Z., Zhou, F., Wang, H., Liu, J., Wang, R., ... & Tang, L. (2019). Effect of levothyroxine supplementation on pregnancy loss and preterm birth in women with subclinical hypothyroidism and thyroid autoimmunity: a systematic review and meta-analysis. Human Reproduction Update, 25(3), 344-361.

Stagnaro-Green A. Thyroid antibodies and miscarriage: where are we at a generation later? J Thyroid Res. 2011; 2011:841949.

Toulis KA, Goulis DG, Venetis CA, Kolibianakis EM, Negro R, Tarlatzis BC, Papadimas I. Risk of spontaneous miscarriage in euthyroid women with thyroid autoimmunity undergoing IVF: a meta-analysis. Eur J Endocrinol. 2010 Apr;162(4):643-52; Prummel MF, Wiersinga WM. Thyroid autoimmunity and miscarriage. Eur J Endocrinol. 2004 Jun;150(6):751-5; Negro R, Schwartz A, Gismondi R, Tinelli A, Mangieri T, Stagnaro-Green A. Increased pregnancy loss rate in thyroid antibody negative women with TSH levels between 2.5 and 5.0 in the first trimester of pregnancy. J Clin Endocrinol Metab. 2010 Sep;95(9):E44-8. ("Negro 2010").

36 Yoshioka, W., Amino, N., Ide, A., Kang, S., Kudo, T., Nishihara, E., ... & Miyauchi, A. (2015). Thyroxine treatment may be useful for subclinical hypothyroidism in patients with female infertility. Endocrine journal, 62(1), 87-92.

37 Kim, C. H., Ahn, J. W., Kang, S. P., Kim, S. H., Chae, H. D., & Kang, B. M. (2011). Effect of levothyroxine treatment on in vitro fertilization and pregnancy outcome in infertile women with subclinical hypothyroidism undergoing in vitro fertilization/intracytoplasmic sperm injection. Fertility and sterility, 95(5), 1650-1654.

Maraka, S., Mwangi, R., McCoy, R. G., Yao, X., Sangaralingham, L. R., Ospina, N. M. S., ... & Montori, V. M. (2017). Thyroid hormone treatment among pregnant women with subclinical hypothyroidism: US national assessment. Bmj, 356

38 Bliddal, S., Feldt-Rasmussen, U., Rasmussen, Å. K., Kolte, A. M., Hilsted, L. M., Christiansen, O. B., ... & Nielsen, H. S. (2019). Thyroid peroxidase antibodies and prospective live birth rate: a cohort study of women with recurrent pregnancy loss. Thyroid, 29(10), 1465-1474.

39 Negro R, Formoso G, Mangieri T, Pezzarossa A, Dazzi D, Hassan H. Levothyroxine treatment in euthyroid pregnant women with autoimmune thyroid disease: effects on obstetrical complications. J Clin Endocrinol Metab. 2006 Jul;91(7):2587-91.

Bliddal, S., Feldt-Rasmussen, U., Rasmussen, Å. K., Kolte, A. M., Hilsted, L. M., Christiansen, O. B., ... & Nielsen, H. S. (2019). Thyroid peroxidase antibodies and prospective live birth rate: a cohort study of women with recurrent pregnancy loss. Thyroid, 29(10), 1465-1474

40 van Dijk, M. M., Vissenberg, R., Fliers, E., van der Post, J. A., Van der Hoorn, M. L. P., de Weerd, S., ... & Goddijn, M. (2022). Levothyroxine in euthyroid thyroid peroxidase antibody positive women with recurrent pregnancy loss (T4LIFE trial): a multicentre, randomised, double-blind, placebo-controlled, phase 3 trial. The lancet Diabetes & endocrinology, 10(5), 322-329.

Dhillon-Smith, R. K., Middleton, L. J., Sunner, K. K., Cheed, V., Baker, K., Farrell-Carver, S., ... & Coomarasamy, A. (2019). Levothyroxine in women with thyroid peroxidase antibodies before conception. New England Journal of Medicine, 380(14), 1316-1325.

Wang, H., Gao, H., Chi, H., Zeng, L., Xiao, W., Wang, Y., ... & Qiao, J. (2017). Effect of levothyroxine on miscarriage among women with normal thyroid function and thyroid autoimmunity undergoing in vitro fertilization and embryo transfer: a randomized clinical trial. Jama, 318(22), 2190-2198

41 Anagnostis, P., Lefkou, E., & Goulis, D. G. (2017). Re:"Guidelines of the American Thyroid Association for the diagnosis and management of thyroid disease during pregnancy and the postpartum" by Alexander et al.(Thyroid 2017; 27: 315–389). Thyroid, 27(9), 1209-1210.

42 Ott, J., Pecnik, P., Promberger, R., Pils, S., Seemann, R., Hermann, M., & Frigo, P. (2014). Dehydroepiandrosterone in women with premature ovarian failure and Hashimoto's thyroiditis. Climacteric, 17(1), 92-96.

43 Krysiak, R., Szkróbka, W., & Okopień, B. (2021). Impact of dehydroepiandrosterone on thyroid autoimmunity and function in men with autoimmune hypothyroidism. International Journal of Clinical Pharmacy, 43, 998-1005.

Ott, J., Pecnik, P., Promberger, R., Pils, S., Seemann, R., Hermann, M., & Frigo, P. (2014). Dehydroepiandrosterone in women with premature ovarian failure and Hashimoto's thyroiditis. Climacteric, 17(1), 92-96.

Chapter 4: Hormone Lab Tests

1   Harris, BS, Jukic, AM, Truong, T., Nagle, CT, Erkanli, A., & Steiner, AZ (2023). Markers of ovarian reserve as predictors of future fertility. Fertility and Sterility , 119 (1), 99-106.

2   Moridi, I., Chen, A., Tal, O., & Tal, R. (2020). The association between vitamin D and anti-müllerian hormone: A systematic review and meta-analysis. Nutrients, 12(6), 1567.

Yilmaz, N., Uygur, D., Inal, H., Gorkem, U., Cicek, N., & Mollamahmutoglu, L. (2013). Dehydroepiandrosterone supplementation improves predictive markers for diminished ovarian reserve: serum

AMH, inhibin B and antral follicle count. European Journal of Obstetrics & Gynecology and Reproductive Biology, 169(2), 257-260.

3   Ozay, A. C., Emekci Ozay, O., Okyay, R. E., Cagliyan, E., Kume, T., & Gulekli, B. (2016). Different effects of myoinositol plus folic acid versus combined oral treatment on androgen levels in PCOS women. International Journal of Endocrinology, 2016.

4   Abdalla, H., & Thum, M. Y. (2004). An elevated basal FSH reflects a quantitative rather than qualitative decline of the ovarian reserve. Human Reproduction, 19(4), 893-898.

5   Wang, S., Zhang, Y., Mensah, V., Huber, W. J., Huang, Y. T., & Alvero, R. (2018). Discordant anti-müllerian hormone (AMH) and follicle stimulating hormone (FSH) among women undergoing in vitro fertilization (IVF): which one is the better predictor for live birth?. Journal of ovarian research, 11(1), 1-8.

6   Hurjahan-Banu, S. M. M., Nazma-Akhtar, T. S., & Afroza-Begum, M. Z. (2021). Total testosterone significantly correlates with insulin resistance in polycystic ovary syndrome. Gynecol Reprod Endocrinol Metab, 2(2), 106-11.

7   Gleicher, N., Kushnir, V. A., Darmon, S. K., Wang, Q., Zhang, L., Albertini, D. F., & Barad, D. H. (2017). New PCOS-like phenotype in older infertile women of likely autoimmune adrenal etiology with high AMH but low androgens. The Journal of Steroid Biochemistry and Molecular Biology, 167, 144-152.

8   Nayar, K. D., Gupta, S., Bhattacharya, R., Mehra, P., Mishra, J., Kant, G., & Nayar, K. (2021). P–612 Transdermal testosterone vs. Placebo (lubricant gel) pre-treatment in improving IVF outcomes in diminished ovarian reserve patients (POSEIDON group 3 and 4): a randomised controlled trial. Human Reproduction, 36(Supplement_1), deab130-611. Katsika, E. T., Bosdou, J. K., Goulis, D. G., Grimbizis, G. F., & Kolibianakis, E. M. (2022). Higher probability of live birth after transdermal testosterone pretreatment in women with poor ovarian response undergoing IVF: a systematic review and meta-analysis: Primary Outcome. Reproductive BioMedicine Online.

9   Xu, S., Liu, Y., Xue, K., Liu, X., Jia, G., Zeng, Y., & Chen, Y. (2022). Diagnostic value of total testosterone and free androgen index measured by LC–MS/MS for PCOS and insulin resistance. Journal of Clinical Laboratory Analysis, 36(11), e24739.

10   Chimote, B. N., & Chimote, N. M. (2021). Dehydroepiandrosterone sulphate (DHEAS) concentrations stringently regulate fertilisation, embryo development and IVF outcomes: are we looking at a potentially compelling 'oocyte-related factor'in oocyte activation?. Journal of Assisted Reproduction and Genetics, 38(1), 193-202.

11   Jordan, J., Craig, K., Clifton, D. K., & Soules, M. R. (1994). Luteal phase defect: the sensitivity and specificity of diagnostic methods in common clinical use. Fertility and sterility, 62(1), 54-62.

12 Beardsley, R. D., & Holden, J. P. (2017). A novel definition of insulin resistance helps elucidate luteal phase defects. Fertility and Sterility, 108(3), e250.

13 Mumford, S. L., Browne, R. W., Schliep, K. C., Schmelzer, J., Plowden, T. C., Michels, K. A., ... & Schisterman, E. F. (2016). Serum antioxidants are associated with serum reproductive hormones and ovulation among healthy women. The Journal of nutrition, 146(1), 98-106.
Taketani, T., Tamura, H., Takasaki, A., Lee, L., Kizuka, F., Tamura, I., ... & Sugino, N. (2011). Protective role of melatonin in progesterone production by human luteal cells. Journal of pineal research, 51(2), 207-213.

14 Coomarasamy, A., Williams, H., Truchanowicz, E., Seed, P. T., Small, R., Quenby, S., ... & Rai, R. (2016). PROMISE: first-trimester progesterone therapy in women with a history of unexplained recurrent miscarriages-a randomised, double-blind, placebo-controlled, international multicentre trial and economic evaluation. Health technology assessment (Winchester, England), 20(41), 1.

15 Coomarasamy, A., Harb, H. M., Devall, A. J., Cheed, V., Roberts, T. E., Goranitis, I., ... & Middleton, L. J. (2020). Progesterone to prevent miscarriage in women with early pregnancy bleeding: the PRISM RCT. Health Technology Assessment (Winchester, England), 24(33), 1.

Chapter 5: What to Look

1 CDC, ten great public health achievements- United States, 2001-2010. Morb Mortal Wkly Rep 2011: 60-619-23.

2 Prevention of neural tube defects: results of the Medical Research Council Vitamin Study MRC Vitamin Study Research Group. Lancet. 1991 Jul 20;338(8760):131-7.

3 Smithells RW, Sheppard S, Schorah CJ, Seller MJ, Nevin NC, Harris R, Read AP, Fielding DW.Apparent prevention of neural tube defects by periconceptional vitamin supplementation. 1981.Int J Epidemiol. 2011 Oct;40(5):1146-54.

4 Schorah C. Commentary: from controversy and procrastination to primary prevention. Int J Epidemiol. 2011 Oct;40(5):1156-8. ("Schorah 2011").

5 Schorah 2011.

6 Czeizel AE, Dudás I. Prevention of the first occurrence of neural-tube defects by periconceptional vitamin supplementation. N Engl J Med. 1992 Dec 24;327(26):1832-5;
de Bree A, van Dusseldorp M, Brouwer IA, van het Hof KH, Steegers-Theunissen RP. Folate intake in Europe: recommended, actual and desired intake. Eur J Clin Nutr. 1997 Oct;51(10):643-60.

7 http://www.cdc.gov/ncbddd/folicacid/recommendations.html
http://www.nhs.uk/Conditions/vitamins-minerals/Pages/Vitamin-B.aspx

8   Ebisch IM, Thomas CM, Peters WH, Braat DD, Steegers-Theunissen
     RP. The importance of folate, zinc and antioxidants in the
     pathogenesis and prevention of subfertility. Hum Reprod Update. 2007
     Mar-Apr;13(2):163-74 ("Ebisch 2007").

9   Chavarro JE, Rich-Edwards JW, Rosner BA, Willett WC. Use of
     multivitamins, intake of B vitamins, and risk of ovulatory infertility.
     Fertil Steril. 2008 Mar;89(3):668-76.

10   Westphal LM, Polan ML, Trant AS, Mooney SB. A nutritional
     supplement for improving fertility in women: a pilot study. J Reprod
     Med. 2004 Apr;49(4):289-93.
     Czeizel AE, Métneki J, Dudás I. The effect of preconceptional
     multivitamin supplementation on fertility. Int J Vitam Nutr Res.
     1996;66(1):55-8.

11   Gaskins AJ, Mumford SL, Chavarro JE, Zhang C, Pollack AZ,
     Wactawski-Wende J, Perkins NJ, Schisterman EF. The impact of dietary
     folate intake on reproductive function in premenopausal women: a
     prospective cohort study. PLoS One. 2012;7(9):e46276. ("Gaskins 2012").

12   Boxmeer JC, Brouns RM, Lindemans J, Steegers EA, Martini E, Macklon
     NS, Steegers-Theunissen RP. Preconception folic acid treatment affects
     the microenvironment of the maturing oocyte in humans. Fertil Steril.
     2008 Jun;89(6):1766-70. ("Boxmeer 2008").

13   Enciso M, Sarasa J, Xanthopoulou L, Bristow S, Bowles M, Fragouli
     E, Delhanty J, Wells D. Polymorphisms in the MTHFR gene influence
     embryo viability and the incidence of aneuploidy. Human genetics. 2016
     May 1;135(5):555-68.

14   Yang, Y., Luo, Y., Yuan, J., Tang, Y., Xiong, L., Xu, M., ... & Liu, H.
     (2016). Association between maternal, fetal and paternal MTHFR gene
     C677T and A1298C polymorphisms and risk of recurrent pregnancy
     loss: a comprehensive evaluation. Archives of gynecology and obstetrics,
     293(6), 1197-1211.
     Puri, M., Kaur, L., Walia, G. K., Mukhopadhhyay, R., Sachdeva,
     M. P., Trivedi, S. S., ... & Saraswathy, K. N. (2013). MTHFR C677T
     polymorphism, folate, vitamin B12 and homocysteine in recurrent
     pregnancy losses: a case control study among North Indian women.
     Journal of perinatal medicine, 41(5), 549-554.
     Al-Achkar, W., Wafa, A., Ammar, S., Moassass, F., & Jarjour, R. A.
     (2017). Association of methylenetetrahydrofolate reductase C677T and
     A1298C gene polymorphisms with recurrent pregnancy loss in Syrian
     women. Reproductive Sciences, 24(9), 1275-1279.
     Luo, L., Chen, Y., Wang, L., Zhuo, G., Qiu, C., Tu, Q., ... & Wang,
     X. (2015). Polymorphisms of genes involved in the folate metabolic
     pathway impact the occurrence of unexplained recurrent pregnancy loss.
     Reproductive Sciences, 22(7), 845-851.

Chen, H., Yang, X., & Lu, M. (2016). Methylenetetrahydrofolate reductase gene polymorphisms and recurrent pregnancy loss in China: a systematic review and meta-analysis. Archives of gynecology and obstetrics, 293(2), 283-290.

Cao, Y., Xu, J., Zhang, Z., Huang, X., Zhang, A., Wang, J., ... & Du, J. (2013). Association study between methylenetetrahydrofolate reductase polymorphisms and unexplained recurrent pregnancy loss: a meta-analysis. Gene, 514(2), 105-111.

Unfried, G., Griesmacher, A., Weismüller, W., Nagele, F., Huber, J. C., & Tempfer, C. B. (2002). The C677T polymorphism of the methylenetetrahydrofolate reductase gene and idiopathic recurrent miscarriage. Obstetrics & Gynecology, 99(4), 614-619.

15 Dell'Edera, D., L'Episcopia, A., Simone, F., Lupo, M. G., Epifania, A. A., & Allegretti, A. (2018). Methylenetetrahydrofolate reductase gene C677T and A1298C polymorphisms and susceptibility to recurrent pregnancy loss. Biomedical reports, 8(2), 172-175.

16 Zetterberg, H. (2004). Methylenetetrahydrofolate reductase and transcobalamin genetic polymorphisms in human spontaneous abortion: biological and clinical implications. Reproductive Biology and Endocrinology, 2(1), 7.

Govindaiah, V., Naushad, S. M., Prabhakara, K., Krishna, P. C., & Devi, A. R. R. (2009). Association of parental hyperhomocysteinemia and C677T Methylene tetrahydrofolate reductase (MTHFR) polymorphism with recurrent pregnancy loss. Clinical biochemistry, 42(4-5), 380-386.

Dell'Edera, D., L'Episcopia, A., Simone, F., Lupo, M. G., Epifania, A. A., & Allegretti, A. (2018). Methylenetetrahydrofolate reductase gene C677T and A1298C polymorphisms and susceptibility to recurrent pregnancy loss. Biomedical reports, 8(2), 172-175.

17 Dell'Edera, D., Tinelli, A., Milazzo, G. N., Malvasi, A., Domenico, C., Pacella, E., ... & Epifania, A. A. (2013). Effect of multivitamins on plasma homocysteine in patients with the 5, 10 methylenetetrahydrofolate reductase C677T homozygous state. Molecular medicine reports, 8(2), 609-612.

18 Mtiraoui, N., Zammiti, W., Ghazouani, L., Braham, N. J., Saidi, S., Finan, R. R., ... & Mahjoub, T. (2006). Methylenetetrahydrofolate reductase C677T and A1298C polymorphism and changes in homocysteine concentrations in women with idiopathic recurrent pregnancy losses. Reproduction, 131(2), 395-401.

Yang, Y., Luo, Y., Yuan, J., Tang, Y., Xiong, L., Xu, M., ... & Liu, H. (2016). Association between maternal, fetal and paternal MTHFR gene C677T and A1298C polymorphisms and risk of recurrent pregnancy loss: a comprehensive evaluation. Archives of gynecology and obstetrics, 293(6), 1197-1211.

Hwang, K. R., Choi, Y. M., Kim, J. J., Lee, S. K., Yang, K. M., Paik, E. C., ... & Hong, M. A. (2017). Methylenetetrahydrofolate reductase polymorphisms and risk of recurrent pregnancy loss: a case-control study. Journal of Korean medical science, 32(12), 2029-2034.

Al-Achkar, W., Wafa, A., Ammar, S., Moassass, F., & Jarjour, R. A. (2017). Association of methylenetetrahydrofolate reductase C677T and A1298C gene polymorphisms with recurrent pregnancy loss in Syrian women. Reproductive Sciences, 24(9), 1275-1279.

Puri, M., Kaur, L., Walia, G. K., Mukhopadhhyay, R., Sachdeva, M. P., Trivedi, S. S., ... & Saraswathy, K. N. (2013). MTHFR C677T polymorphism, folate, vitamin B12 and homocysteine in recurrent pregnancy losses: a case control study among North Indian women. Journal of perinatal medicine, 41(5), 549-554.

19 Smith, D., Hornstra, J., Rocha, M., Jansen, G., Assaraf, Y., Lasry, I., ... & Smulders, Y. M. (2017). Folic Acid Impairs the Uptake of 5-Methyltetrahydrofolate in Human Umbilical Vascular Endothelial Cells. Journal of cardiovascular pharmacology, 70(4), 271.

20 Hekmatdoost A, Vahid F, Yari Z, Sadeghi M, Eini-Zinab H, Lakpour N, Arefi S. Methyltetrahydrofolate vs Folic Acid Supplementation in Idiopathic Recurrent Miscarriage with Respect to Methylenetetrahydrofolate Reductase C677T and A1298C Polymorphisms: A Randomized Controlled Trial. PloS one. 2015 Dec 2;10(12):e0143569.

21 Kos, B. J., Leemaqz, S. Y., McCormack, C. D., Andraweera, P. H., Furness, D. L., Roberts, C. T., & Dekker, G. A. (2018). The association of parental methylenetetrahydrofolate reductase polymorphisms (MTHFR 677C> T and 1298A> C) and fetal loss: a case–control study in South Australia. The Journal of Maternal-Fetal & Neonatal Medicine, 1-6.

22 Patanwala, I., King, M. J., Barrett, D. A., Rose, J., Jackson, R., Hudson, M., ... & Jones, D. E. (2014). Folic acid handling by the human gut: implications for food fortification and supplementation–. The American journal of clinical nutrition, 100(2), 593-599.

23 Puri, M., Kaur, L., Walia, G. K., Mukhopadhhyay, R., Sachdeva, M. P., Trivedi, S. S., ... & Saraswathy, K. N. (2013). MTHFR C677T polymorphism, folate, vitamin B12 and homocysteine in recurrent pregnancy losses: a case control study among North Indian women. Journal of perinatal medicine, 41(5), 549-554.

24 Crider, K. S., Devine, O., Hao, L., Dowling, N. F., Li, S., Molloy, A. M., ... & Berry, R. J. (2014). Population red blood cell folate concentrations for prevention of neural tube defects: Bayesian model. Bmj, 349.

Daly LE, Kirke PN, Molloy A, Weir DG, Scott JM. Folate levels and neural tube defects. Implications for prevention. JAMA. 1995;274:1698–702.

25 Fazili, Z., Paladugula, N., Zhang, M., & Pfeiffer, C. M. (2021). Folate forms in red blood cell lysates and conventionally prepared whole blood lysates appear stable for up to 2 years at– 70° C and show comparable concentrations. The Journal of nutrition, 151(9), 2852.

26   Lamers, Y., Prinz-Langenohl, R., Brämswig, S., & Pietrzik, K. (2006). Red blood cell folate concentrations increase more after supplementation with [6 S]-5-methyltetrahydrofolate than with folic acid in women of childbearing age. The American journal of clinical nutrition, 84(1), 156-161.

27   Mills, J. L., Lee, Y. J., Conley, M. R., Kirke, P. N., McPartlin, J. M., Weir, D. G., & Scott, J. M. (1995). Homocysteine metabolism in pregnancies complicated by neural-tube defects. The Lancet, 345(8943), 149-151.

28   Venn, B. J., Green, T. J., Moser, R., & Mann, J. I. (2003). Comparison of the effect of low-dose supplementation with L-5-methyltetrahydrofolate or folic acid on plasma homocysteine: a randomized placebo-controlled study. The American journal of clinical nutrition, 77(3), 658-662.

29   Gaskins, A. J., Chiu, Y. H., Williams, P. L., Ford, J. B., Toth, T. L., Hauser, R., ... & EARTH Study Team. (2015). Association between serum folate and vitamin B-12 and outcomes of assisted reproductive technologies. The American journal of clinical nutrition, 102(4), 943-950.

30   Boxmeer JC, Macklon NS, Lindemans J, Beckers NG, Eijkemans MJ, Laven JS, Steegers EA, Steegers-Theunissen RP. IVF outcomes are associated with biomarkers of the homocysteine pathway in monofollicular fluid. Hum Reprod. 2009 May;24(5):1059-66.

31   Ronnenberg, A. G., Venners, S. A., Xu, X., Chen, C., Wang, L., Guang, W., ... & Wang, X. (2007). Preconception B-vitamin and homocysteine status, conception, and early pregnancy loss. American journal of epidemiology, 166(3), 304-312.

32   Safiyeh, F. D., Mojgan, M., Parviz, S., Sakineh, M. A., & Behnaz, S. O. (2021). The effect of selenium and vitamin E supplementation on anti-Mullerian hormone and antral follicle count in infertile women with occult premature ovarian insufficiency: A randomized controlled clinical trial. Complementary Therapies in Medicine, 56, 102533.
      Negro R, Greco G, Mangieri T, Pezzarossa A, Dazzi D, Hassan H (2007) The influence of selenium supplementation on postpartum thyroid status in pregnant women with thyroid peroxidase autoantibodies. J Clin Endocrinol Metab 92(4):1263–1268

Chapter 6: Energize Your Eggs with Coenzyme Q10

1   Dietmar A, Schmidt ME, Siebrecht SC. Ubiquinol supplementation enhances peak power production in trained athletes: a double-blind, placebo controlled study. J Int Soc Sports Nutr. 2013 Apr 29;10(1):24.

2   Bentinger M, Brismar K, Dallner G. The antioxidant role of coenzyme Q. Mitochondrion. 2007 Jun;7 Suppl:S41-50;
      Sohal RS. Coenzyme Q and vitamin E interactions. Methods Enzymol. 2004;378:146-51.

3   Shigenaga MK, Hagen TM, Ames BN.Oxidative damage and mitochondrial decay in aging.Proc Natl Acad Sci U S A. 1994 Nov 8;91(23):10771-8.

Seo AY, Joseph AM, Dutta D, Hwang JC, Aris JP, Leeuwenburgh C.New insights into the role of mitochondria in aging: mitochondrial dynamics and more.J Cell Sci. 2010 Aug 1;123(Pt 15):2533-42 ("Seo 2010").

4 Seo 2010

5 Tatone C, Amicarelli F, Carbone MC, Monteleone P, Caserta D, Marci R, Artini PG, Piomboni P, Focarelli R. Cellular and molecular aspects of ovarian follicle ageing. Hum Reprod Update. 2008 Mar-Apr;14(2):131-42.

6 Wilding M, Dale B, Marino M, di Matteo L, Alviggi C, Pisaturo ML, Lombardi L, De Placido G. Mitochondrial aggregation patterns and activity in human oocytes and preimplantation embryos. Hum Reprod. 2001 May;16(5):909-17 ("Wilding 2001").

7 de Bruin JP, Dorland M, Spek ER, Posthuma G, van Haaften M, Looman CW, te Velde ER. Age-related changes in the ultrastructure of the resting follicle pool in human ovaries. Biol Reprod. 2004 Feb;70(2):419-24 ("deBruin 2004").

8 Wilding 2001.

9 Bentov Y, Casper RF.The aging oocyte—can mitochondrial function be improved? Fertil Steril. 2013 Jan;99(1):18-22. ("Bentov 2013").

10 Bonomi M, Somigliana E, Cacciatore C, Busnelli M, Rossetti R, Bonetti S, Paffoni A, Mari D, Ragni G, Persani L; Italian Network for the study of Ovarian Dysfunctions. Blood cell mitochondrial DNA content and premature ovarian aging. PLoS One. 2012;7(8):e42423

11 Van Blerkom J, Davis PW, Lee J. ATP content of human oocytes and developmental potential and outcome after in-vitro fertilization and embryo transfer. Hum Reprod. 1995 Feb;10(2):415-24

12 Santos TA, El Shourbagy A, St John JC. Mitochondrial content reflects oocyte variability and fertilization outcome. Fertil Steril. 2006;85:584–91; Bentov Y, Esfandiari N, Burstein E, Casper RF.The use of mitochondrial nutrients to improve the outcome of infertility treatment in older patients.Fertil Steril.
2010 Jan;93(1):272-5 ("Bentov 2010").

13 Van Blerkom J. Mitochondrial function in the human oocyte and embryo and their role in developmental competence. Mitochondrion. 2011 Sep;11(5):797-813 ("Van Blerkom 2011").
Dumollard R, Carroll J, Duchen MR, Campbell K, Swann K. Mitochondrial function and redox state in mammalian embryos. Semin Cell Dev Biol. 2009 May;20(3):346-53.

14 Eichenlaub-Ritter U, Vogt E, Yin H, Gosden R. Spindles, mitochondria and redox
potential in ageing oocytes. Reprod Biomed Online. 2004 Jan;8(1):45-58; Van Blerkom 2011; Ge H, Tollner TL, Hu Z, Dai M, Li X, Guan H, Shan D, Zhang X, Lv J, Huang C, Dong Q. The importance of mitochondrial metabolic activity and mitochondrial DNA replication during oocyte

maturation in vitro on oocyte quality and subsequent embryo developmental competence. Mol Reprod Dev. 2012 Jun;79(6):392-401.

15 Wilding M, Placido G, Matteo L, Marino M, Alviggi C, Dale B. Chaotic mosaicism in human preimplantation embryos is correlated with a low mitochondrial membrane potential. Fertil Steril. 2003;79:340–6 ("Wilding 2003").
Zeng HT, Ren Z, Yeung WS, Shu YM, Xu YW, Zhuang GL, Liang XY. Low mitochondrial DNA and ATP contents contribute to the absence of birefringent spindle imaged with PolScope in in vitro matured human oocytes. Hum Reprod. 2007 Jun;22(6):1681-6.

16 Yu Y, Dumollard R, Rossbach A, Lai FA, Swann K. Redistribution of mitochondria leads to bursts of ATP production during spontaneous mouse oocyte maturation. J Cell Physiol. 2010 Sep;224(3):672-80.

17 Wilding 2003.

18 Eichenlaub-Ritter U, Vogt E, Yin H, Gosden R. Spindles, mitochondria and redox potential in ageing oocytes. Reprod Biomed Online. 2004 Jan;8(1):45-58.

19 Bartmann AK, Romao GS, Ramos Eda S, Ferriani RA. Why do older women have poor implantation rates? A possible role of the mitochondria. J Assist Reprod Genet. 2004;21:79–83;
Thundathil J, Filion F, Smith LC.Molecular control of mitochondrial function in
preimplantation mouse embryos.Mol Reprod Dev. 2005 Aug;71(4):405-13.

20 Thouas GA, Trounson AO, Wolvetang EJ, Jones GM. Mitochondrial dysfunction in mouse oocytes results in preimplantation embryo arrest in vitro. Biol Reprod. 2004 Dec;71(6):1936-42; Eichenlaub-Ritter U, Wieczorek M, Lüke S, Seidel T. Age related changes in mitochondrial function and new approaches to study redox regulation in mammalian oocytes in response to age or maturation conditions. Mitochondrion. 2011 Sep;11(5):783-96.

21 Interview with Dr. Bentov, published May 16, 2011, http://www.chatelaine.com/health/what-every-woman-over-30-should-know-about-fertility/

22 Bentov 2010; Bentov 2013.

23 Quinzii CM, Hirano M, DiMauro S. CoQ10 deficiency diseases in adults. Mitochondrion. 2007;7(Suppl):S122–6;
Lopez 2010, Bergamini 2012, Shigenaga MK, Hagen TM, Ames BN. Oxidative damage and mitochondrial decay in aging. Proc Natl Acad Sci U S A. 1994 Nov 8;91(23):10771-8.

24 Perez-Sanchez C, Ruiz-Limon P, Aguirre MA, Bertolaccini ML, Khamashta MA, Rodriguez-Ariza A, Segui P, Collantes-Estevez E, Barbarroja N, Khraiwesh H, Gonzalez-Reyes JA, Villalba JM, Velasco F, Cuadrado MJ, Lopez-Pedrera C. Mitochondrial dysfunction in antiphospholipid syndrome: implications in the pathogenesis of the

disease and effects of coenzyme Q(10) treatment. Blood. 2012 Jun 14;119(24):5859-70.

25 Akarsu, S., Gode, F., Isik, A. Z., Dikmen, Z. G., & Tekindal, M. A. (2017). The association between coenzyme Q10 concentrations in follicular fluid with embryo morphokinetics and pregnancy rate in assisted reproductive techniques. Journal of assisted reproduction and genetics, 34(5), 599-605. Turi A, Giannubilo SR, Brugè F, Principi F, Battistoni S, Santoni F, Tranquilli AL, Littarru G, Tiano L.Coenzyme Q10 content in follicular fluid and its relationship with oocyte fertilization and embryo grading. Arch Gynecol Obstet. 2012 Apr;285(4):1173-6

26 Xu, Y., Nisenblat, V., Lu, C., Li, R., Qiao, J., Zhen, X., & Wang, S. (2018). Pretreatment with coenzyme Q10 improves ovarian response and embryo quality in low-prognosis young women with decreased ovarian reserve: a randomized controlled trial. Reproductive Biology and Endocrinology, 16(1), 29 Giannubilo, S., Orlando, P., Silvestri, S., Cirilli, I., Marcheggiani, F., Ciavattini, A., & Tiano, L. (2018). CoQ10 Supplementation in Patients Undergoing IVF-ET: The Relationship with Follicular Fluid Content and Oocyte Maturity. Antioxidants, 7(10), 141

27 Bentov, Y., Hannam, T., Jurisicova, A., Esfandiari, N., & Casper, R. F. (2014). Coenzyme Q10 supplementation and oocyte aneuploidy in women undergoing IVF-ICSI treatment. Clinical Medicine Insights: Reproductive Health, 8, CMRH-S14681.

28 McGarry, A., McDermott, M., Kieburtz, K., de Blieck, E. A., Beal, F., Marder, K., ... & Guttman, M. (2017). A randomized, double-blind, placebo-controlled trial of coenzyme Q10 in Huntington disease. Neurology, 88(2), 152-159. Yeung, C. K., Billings, F. T., Claessens, A. J., Roshanravan, B., Linke, L., Sundell, M. B., ... & Himmelfarb, J. (2015). Coenzyme Q 10 dose-escalation study in hemodialysis patients: safety, tolerability, and effect on oxidative stress. BMC nephrology, 16(1), 183. Seet, R. C. S., Lim, E. C., Tan, J. J., Quek, A. M., Chow, A. W., Chong, W. L., ... & Halliwell, B. (2014). Does high-dose coenzyme Q10 improve oxidative damage and clinical outcomes in Parkinson's disease?.

29 Aberg F, Appelkvist EL, Dallner G, Ernster L. Distribution and redox state of ubiquinones in rat and human tissues. Arch Biochem Biophys. 1992 Jun;295(2):230-4; Miles MV, Horn PS, Morrison JA, Tang PH, DeGrauw T, Pesce AJ. Plasma coenzyme Q10 reference intervals, but not redox status, are affected by gender and race in self-reported healthy adults. Clin Chim Acta. 2003 Jun;332(1-2):123-32.

30 Zhang, Y., Liu, J., Chen, X. Q., & Chen, C. Y. O. (2018). Ubiquinol is superior to ubiquinone to enhance Coenzyme Q10 status in older men. Food & function.

Langsjoen, P. H., & Langsjoen, A. M. (2014). Comparison study of plasma coenzyme Q10 levels in healthy subjects supplemented with ubiquinol versus ubiquinone. Clinical pharmacology in drug development, 3(1), 13-17

31 Villalba JM, Parrado C, Santos-Gonzalez M, Alcain FJ. Therapeutic use of coenzyme Q10 and coenzyme Q10-related compounds and formulations. Expert Opin Investig Drugs. 2010 Apr;19(4):535-54.

32 Bergamini C, Moruzzi N, Sblendido A, Lenaz G, Fato R. A water soluble CoQ10 formulation improves intracellular distribution and promotes mitochondrial respiration in cultured cells. PLoS One. 2012;7(3):e33712; Chopra RK, Goldman R, Sinatra ST, Bhagavan HN. Relative bioavailability of coenzyme Q10 formulations in human subjects. Int J Vitam Nutr Res. 1998;68(2):109-13., Bhagavan 2006;

33 López-Lluch, G., del Pozo-Cruz, J., Sánchez-Cuesta, A., Cortés-Rodríguez, A. B., & Navas, P. (2019). Bioavailability of coenzyme Q10 supplements depends on carrier lipids and solubilization. Nutrition, 57, 133-140.

34 Singh, R. B., Niaz, M. A., Kumar, A., Sindberg, C. D., Moesgaard, S., & Littarru, G. P. (2005). Effect on absorption and oxidative stress of different oral Coenzyme Q10 dosages and intake strategy in healthy men. Biofactors, 25(1-4), 219-224.

35 Spindler M, Beal MF, Henchcliffe C. Coenzyme Q10 effects in neurodegenerative disease. Neuropsychiatr Dis Treat. 2009;5:597-610 ("Spindler 2009");
Hosoe 2007.

36 Ferrante KL, Shefner J, Zhang H, Betensky R, O'Brien M, Yu H, Fantasia M, Taft J, Beal MF, Traynor B, Newhall K, Donofrio P, Caress J, Ashburn C, Freiberg B, O'Neill C, Paladenech C, Walker T, Pestronk A, Abrams B, Florence J, Renna R, Schierbecker J, Malkus B, Cudkowicz M. Tolerance of high-dose (3,000 mg/day) coenzyme Q10 in ALS. Neurology. 2005 Dec 13;65(11):1834-6; Spindler 2009.

37 Mezawa M, Takemoto M, Onishi S, Ishibashi R, Ishikawa T, Yamaga M, Fujimoto M, Okabe E, He P, Kobayashi K, Yokote K. The reduced form of coenzyme Q10 improves glycemic control in patients with type 2 diabetes: an open label pilot study. Biofactors. 2012 Nov-Dec;38(6):416-21.

38 Teran, E., Hernandez, I., Nieto, B., Tavara, R., Ocampo, J. E., & Calle, A. (2009). Coenzyme Q10 supplementation during pregnancy reduces the risk of pre-eclampsia. International Journal of Gynecology & Obstetrics, 105(1), 43-45.

39 Noia, G., Littarru, G. P., De Santis, M., Oradei, A., Mastromarino, C., Trivellini, C., & Caruso, A. (1996). Coenzyme Q10 in pregnancy. Fetal diagnosis and therapy, 11(4), 264-270.

40 Pérez-Sánchez, C., Aguirre, M. Á., Ruiz-Limón, P., Ábalos-Aguilera, M. C., Jiménez-Gómez, Y., Arias-de la Rosa, I., ... & Collantes-Estévez, E.

(2017). Ubiquinol effects on antiphospholipid syndrome prothrombotic profile: a randomized, placebo-controlled trial. Arteriosclerosis, thrombosis, and vascular biology, ATVBAHA-117

Chapter 7: Melatonin and Other Antioxidants

1   de Bruin JP, Dorland M, Spek ER, Posthuma G, van Haaften M, Looman CW, te Velde ER. Age-related changes in the ultrastructure of the resting follicle pool in human ovaries. Biol Reprod. 2004 Feb;70(2):419-24. ("de Bruin 2004").

2   Tatone C, Carbone MC, Falone S, Aimola P, Giardinelli A, Caserta D, Marci R, Pandolfi A, Ragnelli AM, Amicarelli F. Age-dependent changes in the expression of superoxide dismutases and catalase are associated with ultrastructural modifications in human granulosa cells. Mol Hum Reprod. 2006 Nov;12(11):655-60.
    Carbone MC, Tatone C, Delle Monache S, Marci R, Caserta D, Colonna R, Amicarelli F. Antioxidant enzymatic defences in human follicular fluid: characterization and age-dependent changes. Mol Hum Reprod. 2003 Nov;9(11):639-43.

3   Shigenaga MK, Hagen TM, Ames BN.Oxidative damage and mitochondrial decay in aging. Proc Natl Acad Sci U S A. 1994 Nov 8;91(23):10771-8.

4   Wiener-Megnazi Z, Vardi L, Lissak A, Shnizer S, Reznick AZ, Ishai D, Lahav-Baratz S, Shiloh H, Koifman M, Dirnfeld M. Oxidative stress indices in follicular fluid as measured by the thermochemiluminescence assay correlate with outcome parameters in in vitro fertilization. Fertil Steril. 2004;82(Suppl 3):1171–1176.
    de Bruin 2004, Eichenlaub 2011, premkumar 2012, Carbone 2003, Tatone 2006, Wang LY, Wang DH, Zou XY, Xu CM. Mitochondrial functions on oocytes and preimplantation embryos. J Zhejiang Univ Sci B. 2009 Jul;10(7):483-92

5   Polak G, Koziol-Montewka M, Gogacz M, Blaszkowska I, Kotarski J. Total antioxidant status of peritoneal fluid in infertile women. Eur J Obstet Gynecol Reprod Biol. 2001;94:261–263.
    Wang Y, Sharma RK, Falcone T, Goldberg J, Agarwal A. Importance of reactive oxygen species in the peritoneal fluid of women with endometriosis or idiopathic infertility. Fertil Steril. 1997;68:826–830. ("Wang 1997").
    Paszkowski T, Traub AI, Robinson SY, McMaster D. Selenium dependent glutathione peroxidase activity in human follicular fluid. Clin Chim Acta. 1995;236(2):173–180. doi: 10.1016/0009-8981(95)98130-9. ("Paszkowski 1995").
    Agarwal 2012; Wang 1997.

6   Song, Y., Liu, J., Qiu, Z., Chen, D., Luo, C., Liu, X., ... & Liu, W. (2018). Advanced oxidation protein products from the follicular

microenvironment and their role in infertile women with endometriosis. Experimental and therapeutic medicine, 15(1), 479-486.

Da Broi, M. G., Jordão-Jr, A. A., Ferriani, R. A., & Navarro, P. A. (2018). Oocyte oxidative DNA damage may be involved in minimal/ mild endometriosis-related infertility. Molecular reproduction and development, 85(2), 128-136.

7   Victor VM, Rocha M, Banuls C, Alvarez A, de Pablo C, Sanchez-Serrano M, Gomez M, Hernandez-Mijares A. Induction of oxidative stress and human leukocyte/endothelial cell interactions in polycystic ovary syndrome patients with insulin resistance. J Clin Endocrinol Metab. 2011;96:3115–3122. ("Victor 2011").

8   Shaum KM, Polotsky AJ.Nutrition and reproduction: is there evidence to support a "Fertility Diet" to improve mitochondrial function? Maturitas. 2013 Apr;74(4):309-12
    Ruder EH, Hartman TJ, Reindollar RH, Goldman MB. Female dietary antioxidant intake and time to pregnancy among couples treated for unexplained infertility. Fertil Steril. 2013 Dec 17 [Epub ahead of print]. ("Ruder 2014").

9   Aydin Y, Ozatik O, Hassa H, Ulusoy D, Ogut S, Sahin F.Relationship between oxidative stress and clinical pregnancy in assisted reproductive technology treatment cycles. J Assist Reprod Genet. 2013 Jun;30(6):765-72.

10 Ruder 2014.

11 Chemineau P, Guillaume D, Migaud M, Thiéry JC, Pellicer-Rubio MT, Malpaux B. Seasonality of reproduction in mammals: intimate regulatory mechanisms and practical implications. Reprod Domest Anim. 2008 Jul;43 Suppl 2:40-7.

12 Brzezinski A, Seibel MM, Lynch HJ, Deng MH, Wurtman RJ. Melatonin in human preovulatory follicular fluid. J Clin Endocrinol Metab. 1987;64(4):865–867.
    Ronnberg L, Kauppila A, Leppaluoto J, Martikainen H, Vakkuri O. Circadian and seasonal variation in human preovulatory follicular fluid melatonin concentration. J Clin Endocrinol Metab. 1990;71(2):492–496.

13 Tamura H, Takasaki A, Taketani T, Tanabe M, Kizuka F, Lee L, Tamura I, Maekawa R, Aasada H, Yamagata Y, Sugino N. The role of melatonin as an antioxidant in the follicle. J Ovarian Res. 2012 Jan 26;5:5. ("Tamura 2012").
    Nakamura Y, Tamura H, Takayama H, Kato H. Increased endogenous level of melatonin in preovulatory human follicles does not directly influence progesterone production. Fertil Steril. 2003 Oct;80(4):1012-6.

14 Poeggeler B, Reiter RJ, Tan DX, Chen LD, Manchester LC. Melatonin, hydroxyl radical-mediated oxidative damage, and aging: a hypothesis. J Pineal Res. 1993;14(4):151–168.
    Schindler AE, Christensen B, Henkel A, Oettel M, Moore C. High-dose pilot study with the novel progestogen dienogestin patients with endometriosis. Gynecol Endocrinol. 2006;22(1):9–17.

15 Reiter RJ, Tan DX, Manchester LC, Qi W. Biochemical reactivity of
    melatonin with reactive oxygen and nitrogen species: a review of the
    evidence. Cell Biochem Biophys. 2001;34(2):237–256.
    Tan DX, Manchester LC, Reiter RJ, Plummer BF, Limson J, Weintraub
    ST, Qi W. Melatonin directly scavenges hydrogen peroxide: a potentially
    new metabolic pathway of melatonin biotransformation. Free Radic Biol
    Med. 2000;29(11):1177–1185. ("Tan 2000").
16 Sack RL, Lewy AJ, Erb DL, Vollmer WM, Singer CM. Human melatonin
    production decreases with age. J Pineal Res. 1986;3(4):379-88.
17 Tong, J., Sun, Y., Li, H., Li, W. P., Zhang, C., & Chen, Z. (2017).
    Melatonin levels in follicular fluid as markers for IVF outcomes and
    predicting ovarian reserve. Reproduction, REP-16.
    Tamura H, Takasaki A, Miwa I, Taniguchi K, Maekawa R, Asada H,
    Taketani T, Matsuoka A, Yamagata Y, Shimamura K. et al. Oxidative
    stress impairs oocyte quality and melatonin protects oocytes from
    free radical damage and improves fertilization rate. J Pineal Res.
    2008;44(3):280–287 ("Tamura 2008")
    Jahnke G, Marr M, Myers C, Wilson R, Travlos G, Price C. Maternal and
    developmental toxicity evaluation of melatonin administered orally to
    pregnant Sprague-Dawley rats. Toxicol Sci. 1999;50(2):271–279.
    Ishizuka B, Kuribayashi Y, Murai K, Amemiya A, Itoh MT. The effect of
    melatonin on in vitro fertilization and embryo development in mice. J
    Pineal Res. 2000;28(1):48–51 Papis K, Poleszczuk O, Wenta-Muchalska E,
    Modlinski JA. Melatonin effect on bovine embryo development in vitro
    in relation to oxygen concentration. J Pineal Res. 2007;43(4):321–326.
    Shi JM, Tian XZ, Zhou GB, Wang L, Gao C, Zhu SE, Zeng SM, Tian
    JH, Liu GS. Melatonin exists in porcine follicular fluid and improves in
    vitro maturation and parthenogenetic development of porcine oocytes. J
    Pineal Res. 2009;47(4):318–323.
18 Id.
19 Id.
20 Tamura H, Takasaki A, Miwa I, Taniguchi K, Maekawa R, Asada H,
    Taketani T, Matsuoka A, Yamagata Y, Shimamura K. et al. Oxidative
    stress impairs oocyte quality and melatonin protects oocytes from
    free radical damage and improves fertilization rate. J Pineal Res.
    2008;44(3):280–287 ("Tamura 2008")
    Jahnke G, Marr M, Myers C, Wilson R, Travlos G, Price C. Maternal and
    developmental toxicity evaluation of melatonin administered orally to
    pregnant Sprague-Dawley rats. Toxicol Sci. 1999;50(2):271–279.
    Ishizuka B, Kuribayashi Y, Murai K, Amemiya A, Itoh MT. The effect of
    melatonin on in vitro fertilization and embryo development in mice. J
    Pineal Res. 2000;28(1):48–51

Papis K, Poleszczuk O, Wenta-Muchalska E, Modlinski JA. Melatonin effect on bovine embryo development in vitro in relation to oxygen concentration. J Pineal Res. 2007;43(4):321–326.

Shi JM, Tian XZ, Zhou GB, Wang L, Gao C, Zhu SE, Zeng SM, Tian JH, Liu GS. Melatonin exists in porcine follicular fluid and improves in vitro maturation and parthenogenetic development of porcine oocytes. J Pineal Res. 2009;47(4):318–323.

21 Tamura 2008; Tamura 2012.

22 Tamura 2012.

23 Rizzo P, Raffone E, Benedetto V.Effect of the treatment with myo-inositol plus folic acid plus melatonin in comparison with a treatment with myo-inositol plus folic acid on oocyte quality and pregnancy outcome in IVF cycles. A prospective, clinical trial.Eur Rev Med Pharmacol Sci. 2010 Jun;14(6):555-61.

Nishihara, T., Hashimoto, S., Ito, K., Nakaoka, Y., Matsumoto, K., Hosoi, Y., & Morimoto, Y. (2014). Oral melatonin supplementation improves oocyte and embryo quality in women undergoing in vitro fertilization-embryo transfer. Gynecological endocrinology, 30(5), 359-362.

Jahromi, B. N., Sadeghi, S., Alipour, S., Parsanezhad, M. E., & Alamdarloo, S. M. (2017). Effect of melatonin on the outcome of assisted reproductive technique cycles in women with diminished ovarian reserve: A double-blinded randomized clinical trial. Iranian journal of medical sciences, 42(1), 73.

Fernando, S., Wallace, E. M., Vollenhoven, B., Lolatgis, N., Hope, N., Wong, M., … & Thomas, P. (2018). Melatonin in Assisted Reproductive Technology: A Pilot Double-Blind Randomized Placebo-Controlled Clinical Trial. Frontiers in endocrinology, 9.

Eryilmaz, O. G., Devran, A., Sarikaya, E., Aksakal, F. N., Mollamahmutoğlu, L., & Cicek, N. (2011). Melatonin improves the oocyte and the embryo in IVF patients with sleep disturbances, but does not improve the sleeping problems. Journal of assisted reproduction and genetics, 28(9), 815.

Batıoğlu, A. S., Şahin, U., Gürlek, B., Öztürk, N., & Ünsal, E. (2012). The efficacy of melatonin administration on oocyte quality. Gynecological Endocrinology, 28(2), 91-93.

24 Schwertner, A., Dos Santos, C. C. C., Costa, G. D., Deitos, A., de Souza, A., de Souza, I. C. C., … & Caumo, W. (2013). Efficacy of melatonin in the treatment of endometriosis: a phase II, randomized, double-blind, placebo-controlled trial. PAIN®, 154(6), 874-881.

25 Nishihara, T., Hashimoto, S., Ito, K., Nakaoka, Y., Matsumoto, K., Hosoi, Y., & Morimoto, Y. (2014). Oral melatonin supplementation improves oocyte and embryo quality in women undergoing in vitro fertilization-embryo transfer. Gynecological endocrinology, 30(5), 359-362.

26 Jahromi, B. N., Sadeghi, S., Alipour, S., Parsanezhad, M. E., & Alamdarloo, S. M. (2017). Effect of melatonin on the outcome of assisted reproductive technique cycles in women with diminished ovarian reserve: A double-blinded randomized clinical trial. Iranian journal of medical sciences, 42(1), 73.

27 Woo MM, Tai CJ, Kang SK, Nathwani PS, Pang SF, Leung PC.Direct action of melatonin in human granulosa-luteal cells.J Clin Endocrinol Metab. 2001 Oct;86(10):4789-97.
Voordouw, B. C., Euser, R., Verdonk, R. E., Alberda, B. T., de Jong, F. H., Drogendijk, A. C., ... & Cohen, M. (1992). Melatonin and melatonin-progestin combinations alter pituitary-ovarian function in women and can inhibit ovulation. The Journal of Clinical Endocrinology & Metabolism, 74(1), 108-117.

28 Chaudhary, A., Agarwal, A., Tanwar, M., Singh, P., & Negi, P. (2021). Effect of melatonin addition in ovulation induction protocols with clomiphene citrate in management of infertility. International Journal of Reproduction, Contraception, Obstetrics and Gynecology, 10(12), 4438-4443.
Singh, M., & Kumari, S. (2020). Comparison of fertility rates of combination of enclomiphene citrate and melatonin with fertility rates of plain enclomiphene citrate in cases of dysovulatory infertility. International Journal of Reproduction, Contraception, Obstetrics and Gynecology, 9(4), 1700-1705.

29 Tagliaferri, V., Romualdi, D., Scarinci, E., Cicco, S. D., Florio, C. D., Immediata, V., ... & Apa, R. (2018). Melatonin treatment may be able to restore menstrual cyclicity in women with PCOS: a pilot study. Reproductive Sciences, 25(2), 269-275..

30 Bellipanni, G., Bianchi, P., Pierpaoli, W., Bulian, D., & Ilyia, E. (2001). Effects of melatonin in perimenopausal and menopausal women: a randomized and placebo controlled study. Experimental gerontology, 36(2), 297-310.

31 Tamura H, Takasaki A, Miwa I, Taniguchi K, Maekawa R, Asada H, Taketani T, Matsuoka A, Yamagata Y, Shimamura K, Morioka H, Ishikawa H, Reiter RJ, Sugino N. Oxidative stress impairs oocyte quality and melatonin protects oocytes from free radical damage and improves fertilization rate. J Pineal Res. 2008 Apr;44(3):280-7.

32 Evans H. The pioneer history of vitamin E. Vitam Horm. 1963;20:379–387.

33 Bahadori, M. H., Sharami, S. H., Fakor, F., Milani, F., Pourmarzi, D., & Dalil-Heirati, S. F. (2017). Level of vitamin e in follicular fluid and serum and oocyte morphology and embryo quality in patients undergoing ivf treatment. Journal of Family & Reproductive Health, 11(2), 74.

34 Yeh J, Bowman MJ, Browne RW, Chen N. Reproductive aging results in a reconfigured ovarian antioxidant defense profile in rats. Fertil Steril. 2005 Oct;84 Suppl 2:1109-13; Ruder 2014.

35 Amini, L., Chekini, R., Nateghi, M. R., Haghani, H., Jamialahmadi, T., Sathyapalan, T., & Sahebkar, A. (2021). The effect of combined vitamin C and vitamin E supplementation on oxidative stress markers in women with endometriosis: a randomized, triple-blind placebo-controlled clinical trial. Pain Research and Management, 2021.

36 Ruder EH, Hartman TJ, Reindollar RH, Goldman MB. Female dietary antioxidant intake and time to pregnancy among couples treated for unexplained infertility. Fertil Steril. 2013 Dec 17 [Epub ahead of print]. ("Ruder 2014").

37 Safiyeh, F. D., Mojgan, M., Parviz, S., Sakineh, M. A., & Behnaz, S. O. (2021). The effect of selenium and vitamin E supplementation on anti-Mullerian hormone and antral follicle count in infertile women with occult premature ovarian insufficiency: A randomized controlled clinical trial. Complementary Therapies in Medicine, 56, 102533.

38 Murray, A. A., Molinek, M. D., Baker, S. J., Kojima, F. N., Smith, M. F., Hillier, 1. S., & Spears, N. (2001). Role of ascorbic acid in promoting follicle integrity and survival in intact mouse ovarian follicles in vitro. REPRODUCTION-CAMBRIDGE-, 121(1), 89-96.

39 Henmi, H., Endo, T., Kitajima, Y., Manase, K., Hata, H., & Kudo, R. (2003). Effects of ascorbic acid supplementation on serum progesterone levels in patients with a luteal phase defect. Fertility and Sterility, 80(2), 459-461.

40 Lu, X., Wu, Z., Wang, M., & Cheng, W. (2018). Effects of vitamin C on the outcome of in vitro fertilization–embryo transfer in endometriosis: A randomized controlled study. Journal of International Medical Research, 46(11), 4624-4633.

41 Packer L, Witt EH, Tritschler HJ: -Lipoic acid as a biological antioxidant. Free Radic Biol Med, 1995, 19, 227–250.

42 Arivazhagan P, Ramanathan K, Panneerselvam C: Effect of DL—lipoic acid on mitochondrial enzymes in aged rats. Chem Biol Interact, 2001, 138, 189–198.
Mc Carthy MF, Barroso-Aranda J, Contreras F: The "rejuvenatory" impact of lipoic acid on mitochondrial function in aging rats may reflect induction and activation of PPAR-coactivator-1. Med Hypotheses, 2009, 72, 29–33

43 Rago, R., Marcucci, I., Leto, G., Caponecchia, L., Salacone, P., Bonanni, P., ... & Sebastianelli, A. (2015). Effect of myo-inositol and alpha-lipoic acid on oocyte quality in polycystic ovary syndrome non-obese women undergoing in vitro fertilization: a pilot study. J Biol Regul Homeost Agents, 29(4), 913-923.

44 De Cicco, S., Immediata, V., Romualdi, D., Policola, C., Tropea, A., Di Florio, C., ... & Apa, R. (2017). Myoinositol combined with alpha-lipoic acid may improve the clinical and endocrine features of polycystic

ovary syndrome through an insulin-independent action. Gynecological Endocrinology, 33(9), 698-701.

Masharani U, Gjerde C, Evans JL, Youngren JF, Goldfine ID. Effects of controlled-release alpha lipoic acid in lean, nondiabetic patients with polycystic ovary syndrome. J Diabetes Sci Technol. 2010 Mar 1;4(2):359-64.

45 Haghighian, H. K., Haidari, F., Mohammadi-asl, J., & Dadfar, M. (2015). Randomized, triple-blind, placebo-controlled clinical trial examining the effects of alpha-lipoic acid supplement on the spermatogram and seminal oxidative stress in infertile men. Fertility and sterility, 104(2), 318-324

46 Pınar, N., Soylu Karapınar, O., Özcan, O., Özgür, T., & Bayraktar, S. (2017). Effect of alpha-lipoic acid on endometrial implants in an experimental rat model. Fundamental & clinical pharmacology, 31(5), 506-512.

Lete, I., Mendoza, N., de la Viuda, E., & Carmona, F. (2018). Effectiveness of an antioxidant preparation with N-acetyl cysteine, alpha lipoic acid and bromelain in the treatment of endometriosis-associated pelvic pain: LEAP study. European Journal of Obstetrics & Gynecology and Reproductive Biology, 228, 221-224.

47 Segermann J, Hotze A, Ulrich H, et al. Effect of alpha-lipoic acid on the peripheral conversion of thyroxine to triiodothyronine and on serum lipid-, protein- and glucose levels. Arzneimittelforschung. 1991;41:1294-1298.

48 Xiang, G. D., Pu, J. H., Sun, H. L., & Zhao, L. S. (2010). Alpha-lipoic acid improves endothelial dysfunction in patients with subclinical hypothyroidism. Experimental and clinical endocrinology & diabetes, 118(09), 625-629.

49 Porasuphatana S, Suddee S, Nartnampong A, et al. Gylcemic and oxidative status of patients with type 2 diabetes mellitus following oral administration of alpha-lipoic acid: a randomized double-blinded placebo-controlled study. *Asia Pac J Clin Nutr* 2012;21(1):12-21.
Golbidi S, Badran M, Laher I. Diabetes and alpha lipoic Acid. Front Pharmacol. 2011;2:69.

50 Atkuri KR, Mantovani JJ, Herzenberg LA, Herzenberg LA.N-Acetylcysteine—a safe antidote for cysteine/glutathione deficiency.Curr Opin Pharmacol. 2007 Aug;7(4):355-9. ("Atkuri 2007").

51 Li, Q., & Zhao, Z. (2019). Influence of N-acetyl-L-cysteine against bisphenol a on the maturation of mouse oocytes and embryo development: in vitro study. BMC Pharmacology and Toxicology, 20(1), 1-9.

52 Fan, L., Guan, F., Ma, Y., Zhang, Y., Li, L., Sun, Y., … & He, M. (2022). N-Acetylcysteine improves oocyte quality through modulating the Nrf2 signaling pathway to ameliorate oxidative stress caused by repeated controlled ovarian hyperstimulation. Reproduction, Fertility and Development.

53 Bedaiwy, M. A., Al Inany, A. R., & Falcone, T. (2004). N-acetyl cystein improves pregnancy rate in long standing unexplained infertility: A novel mechanism of ovulation induction. Fertility and Sterility, 82, S228.

54 Hebisha, S. A., Omran, M. S., Sallam, H. N., & Ahmed, A. I. (2015). Follicular fluid homocysteine levels with N-Acetyl cysteine supplemented controlled ovarian hyperstimulation, correlation with oocyte yield and ICSI cycle outcome. Fertility and Sterility, 104(3), e324.:

55 Thakker, D., Raval, A., Patel, I., & Walia, R. (2015). N-acetylcysteine for polycystic ovary syndrome: a systematic review and meta-analysis of randomized controlled clinical trials. Obstetrics and gynecology international, 2015.
Mostajeran, F., Tehrani, H. G., & Rahbary, B. (2018). N-Acetylcysteine as an Adjuvant to Letrozole for Induction of Ovulation in Infertile Patients with Polycystic Ovary Syndrome. Advanced biomedical research, 7.
Cheraghi, E., Mehranjani, M. S., Shariatzadeh, M. A., Esfahani, M. H. N., & Ebrahimi, Z. (2016). N-Acetylcysteine improves oocyte and embryo quality in polycystic ovary syndrome patients undergoing intracytoplasmic sperm injection: an alternative to metformin. Reproduction, Fertility and Development, 28(6), 723-731
Nasr A. Effect of N-acetyl-cysteine after ovarian drilling in clomiphene citrate-resistant PCOS women: a pilot study.Reprod Biomed Online. 2010 Mar;20(3):403-9. ("Nasr 2010").

56 Salehpour S, Sene AA, Saharkhiz N, Sohrabi MR, Moghimian F.N-Acetylcysteine as an adjuvant to clomiphene citrate for successful induction of ovulation in infertile patients with polycystic ovary syndrome.J Obstet Gynaecol Res. 2012 Sep;38(9):1182-6.

57 Amin AF, Shaaban OM, Bediawy MA.N-acetyl cysteine for treatment of recurrent unexplained pregnancy loss. Reprod Biomed Online. 2008 Nov;17(5):722-6.

58 Nasr 2010.

59 Giorgi, V. S., Da Broi, M. G., Paz, C. C., Ferriani, R. A., & Navarro, P. A. (2016). N-acetyl-cysteine and L-carnitine prevent meiotic oocyte damage induced by follicular fluid from infertile women with mild endometriosis. Reproductive Sciences, 23(3), 342-351.

60 Porpora, M. G., Brunelli, R., Costa, G., Imperiale, L., Krasnowska, E. K., Lundeberg, T., ... & Parasassi, T. (2013). A promise in the treatment of endometriosis: an observational cohort study on ovarian endometrioma reduction by N-acetylcysteine. Evidence-based Complementary and Alternative Medicine, 2013.

61 Dodd 2008, Atkuri 2007

62 Lynch RM, Robertson R. Anaphylactoid reactions to intravenous N-acetylcysteine: a prospective case controlled study.Accid Emerg Nurs. 2004 Jan;12(1):10-5.

63 Ismail, A. M., Hamed, A. H., Saso, S., & Thabet, H. H. (2014). Adding L-carnitine to clomiphene resistant PCOS women improves the quality of ovulation and the pregnancy rate. A randomized clinical trial. European Journal of Obstetrics & Gynecology and Reproductive Biology, 180, 148-152. Latifian, S., Hamdi, K., & Totakneh, R. (2015). Effect of addition of l-carnitine in polycystic ovary syndrome (PCOS) patients with clomiphene citrate and gonadotropin resistant. Int J Curr Res Acad Rev, 3, 469-76.

64 Fenkci, S. M., Fenkci, V., Oztekin, O., Rota, S., & Karagenc, N. (2008). Serum total L-carnitine levels in non-obese women with polycystic ovary syndrome. Human reproduction, 23(7), 1602-1606.

65 Agarwal, A., Sengupta, P., & Durairajanayagam, D. (2018). Role of L-carnitine in female infertility. Reproductive Biology and Endocrinology, 16(1), 5.
Dionyssopoulou, E., Vassiliadis, S., Evangeliou, A., Koumantakis, E. E., & Athanassakis, I. (2005). Constitutive or induced elevated levels of L-carnitine correlate with the cytokine and cellular profile of endometriosis. Journal of reproductive immunology, 65(2), 159-170.
Christiana, K., George, T., George, F., Margarita, T., Anna, T., Costas, F., & Irene, A. (2014). L-carnitine alters lipid body content in pre-implantation embryos leading to infertility. J Reprod Immunol, 101, 18-39.

66 Kitano, Y., Hashimoto, S., Matsumoto, H., Yamochi, T., Yamanaka, M., Nakaoka, Y., ... & Morimoto, Y. (2018). Oral administration of l-carnitine improves the clinical outcome of fertility in patients with IVF treatment. Gynecological Endocrinology, 1-5.

67 Lim J, Luderer U. Oxidative damage increases and antioxidant gene expression decreases with aging in the mouse ovary. Biol Reprod. 2011 Apr;84(4):775-82; Liu 2012.

Chapter 8: Restoring Ovulation with Myo-Inositol

1 Lisi F, Carfagna P, Oliva MM, Rago R, Lisi R, Poverini R, Manna C, Vaquero E, Caserta D, Raparelli V, Marci R, Moscarini M.Pretreatment with myo-inositol in non polycystic ovary syndrome patients undergoing multiple follicular stimulation for IVF: a pilot study. Reprod Biol Endocrinol. 2012 Jul 23;10:52. ("Lisi 2012").
Caprio, F., D'Eufemia, M. D., Trotta, C., Campitiello, M. R., Ianniello, R., Mele, D., & Colacurci, N. (2015). Myo-inositol therapy for poor-responders during IVF: a prospective controlled observational trial. Journal of ovarian research, 8(1), 37
Nazari, L., Salehpour, S., Hosseini, S., Saharkhiz, N., Azizi, E., Hashemi, T., & Ghodssi-Ghassemabadi, R. (2020). Effect of myo-inositol supplementation on ICSI outcomes among poor ovarian responder patients: A randomized controlled trial. Journal of Gynecology Obstetrics and Human Reproduction, 49(5), 101698.

Mohammadi, S., Eini, F., Bazarganipour, F., Taghavi, S. A., & Kutenaee, M. A. (2021). The effect of Myo-inositol on fertility rates in poor ovarian responder in women undergoing assisted reproductive technique: a randomized clinical trial. Reproductive Biology and Endocrinology, 19(1), 1-7.

2 Mohammadi, S., Eini, F., Bazarganipour, F., Taghavi, S. A., & Kutenaee, M. A. (2021). The effect of Myo-inositol on fertility rates in poor ovarian responder in women undergoing assisted reproductive technique: a randomized clinical trial. Reproductive Biology and Endocrinology, 19(1), 1-7.

3 Papaleo E, Unfer V, Baillargeon JP, Fusi F, Occhi F, De Santis L.Myo-inositol may improve oocyte quality in intracytoplasmic sperm injection cycles. A prospective, controlled, randomized trial. Fertil Steril. 2009 May;91(5):1750-4; ("Papaleo 2009").

Genazzani AD, Lanzoni C, Ricchieri F, Jasonni VM. Myo-inositol administration positively affects hyperinsulinemia and hormonal parameters in overweight patients with polycystic ovary syndrome. Gynecol Endocrinol. 2008 Mar;24(3):139-44. ("Genazzani 2008").

4 Baptiste CG, Battista MC, Trottier A, Baillargeon JP. Insulin and hyperandrogenism in women with polycystic ovary syndrome. J Steroid Biochem Mol Biol. 2010 Oct;122(1-3):42-52.

Filicori M, Flamigni C, Campaniello E, Meriggiola MC, Michelacci L, Valdiserri A, Ferrari P. Polycystic ovary syndrome: abnormalities and management with pulsatile gonadotropin-releasing hormone and gonadotropin-releasing hormone analogs. Am J Obstet Gynecol. 1990 Nov;163(5 Pt 2):1737-42.

5 Baillargeon JP, Diamanti-Kandarakis E, Ostlund RE Jr, Apridonidze T, Iuorno MJ, Nestler JE. Altered D-chiro-inositol urinary clearance in women with polycystic ovary syndrome. Diabetes Care. 2006 Feb;29(2):300-5; Constantino 2009.

Chiu TT, Rogers MS, Briton-Jones C, Haines C. Effects of myo-inositol on the in-vitro maturation and subsequent development of mouse oocytes. Hum Reprod. 2003 Feb;18(2):408-16.

6 Papaleo E, Unfer V, Baillargeon JP, De Santis L, Fusi F, Brigante C, Marelli G, Cino I, Redaelli A, Ferrari A. Myo-inositol in patients with polycystic ovary syndrome: a novel method for ovulation induction. Gynecol Endocrinol. 2007 Dec;23(12):700-3.

7 Genazzani 2008; Costantino D, Minozzi G, Minozzi E, Guaraldi C.Metabolic and hormonal effects of myo-inositol in women with polycystic ovary syndrome: a double-blind trial.Eur Rev Med Pharmacol Sci. 2009 Mar-Apr;13(2):105-10.

8 Papaleo 2009

9 Ciotta L, Stracquadanio M, Pagano I, Carbonaro A, Palumbo M, Gulino F.Effects of myo-inositol supplementation on oocyte's quality in

PCOS patients: a double blind trial.Eur Rev Med Pharmacol Sci. 2011 May;15(5):509-14.

10   Unfer V, Carlomagno G, Rizzo P, Raffone E, Roseff S. Myo-inositol rather than D-chiro-inositol is able to improve oocyte quality in intracytoplasmic sperm injection cycles. A prospective, controlled, randomized trial. Eur Rev Med Pharmacol Sci. 2011 Apr;15(4):452-7.

11   Pacchiarotti, A., Carlomagno, G., Antonini, G., & Pacchiarotti, A. (2016). Effect of myo-inositol and melatonin versus myo-inositol, in a randomized controlled trial, for improving in vitro fertilization of patients with polycystic ovarian syndrome. Gynecological endocrinology, 32(1), 69-73.

12   D'Anna R, Di Benedetto V, Rizzo P, Raffone E, Interdonato ML, Corrado F, Di Benedetto A. Myo-inositol may prevent gestational diabetes in PCOS women. Gynecol Endocrinol. 2012 Jun;28(6):440-2

13   Crawford, T. J., Crowther, C. A., Alsweiler, J., & Brown, J. (2015). Antenatal dietary supplementation with myo-inositol in women during pregnancy for preventing gestational diabetes. Cochrane Database of Systematic Reviews, (12).

14   Craig LB, Ke RW, Kutteh WH.Increased prevalence of insulin resistance in women with a history of recurrent pregnancy loss. Fertil Steril. 2002 Sep;78(3):487-90. ("Craig 2002").

15   Craig 2002.

16   Vega, M., Mauro, M., & Williams, Z. (2019). Direct toxicity of insulin on the human placenta and protection by metformin. Fertility and Sterility, 111(3), 489-496.

17   Fatima, K., Jamil, Z., Faheem, S., Adnan, A., Javaid, S. S., Naeem, H., ... & Ochani, S. (2023). Effects of myo-inositol vs. metformin on hormonal and metabolic parameters in women with PCOS: a meta-analysis. Irish Journal of Medical Science (1971-), 1-8.

18   Lisi 2012; Carlomagno G, Unfer V.Inositol safety: clinical evidences. Eur Rev Med Pharmacol Sci. 2011 Aug;15(8):931-6.

19   Mitchell Bebel Stargrove, Jonathan Treasure, Dwight L. McKee. Herb, Nutrient, and Drug Interactions: Clinical Implications and Therapeutic Strategies, Health Sciences, 2008, p. 765.

20   Isabella R, Raffone E. Does ovary need D-chiro-inositol? J Ovarian Res. 2012 May 15;5(1):14. ("Isabella 2012").

21   Galletta M, Grasso S, Vaiarelli A, Roseff SJ. Bye-bye chiro-inositol - myo-inositol: true progress in the treatment of polycystic ovary syndrome and ovulation induction. Eur Rev Med Pharmacol Sci. 2011 Oct;15(10):1212-4.

22   Isabella 2012

23   Kalra, B., Kalra, S., & Sharma, J. B. (2016). The inositols and polycystic ovary syndrome. Indian journal of endocrinology and metabolism, 20(5), 720.

24   Carlomagno G, Unfer V, Roseff S.The D-chiro-inositol paradox in the ovary.Fertil Steril. 2011 Jun 30;95(8):2515-6.

25 Nordio, M., & Proietti, E. (2012). The combined therapy with myo-inositol and D-chiro-inositol reduces the risk of metabolic disease in PCOS overweight patients compared to myo-inositol supplementation alone. Eur Rev Med Pharmacol Sci, 16(5), 575-81.

Chapter 9. DHEA for Low Ovarian Reserve

1   Harper AJ, Buster JE, Casson PR. Changes in adrenocortical function with aging and therapeutic implications. Semin Reprod Endocrinol. 1999;17(4):327-38.

2   Doldi, N., Belvisi, L., Bassan, M., Fusi, F. M., & Ferrari, A. (1998). Premature ovarian failure: steroid synthesis and autoimmunity. Gynecological Endocrinology, 12(1), 23-28.
    Gleicher, N., Kushnir, V. A., Weghofer, A., & Barad, D. H. (2016). The importance of adrenal hypoandrogenism in infertile women with low functional ovarian reserve: a case study of associated adrenal insufficiency. Reproductive Biology and Endocrinology, 14(1), 23.

3   Chen, S. N., Tsui, K. H., Wang, P. H., Chern, C. U., Wen, Z. H., & Lin, L. T. (2019). Dehydroepiandrosterone supplementation improves the outcomes of in vitro fertilization cycles in older patients with diminished ovarian reserve. Frontiers in Endocrinology, 10, 800.
    Wiser, A., Gonen, O., Ghetler, Y., Shavit, T., Berkovitz, A., & Shulman, A. (2010). Addition of dehydroepiandrosterone (DHEA) for poor-responder patients before and during IVF treatment improves the pregnancy rate: a randomized prospective study. Human Reproduction, 25(10), 2496-2500.
    Kotb, M. M., Hassan, A. M., & AwadAllah, A. M. (2016). Does dehydroepiandrosterone improve pregnancy rate in women undergoing IVF/ICSI with expected poor ovarian response according to the Bologna criteria? A randomized controlled trial. European Journal of Obstetrics & Gynecology and Reproductive Biology, 200, 11-15.
    Moawad, A., & Shaeer, M. (2012). Long-term androgen priming by use of dehydroepiandrosterone (DHEA) improves IVF outcome in poor-responder patients. A randomized controlled study. Middle East Fertility Society Journal, 17(4), 268-274.

4   Casson PR, Lindsay MS, Pisarska MD, Carson SA, Buster JE. Dehydroepiandrosterone supplementation augments ovarian stimulation in poor responders: a case series. Hum Reprod 2000;15:2129-2132.

5   Barad DH, et al, Update on the use of dehydroepiandrosterone supplementation among women with diminished ovarian reserve. J Assist Reprod Genet 2007;24(12):629-34.

6   http://www.centerforhumanreprod.com/dhea.html, interview with CBS News.

7   Gleicher N, Barad DH. Dehydroepiandrosterone (DHEA) supplementation in diminished ovarian reserve (DOR). Reprod Biol Endocrinol. 2011 May 17;9:67 ("Gleicher 2011").

8   Kotb, M. M., Hassan, A. M., & AwadAllah, A. M. (2016). Does
     dehydroepiandrosterone improve pregnancy rate in women undergoing
     IVF/ICSI with expected poor ovarian response according to the Bologna
     criteria? A randomized controlled trial. European Journal of Obstetrics
     & Gynecology and Reproductive Biology, 200, 11-15.
     Wiser, A., Gonen, O., Ghetler, Y., Shavit, T., Berkovitz, A., & Shulman, A.
     (2010). Addition of dehydroepiandrosterone (DHEA) for poor-responder
     patients before and during IVF treatment improves the pregnancy rate: a
     randomized prospective study. Human Reproduction, 25(10), 2496-2500.
     Moawad, A., & Shaeer, M. (2012). Long-term androgen priming by use
     of dehydroepiandrosterone (DHEA) improves IVF outcome in poor-
     responder patients. A randomized controlled study. Middle East Fertility
     Society Journal, 17(4), 268-274.
9   Kotb, M. M., Hassan, A. M., & AwadAllah, A. M. (2016). Does
     dehydroepiandrosterone improve pregnancy rate in women undergoing
     IVF/ICSI with expected poor ovarian response according to the Bologna
     criteria? A randomized controlled trial. European Journal of Obstetrics
     & Gynecology and Reproductive Biology, 200, 11-15.
10   Chern, C. U., Tsui, K. H., Vitale, S. G., Chen, S. N., Wang, P. H.,
     Cianci, A., ... & Lin, L. T. (2018). Dehydroepiandrosterone (DHEA)
     supplementation improves in vitro fertilization outcomes of poor
     ovarian responders, especially in women with low serum concentration
     of DHEA-S: a retrospective cohort study. Reproductive Biology and
     Endocrinology, 16(1), 90.
11   Wang, Z., Yang, A., Bao, H., Wang, A., Deng, X., Xue, D., ... & Shi, Y.
     (2022). Effect of dehydroepiandrosterone administration before in vitro
     fertilization on the live birth rate in poor ovarian responders according
     to the Bologna criteria: A randomised controlled trial. BJOG: An
     International Journal of Obstetrics & Gynaecology, 129(7), 1030-1038.
12   Perelló, M. A., Moreno, J. A., Crespo, M., Espinós, J. J., & Checa, M.
     Á. (2022). Does Dehydroepiandrosterone supplementation improve
     reproductive outcomes in patients with normal ovarian reserve
     undergoing in vitro fertilization? A systematic review and meta-analysis.
     Medicina Reproductiva y Embriología Clínica, 9(3), 100120.
     Neves, A. R., Montoya-Botero, P., & Polyzos, N. P. (2022). Androgens and
     diminished ovarian reserve: the long road from basic science to clinical
     implementation. A comprehensive and systematic review with meta-
     analysis. American Journal of Obstetrics and Gynecology.
     Richardson, A., & Jayaprakasan, K. (2021, November). The Use
     of Androgen Priming in Women with Reduced Ovarian Reserve
     Undergoing Assisted Reproductive Technology. In Seminars in
     Reproductive Medicine (Vol. 39, No. 05/06, pp. 207-219). Thieme Medical
     Publishers, Inc.

Zhang, Y., Zhang, C., Shu, J., Guo, J., Chang, H. M., Leung, P. C., ... & Huang, H. (2020). Adjuvant treatment strategies in ovarian stimulation for poor responders undergoing IVF: a systematic review and network meta-analysis. Human Reproduction Update, 26(2), 247-263.

Xu L, Hu C, Liu Q, Li Y. The Effect of Dehydroepiandrosterone (DHEA) Supplementation on IVF or ICSI: A Meta-Analysis of Randomized Controlled Trials. Geburtshilfe Frauenheilkd (2019) 79(7):705–12. doi: 10.1055/a-0882-3791

de Souza Monteiro, C., Scheffer, B. B., de Carvalho, R. F., & Scheffer, J. B. (2019). The impact of dehydroepiandrosterone in poor ovarian responders on assisted reproduction technology treatment. JBRA Assisted Reproduction, 23(4), 414

Schwarze JE, Canales J, Crosby J, Ortega-Hrepich C, Villa S, Pommer R. DHEA Use to Improve Likelihood of IVF/ICSI Success in Patients With Diminished Ovarian Reserve: A Systematic Review and Meta-Analysis. J Bras Reprod Assist (2018) 22(4):369–74

Liu Y, Hu L, Fan L, Wang F. Efficacy of Dehydroepiandrosterone (DHEA) Supplementation for in Vitro Fertilization and Embryo Transfer Cycles: A Systematic Review and Meta-Analysis. Gynecol Endocrinol (2017) 34(3):178–83.

Lin, J., Dang, Y., Guo, G., & Wang, Z. (2017). The influence of dehydroepiandrosterone (DHEA) supplementation for in vitro fertilization in women with diminished ovarian reserve: a meta-analysis of randomized controlled trials. Int J Clin Exp Med, 10(12), 15878-15885.

Qin JC, Fan L, Qin AP. The Effect of Dehydroepiandrosterone (DHEA) Supplementation on Women With Diminished Ovarian Reserve (DOR) in IVF Cycle: Evidence From a Meta-Analysis. J Gynecol Obstet Hum Reprod (2016) 46(1):1–7.

Li, J., Yuan, H., Chen, Y., Wu, H., Wu, H., & Li, L. (2015). A meta-analysis of dehydroepiandrosterone supplementation among women with diminished ovarian reserve undergoing in vitro fertilization or intracytoplasmic sperm injection. International Journal of Gynecology & Obstetrics, 131(3), 240-245.

Narkwichean A, Maalouf W, Campbell BK, Jayaprakasan K. Efficacy of Dehydroepiandrosterone to Improve Ovarian Response in Women With Diminished Ovarian Reserve: A Meta-Analysis. Reprod Biol Endocrinol (2013) 11:1–8. doi: 10.1186/1477-7827-11-44

13   Neves, A. R., Montoya-Botero, P., & Polyzos, N. P. (2021). The role of androgen supplementation in women with diminished ovarian reserve: time to randomize, not meta-analyze. Frontiers in Endocrinology, 12, 653857.

14   Chern, C. U., Tsui, K. H., Vitale, S. G., Chen, S. N., Wang, P. H., Cianci, A., ... & Lin, L. T. (2018). Dehydroepiandrosterone (DHEA) supplementation improves in vitro fertilization outcomes of poor

ovarian responders, especially in women with low serum concentration of DHEA-S: a retrospective cohort study. Reproductive Biology and Endocrinology, 16(1), 90.

15 Chimote, B. N., & Chimote, N. M. (2021). Dehydroepiandrosterone sulphate (DHEAS) concentrations stringently regulate fertilisation, embryo development and IVF outcomes: are we looking at a potentially compelling 'oocyte-related factor'in oocyte activation?. Journal of Assisted Reproduction and Genetics, 38(1), 193-202.

16 Malik, N., Kriplani, A., Agarwal, N., Bhatla, N., Kachhawa, G., & Yadav, R. K. (2015). Dehydroepiandrosterone as an adjunct to gonadotropins in infertile Indian women with premature ovarian aging: A pilot study. Journal of human reproductive sciences, 8(3), 135.

17 Bedaiwy MA, Ryan E, Shaaban O, Claessens EA, Blanco-Mejia S, Casper RF: Follicular conditioning with dehydroepiandrosterone co-treatment improves IUI outcome in clomiphene citrate patients. 55th Annual Meeting of the Canadian Fertility and Andrology Society, Montreal, Canada, November 18-21, 2009.

18 Ozcil, M. D. (2020). Dehydroepiandrosterone supplementation improves ovarian reserve and pregnancy rates in poor responders. European review for medical and pharmacological sciences, 24(17), 9104-9111.

19 Fusi FM, Ferrario M, Bosisio C, Arnoldi M, Zanga L. DHEA supplementation positively affects spontaneous pregnancies in women with diminished ovarian function. Gynecol Endocrinol. 2013 Oct;29(10):940-3 ("Fusi 2013").

20 Barad 2007.

21 Barad 2007; Fusi 2013.

22 Chatterjee, S., Chowdhury, R. G., Dey, S., & Ganguly, D. (2015). Pregnancy in a lady with premature ovarian failure following dehydroepiandrosterone (DHEA) treatment. Fertility Science and Research, 2(1), 40.

23 Mamas, L., & Mamas, E. (2009). Premature ovarian failure and dehydroepiandrosterone. Fertility and sterility, 91(2), 644-646.

24 Wong, Q. H. Y., Yeung, T. W. Y., Yung, S. S. F., Ko, J. K. Y., Li, H. W. R., & Ng, E. H. Y. (2018). The effect of 12-month dehydroepiandrosterone supplementation on the menstrual pattern, ovarian reserve markers, and safety profile in women with premature ovarian insufficiency. Journal of Assisted Reproduction and Genetics, 35, 857-862.

25 Gleicher N, et al, Miscarriage rates after dehydroepiandrosterone (DHEA) supplementation in women with diminished ovarian reserve: a case control study. Reprod Biol Endocrinol 2009;7(7):108 ("Gleicher 2009").

26 Gleicher 2010a.

27 Grunwald, K., Feldmann, K., Melsheimer, P., Rabe, T., Neulen, J., & Runnebaum, B. (1998). Aneuploidy in human granulosa lutein cells obtained from gonadotrophin-stimulated follicles and its relation to

intrafollicular hormone concentrations. Human reproduction (Oxford, England), 13(10), 2679-2687.

28 Zhang, M., Niu, W., Wang, Y., Xu, J., Bao, X., Wang, L., ... & Sun, Y. (2016). Dehydroepiandrosterone treatment in women with poor ovarian response undergoing IVF or ICSI: a systematic review and meta-analysis. Journal of assisted reproduction and genetics, 33(8), 981-991.
Schwarze, J. E., Canales, J., Crosby, J., Ortega-Hrepich, C., Villa, S., & Pommer, R. (2018). DHEA use to improve likelihood of IVF/ICSI success in patients with diminished ovarian reserve: A systematic review and meta-analysis. JBRA assisted reproduction, 22(4), 369.
Perelló, M. A., Moreno, J. A., Crespo, M., Espinós, J. J., & Checa, M. Á. (2022). Does Dehydroepiandrosterone supplementation improve reproductive outcomes in patients with normal ovarian reserve undergoing in vitro fertilization? A systematic review and meta-analysis. Medicina Reproductiva y Embriología Clínica, 9(3), 100120.

29 Rao, K. A. (2018). DHEA supplementation in a woman with endometriosis desiring pregnancy. MEDICINE, 25(9), 24.; https://www.centerforhumanreprod.com/fertility/endometriosis-infertility-monthly-case-report/

30 Zhang, Y., Li, M., Li, L., Xiao, J., & Chen, Z. (2021). Randomized Controlled Study of the Effects of DHEA on the Outcome of IVF in Endometriosis. Evidence-Based Complementary and Alternative Medicine, 2021.

31 Gleicher, N., Kushnir, V. A., Darmon, S. K., Wang, Q., Zhang, L., Albertini, D. F., & Barad, D. H. (2017). New PCOS-like phenotype in older infertile women of likely autoimmune adrenal etiology with high AMH but low androgens. The Journal of steroid biochemistry and molecular biology, 167, 144-152.

32 Gleicher 2011; Wiser 2010.

33 Sen A, Hammes SR: Granulosa cell-specific androgen receptors are critical regulators of development and function. Mol Endocrinol 2010, 24:1393-1403.

34 Saharkhiz, N., Zademodares, S., Salehpour, S., Hosseini, S., Nazari, L., & Tehrani, H. G. (2018). The effect of testosterone gel on fertility outcomes in women with a poor response in in vitro fertilization cycles: a pilot randomized clinical trial. Journal of research in medical sciences: the official journal of Isfahan University of Medical Sciences, 23.
Katsika, E. T., Bosdou, J. K., Goulis, D. G., Grimbizis, G. F., & Kolibianakis, E. M. (2022). Higher probability of live birth after transdermal testosterone pretreatment in women with poor ovarian response undergoing IVF: a systematic review and meta-analysis: Primary Outcome. Reproductive BioMedicine Online.
Fabregues, F., Penarrubia, J., Creus, M., Manau, D., Casals, G., Carmona, F., & Balasch, J. (2009). Transdermal testosterone may improve

ovarian response to gonadotrophins in low-responder IVF patients: a randomized, clinical trial. Human Reproduction, 24(2), 349-359.

Subirá, J., Algaba, A., Vázquez, S., Dasí, R. T., Robles, G. M., Fabuel, S. M., ... & Rubio, J. M. R. (2021). Testosterone does not improve ovarian response in Bologna poor responders: a randomized controlled trial (TESTOPRIM). Reproductive BioMedicine Online, 43(3), 466-474.

Nayar, K. D., Gupta, S., Bhattacharya, R., Mehra, P., Mishra, J., Kant, G., & Nayar, K. (2021). P–612 Transdermal testosterone vs. Placebo (lubricant gel) pre-treatment in improving IVF outcomes in diminished ovarian reserve patients (POSEIDON group 3 and 4): a randomised controlled trial. Human Reproduction, 36(Supplement_1), deab130-611.

35   Gleicher 2011.

36   Gleicher 2011

37   Wiser 2010.

38   Panjari M, Bell RJ, Jane F, Adams J, Morrow C, Davis SR: The safety of 52 weeks of oral DHEA therapy for postmenopausal women. Maturitas 2009, 63:240-245.

39   Franasiak, J. M., Thomas, S., Ng, S., Fano, M., Ruiz, A., Scott, R. T., & Forman, E. J. (2016). Dehydroepiandrosterone (DHEA) supplementation results in supraphysiologic DHEA-S serum levels and progesterone assay interference that may impact clinical management in IVF. Journal of assisted reproduction and genetics, 33(3), 387-391.

Chapter 10: Supplements to Avoid

1   Ragonese, F., Monarca, L., De Luca, A., Mancinelli, L., Mariani, M., Corbucci, C., ... & Fioretti, B. (2021). Resveratrol depolarizes the membrane potential in human granulosa cells and promotes mitochondrial biogenesis. Fertility and Sterility , 115 (4), 1063-1073.

2   Ochiai, A., Kuroda, K., Ikemoto, Y., Ozaki, R., Nakagawa, K., Nojiri, S., ... & Sugiyama, R. (2019). Influence of resveratrol supplementation on IVF–embryo transfer cycle outcomes. Reproductive BioMedicine Online, 39(2), 205-210.

3   Ochiai, A., Kuroda, K., Ozaki, R., Ikemoto, Y., Murakami, K., Muter, J., ... & Takeda, S. (2019). Resveratrol inhibits decidualization by accelerating downregulation of the CRABP2-RAR pathway in differentiating human endometrial stromal cells. Cell Death & Disease, 10(4), 276.

4   Igarashi, H., Aono, N., Nakajo, Y., Hattori, H., Takahashi, M., Koizumi, M., ... & Kyono, K. (2018). Effects of melatonin and resveratrol on embryo development and clinical outcomes in poor-prognosis IVF patients. Fertility and Sterility, 110(4), e195-e196.

Gerli, S., Della Morte, C., Ceccobelli, M., Mariani, M., Favilli, A., Leonardi, L., ... & Fioretti, B. (2022). Biological and clinical effects of a resveratrol-based multivitamin supplement on intracytoplasmic sperm injection cycles: A single-center, randomized controlled trial. The Journal of Maternal-Fetal & Neonatal Medicine, 35(25), 7640-7648.

5   Igarashi, H., Aono, N., Nakajo, Y., Hattori, H., Takahashi, M., Koizumi, M., ... & Kyono, K. (2018). Effects of melatonin and resveratrol on embryo development and clinical outcomes in poor-prognosis IVF patients. Fertility and Sterility, 110(4), e195-e196.

6   Ochiai, A., Kuroda, K., Ikemoto, Y., Ozaki, R., Nakagawa, K., Nojiri, S., ... & Sugiyama, R. (2019). Influence of resveratrol supplementation on IVF–embryo transfer cycle outcomes. Reproductive BioMedicine Online, 39(2), 205-210.

7   Rajuddin, R.., Wiweko, B., & Nugroho, L. (2019). The effects of curcumin administration on expression patterns of VEGF and COX-2 in fertile endometrium: A randomised clinical trial.
Mohajeri, M., Bianconi, V., Ávila-Rodriguez, M. F., Barreto, G. E., Jamialahmadi, T., Pirro, M., & Sahebkar, A. (2020). Curcumin: a phytochemical modulator of estrogens and androgens in tumors of the reproductive system. Pharmacological Research, 156, 104765.
Busman, H., Farisi, S., & Fahrumnisa, A. R. (2022). Turmeric Rhizome's Extract Reduce Epithelium Cells and Endometrium Layer Thickness of Female Rats. Biomedical and Pharmacology Journal, 15(1), 299-304.

8   O'Connell, A. A., Abdalla, T. E., Radulovich, A. A., Best, J. C., Wood, E. G., O'Connell, A., ... & Wood, E. (2021). Curcumin Supplementation and Endometrial Lining: Examining the Role and Pathophysiology of Use During Frozen-Thawed Embryo Transfer. Cureus, 13(12).

9   Chen, C. C., & Chan, W. H. (2012). Injurious effects of curcumin on maturation of mouse oocytes, fertilization and fetal development via apoptosis. International journal of molecular sciences, 13(4), 4655-4672.

10 Souto, E. B., Durazzo, A., Nazhand, A., Lucarini, M., Zaccardelli, M., Souto, S. B., ... & Santini, A. (2020). Vitex agnus-castus L.: main features and nutraceutical perspectives. Forests, 11(7), 761.

11 Souto, E. B., Durazzo, A., Nazhand, A., Lucarini, M., Zaccardelli, M., Souto, S. B., ... & Santini, A. (2020). Vitex agnus-castus L.: main features and nutraceutical perspectives. Forests, 11(7), 761.

12 Wuttke, W., Jarry, H., Christoffel, V., Spengler, B., & Seidlova-Wuttke, D. (2003). Chaste tree (Vitex agnus-castus)–pharmacology and clinical indications. Phytomedicine, 10(4), 348-357.
Milewicz, A., Gejdel, E., Sworen, H., Sienkiewicz, K., Jedrzejak, J., Teucher, T., & Schmitz, H. (1993). Vitex agnus castus extract in the treatment of luteal phase defects due to latent hyperprolactinemia. Results of a randomized placebo-controlled double-blind study. Arzneimittel-forschung, 43(7), 752-756.
Hossein-Rashidi, B., & Nemati, M. (2017). Effects of Vitex agnus-castus extract on the secretory function of pituitary-gonadal axis and

pregnancy rate in patients with premature ovarian aging (POA). Journal of herbal medicine, 10, 24-30.

Westphal, L. M., Polan, M. L., Trant, A. S., & Mooney, S. B. (2004). A nutritional supplement for improving fertility in women. J Reprod Med, 49(4), 289-93.

13 Najib, F. S., Poordast, T., Mahmudi, M. S., Shiravani, Z., Namazi, N., & Omrani, G. R. (2022). Does Vitex Agnus-Castus L. Have Deleterious Effect on Fertility and Pregnancy Outcome? An Experimental Study on Rats for Prediction of Its Safety. Journal of Pharmacopuncture, 25(2), 106.

14 Beharry, S., & Heinrich, M. (2018). Is the hype around the reproductive health claims of maca (Lepidium meyenii Walp.) justified?. Journal of Ethnopharmacology, 211, 126-170.

Melnikovova, I., Tomas, F., Huml, L., Kolarova, M., Lapcik, O., & Cusimamani, E. (2014). Effect of Lepidium meyenii on semen quality and reproductive hormones level in healthy adult men. Climacteric, 17(1), 87.

Poveda, C., Rodriguez, R., Chu, E. E., Aparicio, L. E., Gonzales, I. G., & Moreno, C. J. (2013). A placebo-controlled double-blind randomized trial of the effect of oral supplementation with spermotrend, maca extract (Lepidium meyenii) or L-carnitine in semen parameters of infertile men. Fertility and Sterility, 100(3), S440.

15 Meissner, H. O., Kapczynski, W., Mscisz, A., & Lutomski, J. (2005). Use of gelatinized maca (lepidium peruvianum) in early postmenopausal women. International journal of biomedical science: IJBS, 1(1), 33.

16 Takewaka, T., & Hara, K. (2019). Clinical effect of oral administration of maca (Lepidium meyenii) extract on japanese peri-menopausal women subjects: A randomized, double-blind, placebo-controlled study. International Journal of Biomedical Science,, 15, 11-18.

Meissner, H. O., Reich-Bilinska, H., Mscisz, A., & Kedzia, B. (2006). Therapeutic Effects of Pre-Gelatinized Maca (Lepidium peruvianum Chacon) used as a non-hormonal alternative to HRT in perimenopausal women-Clinical Pilot Study. International journal of biomedical science: IJBS, 2(2), 143.

Brooks, N. A., Wilcox, G., Walker, K. Z., Ashton, J. F., Cox, M. B., & Stojanovska, L. (2008). Beneficial effects of Lepidium meyenii (Maca) on psychological symptoms and measures of sexual dysfunction in postmenopausal women are not related to estrogen or androgen content. Menopause, 15(6), 1157-1162.

17 Mendoza, E. O., Cuadrado, W., Yallico, L., Zárate, R., Quispe-Melgar, H. R., Limaymanta, C. H., ... & Bao-Cóndor, D. (2021). Heavy metals in soils and edible tissues of Lepidium meyenii (maca) and health risk assessment in areas influenced by mining activity in the Central region of Peru. Toxicology Reports, 8, 1461-1470.

18 Blank S, Bantleon FI, McIntyre M, Ollert M, Spillner E. The major royal jelly proteins 8 and 9 (Api m 11) are glycosylated components of Apis

mellifera venom with allergenic potential beyond carbohydrate-based reactivity. Clin Exp Allergy. 2012 Jun;42(6):976-85.

19 Morita H, Ikeda T, Kajita K, Fujioka K, Mori I, Okada H, Uno Y, Ishizuka T. Effect of royal jelly ingestion for six months on healthy volunteers. Nutr J. 2012 Sep 21;11:77.

20 Battaglia C, Salvatori M, Maxia N, Petraglia F, Facchinetti F, Volpe A. Adjuvant L-arginine treatment for in-vitro fertilization in poor responder patients. Hum Reprod. 1999 Jul;14(7):1690-7. ("Battaglia 1999").

21 Battaglia 1999.

22 Battaglia C, Regnani G, Marsella T, Facchinetti F, Volpe A, Venturoli S, Flamigni C. Adjuvant L-arginine treatment in controlled ovarian hyperstimulation: a double-blind, randomized study.Hum Reprod. 2002 Mar;17(3):659-65.

23 Bódis J, Várnagy A, Sulyok E, Kovács GL, Martens-Lobenhoffer J, Bode-Böger SM.Negative association of L-arginine methylation products with oocyte numbers.Hum Reprod. 2010 Dec;25(12):3095-100. doi: 10.1093/humrep/deq257. Epub 2010 Sep 24.

24 So, S., Yamaguchi, W., Murabayashi, N., Miyano, N., Tawara, F., & Kanayama, N. (2020). Beneficial effect of l-arginine in women using assisted reproductive technologies: a small-scale randomized controlled trial. Nutrition Research, 82, 67-73.

Chapter 12: The Egg Quality Diet

1 Hjollund NHI, Jensen TK, Bonde JPE, Henriksen NE, Andersson AM, Skakkebaek NE. Is glycosilated haemoglobin a marker of fertility? A follow-up study of first-pregnancy planners. Hum Reprod. 1999;14:1478–1482 ("Hjolland 1999").

2 Chavarro JE, Rich-Edwards JW, Rosner BA, Willett WC. A prospective study of dietary carbohydrate quantity and quality in relation to risk of ovulatory infertility. Eur J Clin Nutr. 2009 Jan;63(1):78-86 ("Chavarro 2009a").

3 Dumesic DA, Abbott DH. Implications of polycystic ovary syndrome on oocyte development. Semin Reprod Med. 2008 Jan;26(1):53-61.

4 Jinno 2011.

5 Jinno, M., Takeuchi, M., Watanabe, A., Teruya, K., Hirohama, J., Eguchi, N., & Miyazaki, A. (2011). Advanced glycation end-products accumulation compromises embryonic development and achievement of pregnancy by assisted reproductive technology. Human reproduction, 26(3), 604-610.

6 Abuarab, N., Munsey, T. S., Jiang, L. H., Li, J., & Sivaprasadarao, A. (2017). High glucose–induced ROS activates TRPM2 to trigger lysosomal

membrane permeabilization and Zn2+-mediated mitochondrial fission. Science Signaling, 10(490), eaal4161.

7   Tatone C, Amicarelli F, Carbone MC, Monteleone P, Caserta D, Marci R, Artini PG, Piomboni P, Focarelli R. Cellular and molecular aspects of ovarian follicle ageing. Hum Reprod Update. 2008 Mar-Apr;14(2):131-42.

8   Wang Q, Moley KH. Maternal diabetes and oocyte quality. Mitochondrion. 2010 Aug;10(5):403-10 ("Wang 2010").

9   Craig LB, Ke RW, Kutteh WH. Increased prevalence of insulin resistance in women with a history of recurrent pregnancy loss. Fertil Steril. 2002 Sep;78(3):487-90.
    Chakraborty P, Goswami SK, Rajani S, Sharma S, Kabir SN, Chakravarty B, Jana K. Recurrent pregnancy loss in polycystic ovary syndrome: role of hyperhomocysteinemia and insulin resistance. PLoS One. 2013 May 21;8(5):e64446; Tian L, Shen H, Lu Q, Norman RJ, Wang J. Insulin resistance increases the risk of spontaneous abortion after assisted reproduction technology treatment. J Clin Endocrinol Metab. 2007 Apr;92(4):1430-3.

10 Russell, J. B., Abboud, C., Williams, A., Gibbs, M., Pritchard, S., & Chalfant, D. (2012). Does changing a patient's dietary consumption of proteins and carbohydrates impact blastocyst development and clinical pregnancy rates from one cycle to the next?. Fertility and Sterility, 98(3), S47.

11 McGrice, M., & Porter, J. (2017). The effect of low carbohydrate diets on fertility hormones and outcomes in overweight and obese women: a systematic review. Nutrients, 9(3), 204.

12 Machtinger, R., Gaskins, A. J., Mansur, A., Adir, M., Racowsky, C., Baccarelli, A. A., ... & Chavarro, J. E. (2017). Association between preconception maternal beverage intake and in vitro fertilization outcomes. Fertility and sterility, 108(6), 1026-1033. Hatch, E. E., Wesselink, A. K., Hahn, K. A., Michiel, J. J., Mikkelsen, E. M., Sorensen, H. T., ... & Wise, L. A. (2018). Intake of Sugar-sweetened Beverages and Fecundability in a North American Preconception Cohort. Epidemiology, 29(3), 369-378.

13 Melanson KJ, Zukley L, Lowndes J, Nguyen V, Angelopoulos TJ, Rippe JM. Effects of high-fructose corn syrup and sucrose consumption on circulating glucose, insulin, leptin, and ghrelin and on appetite in normal-weight women. Nutrition. 2007;23:103–112.
    Stanhope KL, Griffen SC, Bair BR, Swarbrick MM, Keim NL, Havel PJ. Twenty-four-hour endocrine and metabolic profiles following consumption of high-fructose corn syrup-, sucrose-, fructose-, and glucose-sweetened beverages with meals. Am J Clin Nutr. 2008;87:1194–1203

14 Shukla, A. P., Iliescu, R. G., Thomas, C. E., & Aronne, L. J. (2015). Food order has a significant impact on postprandial glucose and insulin levels. Diabetes care, 38(7), e98-e99.

Nishino, K., Sakurai, M., Takeshita, Y., & Takamura, T. (2018). Consuming carbohydrates after meat or vegetables lowers postprandial excursions of glucose and insulin in nondiabetic subjects. Journal of nutritional science and vitaminology, 64(5), 316-320.

Tricò, D., Filice, E., Trifirò, S., & Natali, A. (2016). Manipulating the sequence of food ingestion improves glycemic control in type 2 diabetic patients under free-living conditions. Nutrition & diabetes, 6(8), e226-e226.

15 Santos, H. O., de Moraes, W. M., da Silva, G. A., Prestes, J., & Schoenfeld, B. J. (2019). Vinegar (acetic acid) intake on glucose metabolism: A narrative review. Clinical nutrition ESPEN, 32, 1-7.

Shishehbor, F., Mansoori, A., & Shirani, F. (2017). Vinegar consumption can attenuate postprandial glucose and insulin responses; a systematic review and meta-analysis of clinical trials. diabetes research and clinical practice, 127, 1-9.

Mitrou, P., Petsiou, E., Papakonstantinou, E., Maratou, E., Lambadiari, V., Dimitriadis, P., ... & Dimitriadis, G. (2015). Vinegar consumption increases insulin-stimulated glucose uptake by the forearm muscle in humans with type 2 diabetes. Journal of diabetes research, 2015.

16 Santos, H. O., de Moraes, W. M., da Silva, G. A., Prestes, J., & Schoenfeld, B. J. (2019). Vinegar (acetic acid) intake on glucose metabolism: A narrative review. Clinical nutrition ESPEN, 32, 1-7.

17 Wu, D., Kimura, F., Takashima, A., Shimizu, Y., Takebayashi, A., Kita, N., ... & Murakami, T. (2013). Intake of vinegar beverage is associated with restoration of ovulatory function in women with polycystic ovary syndrome. The Tohoku Journal of Experimental Medicine, 230(1), 17-23.

18 Bellini, A., Nicolò, A., Rocchi, J. E., Bazzucchi, I., & Sacchetti, M. (2023). Walking Attenuates Postprandial Glycemic Response: What Else Can We Do without Leaving Home or the Office?. International Journal of Environmental Research and Public Health, 20(1), 253.

Li, Z., Hu, Y., Yan, R., Zhang, D., Li, H., Li, F., ... & Ma, J. (2018). Twenty minute moderate-intensity post-dinner exercise reduces the postprandial glucose response in Chinese patients with type 2 diabetes. Medical Science Monitor: International Medical Journal of Experimental and Clinical Research, 24, 7170.

19 Heden, T. D., Winn, N. C., Mari, A., Booth, F. W., Rector, R. S., Thyfault, J. P., & Kanaley, J. A. (2015). Postdinner resistance exercise improves postprandial risk factors more effectively than predinner resistance exercise in patients with type 2 diabetes. Journal of Applied Physiology, 118(5), 624-634.

20 Afeiche, M. C., Chiu, Y. H., Gaskins, A. J., Williams, P. L., Souter, I., Wright, D. L., ... & Chavarro, J. E. (2016). Dairy intake in relation to in vitro fertilization outcomes among women from a fertility clinic. Human Reproduction, 31(3), 563-571.

21 Estruch, R., Ros, E., Salas-Salvadó, J., Covas, M. I., Corella, D., Arós, F., ... & Lamuela-Raventos, R. M. (2013). Primary prevention of cardiovascular disease with a Mediterranean diet. New England Journal of Medicine, 368(14), 1279-1290.

Sofi, F., Abbate, R., Gensini, G. F., & Casini, A. (2010). Accruing evidence on benefits of adherence to the Mediterranean diet on health: an updated systematic review and meta-analysis. The American journal of clinical nutrition, 92(5), 1189-1196.

Schwingshackl, L., & Hoffmann, G. (2014). Adherence to Mediterranean diet and risk of cancer: A systematic review and meta-analysis of observational studies. International journal of cancer, 135(8), 1884-1897.

Tresserra-Rimbau, A., Rimm, E. B., Medina-Remón, A., Martínez-González, M. A., López-Sabater, M. C., Covas, M. I., ... & Arós, F. (2014). Polyphenol intake and mortality risk: a re-analysis of the PREDIMED trial. BMC medicine, 12(1), 77.

Martínez-González, M. Á., De la Fuente-Arrillaga, C., Nuñez-Cordoba, J. M., Basterra-Gortari, F. J., Beunza, J. J., Vazquez, Z., ... & Bes-Rastrollo, M. (2008). Adherence to Mediterranean diet and risk of developing diabetes: prospective cohort study. Bmj, 336(7657), 1348-1351.

22 Chrysohoou, C., Panagiotakos, D. B., Pitsavos, C., Das, U. N., & Stefanadis, C. (2004). Adherence to the Mediterranean diet attenuates inflammation and coagulation process in healthy adults: The ATTICA Study. Journal of the American College of Cardiology, 44(1), 152-158.

Richard, C., Couture, P., Desroches, S., & Lamarche, B. (2013). Effect of the Mediterranean diet with and without weight loss on markers of inflammation in men with metabolic syndrome. Obesity, 21(1), 51-57.

Sköldstam, L., Hagfors, L., & Johansson, G. (2003). An experimental study of a Mediterranean diet intervention for patients with rheumatoid arthritis. Annals of the rheumatic diseases, 62(3), 208-214.

23 Maxia, N., Uccella, S., Ersettigh, G., Fantuzzi, M., Manganini, M., Scozzesi, A., & Colognato, R. (2018). Can unexplained infertility be evaluated by a new immunological four-biomarkers panel? A pilot study. Minerva ginecologica, 70(2), 129-137.

Xie, J., Yan, L., Cheng, Z., Qiang, L., Yan, J., Liu, Y., ... & Hao, C. (2018). Potential effect of inflammation on the failure risk of in vitro fertilization and embryo transfer among infertile women. Human Fertility, 1-9.

Buyuk, E., Asemota, O. A., Merhi, Z., Charron, M. J., Berger, D. S., Zapantis, A., & Jindal, S. K. (2017). Serum and follicular fluid monocyte chemotactic protein-1 levels are elevated in obese women and are associated with poorer clinical pregnancy rate after in vitro fertilization: a pilot study. Fertility and sterility, 107(3), 632-640.

Wagner, M. M., Jukema, J. W., Hermes, W., le Cessie, S., de Groot, C. J., Bakker, J. A., ... & Bloemenkamp, K. W. (2018). Assessment of novel cardiovascular biomarkers in women with a history of recurrent miscarriage. Pregnancy hypertension, 11, 129-135. See also: Ahmed, S. K., Mahmood, N., Malalla, Z. H., Alsobyani, F. M., Al-Kiyumi, I. S., & Almawi, W. Y. (2015). C-reactive protein gene variants associated with recurrent pregnancy loss independent of CRP serum levels: a case-control study. Gene, 569(1), 136-140. Kushnir, V. A., Solouki, S., Sarig-Meth, T., Vega, M. G., Albertini, D. F., Darmon, S. K., ... & Gleicher, N. (2016). Systemic inflammation and autoimmunity in women with chronic endometritis. American Journal of Reproductive Immunology, 75(6), 672-677.

24 Karayiannis, D., Kontogianni, M. D., Mendorou, C., Mastrominas, M., & Yiannakouris, N. (2018). Adherence to the Mediterranean diet and IVF success rate among non-obese women attempting fertility. Human Reproduction, 33(3), 494-502.

25 Vujkovic M, de Vries JH, Lindemans J, Macklon NS, van der Spek PJ, Steegers EA, Steegers-Theunissen RP. The preconception Mediterranean dietary pattern in couples undergoing in vitro fertilization/intracytoplasmic sperm injection treatment increases the chance of pregnancy.Fertil Steril. 2010 Nov;94(6):2096-101 ("Vujkovic 2010").

26 Ebisch IM, Peters WH, Thomas CM, Wetzels AM, Peer PG, Steegers-Theunissen RP. Homocysteine, glutathione and related thiols affect fertility parameters in the (sub)fertile couple.Hum Reprod. 2006 Jul;21(7):1725-33
Chakrabarty P, Goswami SK, Rajani S, Sharma S, Kabir SN, Chakravarty B, Jana K. Recurrent pregnancy loss in polycystic ovary syndrome: role of hyperhomocysteinemia and insulin resistance. PLoS One. 2013 May 21;8(5):e64446
Wouters MG, Boers GH, Blom HJ, Trijbels FJ, Thomas CM, Borm GF, Steegers-Theunissen RP, Eskes TK. Hyperhomocysteinemia: a risk factor in women with unexplained recurrent early pregnancy loss. Fertil Steril. 1993 Nov;60(5):820-5
Koloverou, E., Panagiotakos, D. B., Pitsavos, C., Chrysohoou, C., Georgousopoulou, E. N., Grekas, A., ... & Stefanadis, C. (2016). Adherence to Mediterranean diet and 10-year incidence (2002–2012) of diabetes: correlations with inflammatory and oxidative stress biomarkers in the ATTICA cohort study. Diabetes/metabolism research and reviews, 32(1), 73-81.
Arouca, A., Michels, N., Moreno, L. A., González-Gil, E. M., Marcos, A., Gómez, S., ... & Gottrand, F. (2018). Associations between a Mediterranean diet pattern and inflammatory biomarkers in European adolescents. European journal of nutrition, 57(5), 1747-1760

27 Ronnenberg AG, Venners SA, Xu X, Chen C, Wang L, Guang W, Huang A, Wang X. Preconception B-vitamin and homocysteine status,

conception, and early pregnancy loss.Am J Epidemiol. 2007 Aug 1;166(3):304-12.

28 Vujkovic 2010

29 Mirabi, P., Chaichi, M. J., Esmaeilzadeh, S., Jorsaraei, S. G. A., Bijani, A., Ehsani, M., & hashemi Karooee, S. F. (2017). The role of fatty acids on ICSI outcomes: a prospective cohort study. Lipids in health and disease, 16(1), 18

Moran, L. J., Tsagareli, V., Noakes, M., & Norman, R. (2016). Altered preconception fatty acid intake is associated with improved pregnancy rates in overweight and obese women undertaking in vitro fertilisation. Nutrients, 8(1), 10

Chiu, Y. H., Karmon, A. E., Gaskins, A. J., Arvizu, M., Williams, P. L., Souter, I., ... & EARTH Study Team. (2017). Serum omega-3 fatty acids and treatment outcomes among women undergoing assisted reproduction. Human Reproduction, 33(1), 156-165.)

Hammiche F, Vujkovic M, Wijburg W, de Vries JH, Macklon NS, Laven JS, Steegers-Theunissen RP. Increased preconception omega-3 polyunsaturated fatty acid intake improves embryo morphology. Fertil Steril. 2011 Apr;95(5):1820-3.

30 Chiu, Y. H., Karmon, A. E., Gaskins, A. J., Arvizu, M., Williams, P. L., Souter, I., ... & EARTH Study Team. (2017). Serum omega-3 fatty acids and treatment outcomes among women undergoing assisted reproduction. Human Reproduction, 33(1), 156-165.)

31 Wise, L. A., Wesselink, A. K., Tucker, K. L., Saklani, S., Mikkelsen, E. M., Cueto, H., ... & Rothman, K. J. (2017). Dietary Fat Intake and Fecundability in 2 Preconception Cohort Studies. American journal of epidemiology, 187(1), 60-74.

32 Salas-Huetos, A., Arvizu, M., Mínguez-Alarcón, L., Mitsunami, M., Ribas-Maynou, J., Yeste, M., ... & EARTH Study Team. (2022). Women's and men's intake of omega-3 fatty acids and their food sources and assisted reproductive technology outcomes. American Journal of Obstetrics and Gynecology, 227(2), 246-e1.

33 Stanhiser, J., Jukic, A. M. Z., McConnaughey, D. R., & Steiner, A. Z. (2022). Omega-3 fatty acid supplementation and fecundability. Human Reproduction, 37(5), 1037-1046.

34 Hosseini, B., Nourmohamadi, M., Hajipour, S., Taghizadeh, M., Asemi, Z., Keshavarz, S. A., & Jafarnejad, S. (2019). The effect of omega-3 fatty acids, EPA, and/or DHA on male infertility: a systematic review and meta-analysis. Journal of dietary supplements, 16(2), 245-256.

35 Karayiannis, D., Kontogianni, M. D., Mendorou, C., Mastrominas, M., & Yiannakouris, N. (2018). Adherence to the Mediterranean diet and IVF success rate among non-obese women attempting fertility. Human Reproduction, 33(3), 494-502.

36 Matorras, R., Ruiz, J. I., Mendoza, R., Ruiz, N., Sanjurjo, P., & Rodriguez-Escudero, F. J. (1998). Fatty acid composition of fertilization-failed human oocytes. Human reproduction (Oxford, England), 13(8), 2227-2230.
    Aardema, H., Vos, P. L., Lolicato, F., Roelen, B. A., Knijn, H. M., Vaandrager, A. B., ... & Gadella, B. M. (2011). Oleic acid prevents detrimental effects of saturated fatty acids on bovine oocyte developmental competence. Biology of reproduction, 85(1), 62-69.

37 Mirabi, P., Chaichi, M. J., Esmaeilzadeh, S., Jorsaraei, S. G. A., Bijani, A., Ehsani, M., & hashemi Karooee, S. F. (2017). The role of fatty acids on ICSI outcomes: a prospective cohort study. Lipids in health and disease, 16(1), 18.

38 Moran, L. J., Tsagareli, V., Noakes, M., & Norman, R. (2016). Altered preconception fatty acid intake is associated with improved pregnancy rates in overweight and obese women undertaking in vitro fertilisation. Nutrients, 8(1), 10.

39 Mirabi, P., Chaichi, M. J., Esmaeilzadeh, S., Jorsaraei, S. G. A., Bijani, A., Ehsani, M., & hashemi Karooee, S. F. (2017). The role of fatty acids on ICSI outcomes: a prospective cohort study. Lipids in health and disease, 16(1), 18.
    Braga, D. P. A. F., Halpern, G., Setti, A. S., Figueira, R. C. S., Iaconelli Jr, A., & Borges Jr, E. (2015). The impact of food intake and social habits on embryo quality and the likelihood of blastocyst formation. Reproductive biomedicine online, 31(1), 30-38
    Parisi, F., Rousian, M., Huijgen, N. A., Koning, A. H. J., Willemsen, S. P., de Vries, J. H. M., ... & Steegers-Theunissen, R. P. M. (2017). Periconceptional maternal 'high fish and olive oil, low meat'dietary pattern is associated with increased embryonic growth: The Rotterdam Periconceptional Cohort (Predict) Study. Ultrasound in Obstetrics & Gynecology, 50(6), 709-716

40 Arouca, A., Michels, N., Moreno, L. A., González-Gil, E. M., Marcos, A., Gómez, S., ... & Gottrand, F. (2018). Associations between a Mediterranean diet pattern and inflammatory biomarkers in European adolescents. European journal of nutrition, 57(5), 1747-1760.

41 Wagner, M. M., Jukema, J. W., Hermes, W., le Cessie, S., de Groot, C. J., Bakker, J. A., ... & Bloemenkamp, K. W. (2018). Assessment of novel cardiovascular biomarkers in women with a history of recurrent miscarriage. Pregnancy hypertension, 11, 129-135.
    See also: Ahmed, S. K., Mahmood, N., Malalla, Z. H., Alsobyani, F. M., Al-Kiyumi, I. S., & Almawi, W. Y. (2015). C-reactive protein gene variants associated with recurrent pregnancy loss independent of CRP serum levels: a case-control study. Gene, 569(1), 136-140.
    Kushnir, V. A., Solouki, S., Sarig-Meth, T., Vega, M. G., Albertini, D. F., Darmon, S. K., ... & Gleicher, N. (2016). Systemic inflammation and

autoimmunity in women with chronic endometritis. American Journal of Reproductive Immunology, 75(6), 672-677.

42 Lahoz, C., Castillo, E., Mostaza, J. M., de Dios, O., Salinero-Fort, M. A., González-Alegre, T., ... & Sabín, C. (2018). Relationship of the adherence to a mediterranean diet and its main components with CRP levels in the Spanish population. Nutrients, 10(3), 379.
Arouca, A., Michels, N., Moreno, L. A., González-Gil, E. M., Marcos, A., Gómez, S., ... & Gottrand, F. (2018). Associations between a Mediterranean diet pattern and inflammatory biomarkers in European adolescents. European journal of nutrition, 57(5), 1747-1760.

43 Uhde, M., Ajamian, M., Caio, G., De Giorgio, R., Indart, A., Green, P. H., ... & Alaedini, A. (2016). Intestinal cell damage and systemic immune activation in individuals reporting sensitivity to wheat in the absence of coeliac disease. Gut, 65(12), 1930-1937.

44 Lerner, A., Shoenfeld, Y., & Matthias, T. (2017). Adverse effects of gluten ingestion and advantages of gluten withdrawal in nonceliac autoimmune disease. Nutrition Reviews, 75(12), 1046-1058.

45 Marziali, M., Venza, M., Lazzaro, S., Lazzaro, A., Micossi, C., & Stolfi, V. M. (2012). Gluten-free diet: a new strategy for management of painful endometriosis related symptoms?. Minerva chirurgica, 67(6), 499-504.
Marziali, M., & Capozzolo, T. (2015). Role of Gluten-Free Diet in the Management of Chronic Pelvic Pain of Deep Infiltranting Endometriosis. Journal of minimally invasive gynecology, 22(6), S51-S52.

46 Jensen TK, Hjollund NH, Henriksen TB, Scheike T, Kolstad H, Giwercman A, Ernst E, Bonde JP, Skakkebaek NE, Olsen J. Does moderate alcohol consumption affect fertility? Follow up study among couples planning first pregnancy. BMJ. 1998 Aug 22;317(7157):505-10 ("Jensen 1998a");

47 Juhl M, Nyboe Andersen AM, Grønbaek M, Olsen J. Moderate alcohol consumption and waiting time to pregnancy. Hum Reprod. 2001 Dec;16(12):2705-9;

48 Mikkelsen, E. M., Riis, A. H., Wise, L. A., Hatch, E. E., Rothman, K. J., Cueto, H. T., & Sørensen, H. T. (2016). Alcohol consumption and fecundability: prospective Danish cohort study. bmj, 354, i4262.

49 Rossi BV, Berry KF, Hornstein MD, Cramer DW, Ehrlich S, Missmer SA. Effect of alcohol consumption on in vitro fertilization. Obstet Gynecol. 2011 Jan;117(1):136-42.

50 Vittrup, I., Petersen, G. L., Kamper-Jørgensen, M., Pinborg, A., & Schmidt, L. (2017). Male and female alcohol consumption and live birth after assisted reproductive technology treatment: A nationwide register-based cohort study. Reproductive biomedicine online, 35(2), 152-160.
Abadia, L., Chiu, Y. H., Williams, P. L., Toth, T. L., Souter, I., Hauser, R., ... & EARTH Study Team. (2017). The association between pre-treatment maternal alcohol and caffeine intake and outcomes of assisted

reproduction in a prospectively followed cohort. Human Reproduction, 32(9), 1846-1854.

51 Gaskins, A. J., Rich-Edwards, J. W., Williams, P. L., Toth, T. L., Missmer, S. A., & Chavarro, J. E. (2018). Pre-pregnancy caffeine and caffeinated beverage intake and risk of spontaneous abortion. European journal of nutrition, 57(1), 107-117.

52 Chen, L. W., Wu, Y., Neelakantan, N., Chong, M. F. F., Pan, A., & van Dam, R. M. (2016). Maternal caffeine intake during pregnancy and risk of pregnancy loss: a categorical and dose–response meta-analysis of prospective studies. Public health nutrition, 19(7), 1233-1244.

53 Huang H, Hansen KR, Factor-Litvak P, Carson SA, Guzick DS, Santoro N, Diamond MP, Eisenberg E, Zhang H; National Institute of Child Health and Human Development Cooperative Reproductive Medicine Network. Predictors of pregnancy and live birth after insemination in couples with unexplained or male-factor infertility. Fertil Steril. 2012 Apr;97(4):959-67.

54 Al-Saleh I, El-Doush I, Grisellhi B, Coskun S. The effect of caffeine consumption on the success rate of pregnancy as well various performance parameters of in-vitro fertilization treatment. Med Sci Monit. 2010 Dec;16(12):CR598-605.

Chapter 13: Improving Sperm Quality

1 Esteves SC, Agarwal A. Novel concepts in male infertility. Int Braz J Urol. 2011 Jan-Feb;37(1):5-15.

2 Auger J, Eustache F, Andersen AG, Irvine DS, Jørgensen N, Skakkebaek NE, Suominen J, Toppari J, Vierula M, Jouannet P: Sperm morphological defects related to environment, lifestyle and medical history of 1001 male partners of pregnant women from four European cities. Hum Reprod. 2001; 16: 2710-7.

3 Tang, L., Rao, M., Yang, W., Yao, Y., Luo, Q., Lu, L., … & Zhao, S. (2021). Predictive value of the sperm DNA fragmentation index for low or failed IVF fertilization in men with mild-to-moderate asthenozoospermia. Journal of Gynecology Obstetrics and Human Reproduction, 50(6), 101868. González-Marín, C., Gosálvez, J., & Roy, R. (2012). Types, causes, detection and repair of DNA fragmentation in animal and human sperm cells. International journal of molecular sciences, 13(11), 14026-14052. Deng, C., Li, T., Xie, Y., Guo, Y., Yang, Q. Y., Liang, X., … & Liu, G. H. (2019). Sperm DNA fragmentation index influences assisted reproductive technology outcome: A systematic review and meta-analysis combined with a retrospective cohort study. Andrologia, 51(6), e13263.

4 Simon, L., Zini, A., Dyachenko, A., Ciampi, A., & Carrell, D. T. (2017). A systematic review and meta-analysis to determine the effect of sperm DNA damage on in vitro fertilization and intracytoplasmic sperm injection outcome. Asian journal of andrology, 19(1), 80.

5   Jayasena, C. N., Radia, U. K., Figueiredo, M., Revill, L. F.,
     Dimakopoulou, A., Osagie, M., ... & Dhillo, W. S. (2019). Reduced
     Testicular Steroidogenesis and Increased Semen Oxidative Stress in Male
     Partners as Novel Markers of Recurrent Miscarriage. Clinical Chemistry,
     65(1), 161-169.
     Kumar K, Deka D, Singh A, Mitra DK, Vanitha BR, Dada R. Predictive
     value of DNA integrity analysis in idiopathic recurrent pregnancy
     loss following spontaneous conception. J Assist Reprod Genet. 2012
     Sep;29(9):861-7

6   Oleszczuk, K., Augustinsson, L., Bayat, N., Giwercman, A., & Bungum,
     M. (2013). Prevalence of high DNA fragmentation index in male partners
     of unexplained infertile couples. Andrology, 1(3), 357-360.
     Le, M. T., Nguyen, T. A. T., Nguyen, H. T. T., Nguyen, T. T. T., Nguyen,
     V. T., Le, D. D., ... & Cao, N. T. (2019). Does sperm DNA fragmentation
     correlate with semen parameters?. Reproductive medicine and biology,
     18(4), 390-396.

7   Setti, A. S., Braga, D. P. D. A. F., Provenza, R. R., Iaconelli Jr, A., &
     Borges Jr, E. (2021). Oocyte ability to repair sperm DNA fragmentation:
     the impact of maternal age on intracytoplasmic sperm injection
     outcomes. Fertility and Sterility, 116(1), 123-129.

8   Esteves, S. C., Zini, A., Coward, R. M., Evenson, D. P., Gosálvez, J.,
     Lewis, S. E., ... & Humaidan, P. (2021). Sperm DNA fragmentation
     testing: Summary evidence and clinical practice recommendations.
     Andrologia, 53(2), e13874.
     Setti, A. S., Braga, D. P. D. A. F., Provenza, R. R., Iaconelli Jr, A., &
     Borges Jr, E. (2021). Oocyte ability to repair sperm DNA fragmentation:
     the impact of maternal age on intracytoplasmic sperm injection
     outcomes. Fertility and Sterility, 116(1), 123-129.

9   Pagliuca, C., Cariati, F., Bagnulo, F., Scaglione, E., Carotenuto, C.,
     Farina, F., ... & Salvatore, P. (2021). Microbiological evaluation and
     sperm DNA fragmentation in semen samples of patients undergoing
     fertility investigation. Genes, 12(5), 654.
     Paira, D. A., Olivera, C., Tissera, A. D., Molina, R. I., Olmedo, J. J.,
     Rivero, V. E., ... & Motrich, R. D. (2023). Ureaplasma urealyticum
     and Mycoplasma hominis urogenital infections associate with semen
     inflammation and decreased sperm quality. Journal of Leukocyte
     Biology, 113(1), 18-26.
     Al-Sweih, N. A., Al-Fadli, A. H., Omu, A. E., & Rotimi, V. O.
     (2012). Prevalence of Chlamydia trachomatis, Mycoplasma hominis,
     Mycoplasma genitalium, and Ureaplasma urealyticum infections
     and seminal quality in infertile and fertile men in Kuwait. Journal of
     andrology, 33(6), 1323-1329.

10   Eini, F., Kutenaei, M. A., Zareei, F., Dastjerdi, Z. S., Shirzeyli, M. H., &
     Salehi, E. (2021). Effect of bacterial infection on sperm quality and DNA

fragmentation in subfertile men with Leukocytospermia. BMC Molecular and Cell Biology, 22(1), 1-10.

11 Liu, K. S., Mao, X. D., Pan, F., & An, R. F. (2021). Effect and mechanisms of reproductive tract infection on oxidative stress parameters, sperm DNA fragmentation, and semen quality in infertile males. Reproductive Biology and Endocrinology, 19(1), 1-12.

12 Gallegos, G., Ramos, B., Santiso, R., Goyanes, V., Gosálvez, J., & Fernández, J. L. (2008). Sperm DNA fragmentation in infertile men with genitourinary infection by Chlamydia trachomatis and Mycoplasma. Fertility and sterility, 90(2), 328-334.

13 Tímermans, A., Vázquez, R., Otero, F., Gosálvez, J., Johnston, S., & Fernández, J. L. (2022). Antibiotic toxicity on human spermatozoa assessed using the sperm DNA fragmentation dynamic assay. Andrologia, 54(2), e14328.

14 Pajovic, B., Radojevic, N., Vukovic, M., & Stjepcevic, A. (2013). Semen analysis before and after antibiotic treatment of asymptomatic chlamydia-and ureaplasma-related pyospermia. Andrologia, 45(4), 266-271.
Zhang, Q. F., Zhang, Y. J., Wang, S., Wei, Y., Li, F., & Feng, K. J. (2020). The effect of screening and treatment of Ureaplasma urealyticum infection on semen parameters in asymptomatic leukocytospermia: a case–control study. BMC urology, 20(1), 1-8.

15 Wood, G. J. A., Cardoso, J. P. G., Paluello, D. V., Nunes, T. F., & Cocuzza, M. (2021). Varicocele-associated infertility and the role of oxidative stress on sperm DNA fragmentation. Frontiers in Reproductive Health, 3, 695992.

16 Wang, S. L., Bedrick, B. S., & Kohn, T. P. (2021). What is the role of varicocelectomy in infertile men with clinical varicoceles and elevated sperm DNA fragmentation?. Fertility and Sterility, 116(3), 657-658.

17 Siddighi S, Chan CA, Patton WC, Jacobson JD, Chan PJ: Male age and sperm necrosis in assisted reproductive technologies. Urol Int. 2007; 9: 231-4 ("Siddighi 2007").

18 Singh NP, Muller CH, Berger RE. Effects of age on DNA double-strand breaks and apoptosis in human sperm. Fertil Steril. 2003 Dec;80(6):1420-30;
Wyrobek AJ, Eskenazi B, Young S, Arnheim N, Tiemann-Boege I, Jabs EW, Glaser RL, Pearson FS, Evenson D. Advancing age has differential effects on DNA damage, chromatin integrity, gene mutations, and aneuploidies in sperm. Proc Natl Acad Sci U S A. 2006 Jun 20;103(25):9601-6;
Schmid TE, Eskenazi B, Baumgartner A, Marchetti F, Young S, Weldon R, Anderson D, Wyrobek AJ. The effects of male age on sperm DNA damage in healthy non-smokers. Hum Reprod. 2007 Jan;22(1):180-7.

19 Moskovtsev SI, Willis J, Mullen JB: Age-related decline in sperm deoxyribonucleic acid integrity in patients evaluated for male infertility. Fertil Steril. 2006; 85: 496-9.

20 Robinson L, Gallos ID, Conner SJ, Rajkhowa M, Miller D, Lewis S, Kirkman-Brown J, Coomarasamy A. The effect of sperm DNA fragmentation on miscarriage rates: a systematic review and meta-analysis. Hum Reprod. 2012 Oct;27(10):2908-17 ("Robinson 2012").

21 Levitas, E., Lunenfeld, E., Weisz, N., Friger, M., & Potashnik, G. (2007). Relationship between age and semen parameters in men with normal sperm concentration: analysis of 6022 semen samples. Andrologia, 39(2), 45-50.

Johnson L, Petty CS, Porter JC, Neaves WB: Germ cell degeneration during postprophase of meiosis and serum concentrations of gonadotropins in young adult and older adult men. Biol Reprod. 1984; 31: 779-84.18;

Plastira K, Msaouel P, Angelopoulou R, Zanioti K, Plastiras A, Pothos A, Bolaris S, Paparisteidis N, Mantas D: The effects of age on DNA fragmentation, chromatin packaging and conventional semen parameters in spermatozoa of oligoasthenoteratozoospermic patients. J Assist Reprod Genet. 2007; 24: 437-43.

Siddighi 2007

22 Misell LM, Holochwost D, Boban D, Santi N, Shefi N, Hellerstein MK, Turek PJ: A stable isotope-mass spectrometric method for measuring human spermatogenesis kinetics in vivo. J Urol. 2006; 175: 242-6

23 Armstrong JS, Rajasekaran M, Chamulitrat W, Gatti P, Hellstrom WJ, Sikka SC. Characterization of reactive oxygen species induced effects on human spermatozoa movement and energy metabolism. Free Radic. Biol. Med. 1999; 26: 869–80. 12

Kodama H, Yamaguchi R, Fukuda J, Kasai H, Tanaka T. Increased oxidative deoxyribonucleic acid damage in the spermatozoa of infertile male patients. Fertil. Steril. 1997; 68: 519–24. 13

Barroso G, Morshedi M, Oehninger S. Analysis of DNA fragmentation, plasma membrane translocation of phosphatidylserine and oxidative stress in human spermatozoa. Hum. Reprod. 2000; 15: 1338–44.

24 Mahfouz R, Sharma R, Thiyagarajan A, Kale V, Gupta S, Sabanegh E, Agarwal A. Semen characteristics and sperm DNA fragmentation in infertile men with low and high levels of seminal reactive oxygen species. Fertil Steril. 2010 Nov;94(6):2141-6.

25 Wong EW, Cheng CY. Impacts of environmental toxicants on male reproductive dysfunction. Trends Pharmacol Sci. 2011 May;32(5):290-9.

26 Ross C, Morriss A, Khairy M, Khalaf Y, Braude P, Coomarasamy A, El-Toukhy T. A systematic review of the effect of oral antioxidants on male infertility. Reprod Biomed Online. 2010 Jun;20(6):711-23 ("Ross 2010").

Showell MG, Brown J, Yazdani A, Stankiewicz MT, Hart RJ. Antioxidants for male subfertility. Cochrane Database of Systematic Reviews (Online) 2011;11:CD007411 ("Showell 2011");
Robinson 2012.

27 Agarwal, A., Cannarella, R., Saleh, R., Harraz, A. M., Kandil, H., Salvio, G., ... & Shah, R. (2022). Impact of Antioxidant Therapy on Natural Pregnancy Outcomes and Semen Parameters in Infertile Men: A Systematic Review and Meta-Analysis of Randomized Controlled Trials. The World Journal of Men's Health.

28 Greco E, Romano S, Iacobelli M, Ferrero S, Baroni E, Minasi MG, Ubaldi F, Rienzi L, Tesarik J. ICSI in cases of sperm DNA damage: beneficial effect of oral antioxidant treatment. Hum Reprod. 2005 Sep;20(9):2590-4 ("Greco 2005b").

29 Ross C, Morriss A, Khairy M, Khalaf Y, Braude P, Coomarasamy A, El-Toukhy T. A systematic review of the effect of oral antioxidants on male infertility. Reprod Biomed Online. 2010 Jun;20(6):711-23.

30 Schmid TE, Eskenazi B, Marchetti F, Young S, Weldon RH, Baumgartner A, Anderson D, Wyrobek AJ. Micronutrients intake is associated with improved sperm DNA quality in older men. Fertil Steril. 2012 Nov;98(5):1130-7.e1

31 Young 2008.

32 Kos, B. J., Leemaqz, S. Y., McCormack, C. D., Andraweera, P. H., Furness, D. L., Roberts, C. T., & Dekker, G. A. (2018). The association of parental methylenetetrahydrofolate reductase polymorphisms (MTHFR 677C> T and 1298A> C) and fetal loss: a case–control study in South Australia. The Journal of Maternal-Fetal & Neonatal Medicine, 1-6
Vanilla, S., Dayanand, C. D., Kotur, P. F., Kutty, M. A., & Vegi, P. K. (2015). Evidence of paternal N5, N10-methylenetetrahydrofolate reductase (MTHFR) C677T gene polymorphism in couples with recurrent spontaneous abortions (RSAs) in Kolar District-A South West of India. Journal of clinical and diagnostic research: JCDR, 9(2), BC15.
Govindaiah, V., Naushad, S. M., Prabhakara, K., Krishna, P. C., & Devi, A. R. R. (2009). Association of parental hyperhomocysteinemia and C677T Methylene tetrahydrofolate reductase (MTHFR) polymorphism with recurrent pregnancy loss. Clinical biochemistry, 42(4-5), 380-386.

33 Mancini A, De Marinis L, Oradei A, Hallgass ME, Conte G, Pozza D, Littarru GP. Coenzyme Q10 concentrations in normal and pathological human seminal fluid. J Androl. 1994 Nov-Dec;15(6):591-4.

34 Su, L., Qu, H., Cao, Y., Zhu, J., Zhang, S. Z., Wu, J., & Jiao, Y. Z. (2022). Effect of Antioxidants on Sperm Quality Parameters in Subfertile Men: A Systematic Review and Network Meta-Analysis of Randomized Controlled Trials. Advances in Nutrition, 13(2), 586-594.
Lucignani, G., Jannello, L. M. I., Fulgheri, I., Silvani, C., Turetti, M., Gadda, F., ... & Boeri, L. (2022). Coenzyme Q10 and Melatonin for the

Treatment of Male Infertility: A Narrative Review. Nutrients, 14(21), 4585.

Lafuente R, González-Comadrán M, Solà I, López G, Brassesco M, Carreras R, Checa MA. Coenzyme Q10 and male infertility: a meta-analysis. J Assist Reprod Genet. 2013 Sep;30(9):1147-56;

Nadjarzadeh A, Shidfar F, Amirjannati N, Vafa MR, Motevalian SA, Gohari MR, Nazeri Kakhki SA, Akhondi MM, Sadeghi MR. Effect of Coenzyme Q10 supplementation on antioxidant enzymes activity and oxidative stress of seminal plasma: a double-blind randomised clinical trial. Andrologia. 2013 Jan 7.

Balercia 2009, Safarinejad 12.

35 Alahmar, A. T., Sengupta, P., Dutta, S., & Calogero, A. E. (2021). Coenzyme Q10, oxidative stress markers, and sperm DNA damage in men with idiopathic oligoasthenoteratospermia. Clinical and experimental reproductive medicine, 48(2), 150.

Abad C, Amengual MJ, Gosálvez J, Coward K, Hannaoui N, Benet J, García-Peiró A, Prats J. Effects of oral antioxidant treatment upon the dynamics of human sperm DNA fragmentation and subpopulations of sperm with highly degraded DNA. Andrologia. 2013 Jun;45(3):211-6.

36 Tirabassi, G., Vignini, A., Tiano, L., Buldreghini, E., Brugè, F., Silvestri, S., ... & Balercia, G. (2015). Protective effects of coenzyme Q 10 and aspartic acid on oxidative stress and DNA damage in subjects affected by idiopathic asthenozoospermia. Endocrine, 49(2), 549-552.

Nadjarzadeh A, Shidfar F, Amirjannati N, Vafa MR, Motevalian SA, Gohari MR, Nazeri Kakhki SA, Akhondi MM, Sadeghi MR. Effect of Coenzyme Q10 supplementation on antioxidant enzymes activity and oxidative stress of seminal plasma: a double-blind randomised clinical trial. Andrologia. 2013 Jan 7

37 Sue-Ling, C. B., Abel, W. M., & Sue-Ling, K. (2022). Coenzyme Q10 as adjunctive therapy for cardiovascular disease and hypertension: A systematic review. The Journal of Nutrition, 152(7), 1666-1674.

Fan, L., Feng, Y., Chen, G. C., Qin, L. Q., Fu, C. L., & Chen, L. H. (2017). Effects of coenzyme Q10 supplementation on inflammatory markers: A systematic review and meta-analysis of randomized controlled trials. Pharmacological research, 119, 128-136.

38 Alehagen, U., Aaseth, J., Alexander, J., & Johansson, P. (2018). Still reduced cardiovascular mortality 12 years after supplementation with selenium and coenzyme Q10 for four years: A validation of previous 10-year follow-up results of a prospective randomized double-blind placebo-controlled trial in elderly. PLoS One, 13(4), e0193120.

39 Safarinejad MR, Safarinejad S, Shafiei N, Safarinejad S. Effects of the reduced form of coenzyme Q10 (ubiquinol) on semen parameters in men with idiopathic infertility: a double-blind, placebo controlled, randomized study. J Urol. 2012 Aug;188(2):526-31.

40 Salas-Huetos, A., Rosique-Esteban, N., Becerra-Tomás, N., Vizmanos, B., Bulló, M., & Salas-Salvadó, J. (2018). The Effect of Nutrients and Dietary Supplements on Sperm Quality Parameters: A Systematic Review and Meta-Analysis of Randomized Clinical Trials. Advances in Nutrition, 9(6), 833-848.
Martínez-Soto, J. C., Domingo, J. C., Cordobilla, B., Nicolás, M., Fernández, L., Albero, P., ... & Landeras, J. (2016). Dietary supplementation with docosahexaenoic acid (DHA) improves seminal antioxidant status and decreases sperm DNA fragmentation. Systems biology in reproductive medicine, 62(6), 387-395.
Falsig, A. M., Gleerup, C. S., & Knudsen, U. B. (2019). The influence of omega-3 fatty acids on semen quality markers: a systematic PRISMA review. Andrology, 7(6), 794-803.

41 Martínez-Soto, J. C., Domingo, J. C., Cordobilla, B., Nicolás, M., Fernández, L., Albero, P., ... & Landeras, J. (2016). Dietary supplementation with docosahexaenoic acid (DHA) improves seminal antioxidant status and decreases sperm DNA fragmentation. Systems biology in reproductive medicine, 62(6), 387-395.

42 Haghighian, H. K., Haidari, F., Mohammadi-Asl, J., & Dadfar, M. (2015). Randomized, triple-blind, placebo-controlled clinical trial examining the effects of alpha-lipoic acid supplement on the spermatogram and seminal oxidative stress in infertile men. Fertility and sterility, 104(2), 318-324.
Dong, L., Yang, F., Li, J., Li, Y., Yu, X., & Zhang, X. (2022). Effect of oral alpha-lipoic acid (ALA) on sperm parameters: a systematic review and meta-analysis. Basic and Clinical Andrology, 32(1), 23.

43 Haghighian, H. K., Haidari, F., Mohammadi-asl, J., & Dadfar, M. (2015). Randomized, triple-blind, placebo-controlled clinical trial examining the effects of alpha-lipoic acid supplement on the spermatogram and seminal oxidative stress in infertile men. Fertility and sterility, 104(2), 318-324.

44 Salas-Huetos, A., Rosique-Esteban, N., Becerra-Tomás, N., Vizmanos, B., Bulló, M., & Salas-Salvadó, J. (2018). The Effect of Nutrients and Dietary Supplements on Sperm Quality Parameters: A Systematic Review and Meta-Analysis of Randomized Clinical Trials. Advances in Nutrition, 9(6), 833-848.

45 Vessey, W., McDonald, C., Virmani, A., Almeida, P., Jayasena, C., & Ramsay, J. (2016, October). Levels of reactive oxygen species (ROS) in the seminal plasma predicts the effectiveness of L-carnitine to improve sperm function in men with infertility. In Society for Endocrinology BES 2016 (Vol. 44). BioScientifica.

46 Sofimajidpour, H., Ghaderi, E., & Ganji, O. (2016). Comparison of the effects of varicocelectomy and oral L-carnitine on sperm parameters in infertile men with varicocele. Journal of clinical and diagnostic research: JCDR, 10(4), PC07.

47 Balercia, G., Regoli, F., Armeni, T., Koverech, A., Mantero, F., & Boscaro, M. (2005). Placebo-controlled double-blind randomized trial on the use of L-carnitine, L-acetylcarnitine, or combined L-carnitine and L-acetylcarnitine in men with idiopathic asthenozoospermia. Fertility and sterility, 84(3), 662-671.
Zhou, X., Liu, F., & Zhai, S. D. (2007). Effect of L-carnitine and/or L-acetyl-carnitine in nutrition treatment for male infertility: a systematic review. Asia Pacific journal of clinical nutrition, 16(S1), 383-390.
48 Jannatifar, R., Parivar, K., Roodbari, N. H., & Nasr-Esfahani, M. H. (2019). Effects of N-acetyl-cysteine supplementation on sperm quality, chromatin integrity and level of oxidative stress in infertile men. Reproductive Biology and Endocrinology, 17(1), 1-9
Safarinejad, M. R., & Safarinejad, S. (2009). Efficacy of selenium and/or N-acetyl-cysteine for improving semen parameters in infertile men: a double-blind, placebo controlled, randomized study. The Journal of urology, 181(2), 741-751.
Rafiee, B., & Tabei, S. M. B. (2021). The effect of N-acetyl cysteine consumption on men with abnormal sperm parameters due to positive history of COVID-19 in the last three months. Archivio Italiano di Urologia e Andrologia, 93(4), 465-467.
49 Jannatifar, R., Parivar, K., Roodbari, N. H., & Nasr-Esfahani, M. H. (2019). Effects of N-acetyl-cysteine supplementation on sperm quality, chromatin integrity and level of oxidative stress in infertile men. Reproductive Biology and Endocrinology, 17(1), 1-9.
50 Barekat, F., Tavalaee, M., Deemeh, M. R., Bahreinian, M., Azadi, L., Abbasi, H., ... & Nasr-Esfahani, M. H. (2016). A preliminary study: N-acetyl-L-cysteine improves semen quality following varicocelectomy. International journal of fertility & sterility, 10(1), 120.
51 Kopets, R., Kuibida, I., Chernyavska, I., Cherepanyn, V., Mazo, R., Fedevych, V., & Gerasymov, S. (2020). Dietary supplementation with a novel l-carnitine multi-micronutrient in idiopathic male subfertility involving oligo-, astheno-, teratozoospermia: A randomized clinical study. Andrology, 8(5), 1184-1193.
52 Ciccone, I. M., Costa, E. M., Pariz, J. R., Teixeira, T. A., Drevet, J. R., Gharagozloo, P., ... & Hallak, J. (2021). Serum vitamin D content is associated with semen parameters and serum testosterone levels in men. Asian journal of andrology, 23(1), 52.
Blomberg Jensen, M., Bjerrum, P. J., Jessen, T. E., Nielsen, J. E., Joensen, U. N., Olesen, I. A., ... & Jørgensen, N. (2011). Vitamin D is positively associated with sperm motility and increases intracellular calcium in human spermatozoa. Human reproduction, 26(6), 1307-1317.
53 Ciccone, I. M., Costa, E. M., Pariz, J. R., Teixeira, T. A., Drevet, J. R., Gharagozloo, P., ... & Hallak, J. (2021). Serum vitamin D content is

associated with semen parameters and serum testosterone levels in men. Asian journal of andrology, 23(1), 52.

Wadhwa, L., Priyadarshini, S., Fauzdar, A., Wadhwa, S. N., & Arora, S. (2020). Impact of vitamin D supplementation on semen quality in vitamin D-deficient infertile males with oligoasthenozoospermia. The Journal of Obstetrics and Gynecology of India, 70, 44-49.

54 Wadhwa, L., Priyadarshini, S., Fauzdar, A., Wadhwa, S. N., & Arora, S. (2020). Impact of vitamin D supplementation on semen quality in vitamin D-deficient infertile males with oligoasthenozoospermia. The Journal of Obstetrics and Gynecology of India, 70, 44-49.

55 Patel, A. S., Leong, J. Y., Ramos, L., & Ramasamy, R. (2019). Testosterone is a contraceptive and should not be used in men who desire fertility. The world journal of men's health, 37(1), 45-54.

56 Young SS, Eskenazi B, Marchetti FM, Block G, Wyrobek AJ. The association of folate, zinc and antioxidant intake with sperm aneuploidy in healthy non-smoking men. Hum Reprod. 2008 May;23(5):1014-22 ("Young 2008");

Mendiola J, Torres-Cantero AM, Vioque J, Moreno-Grau JM, Ten J, Roca M, Moreno-Grau S, Bernabeu R. A low intake of antioxidant nutrients is associated with poor semen quality in patients attending fertility clinics. Fertil Steril. 2010;11:1128–1133.

Silver EW, Eskenazi B, Evenson DP, Block G, Young S, Wyrobek AJ. Effect of antioxidant intake on sperm chromatin stability in healthy nonsmoking men. J Androl. 2005 Jul-Aug;26(4):550-6.

Braga DP, Halpern G, Figueira Rde C, Setti AS, Iaconelli A Jr, Borges E Jr. Food intake and social habits in male patients and its relationship to intracytoplasmic sperm injection outcomes. Fertil Steril. 2012 Jan;97(1):53-9.

57 Schmid TE, Eskenazi B, Marchetti F, Young S, Weldon RH, Baumgartner A, Anderson D, Wyrobek AJ. Micronutrients intake is associated with improved sperm DNA quality in older men. Fertil Steril. 2012 Nov;98(5):1130-7.e1.

58 Gupta NP, Kumar R (2002) Lycopene therapy in idiopathic male infertility—a preliminary report. Int Urol Nephrol 34(3):369– 372.

59 Chiu, Y. H., Gaskins, A. J., Williams, P. L., Mendiola, J., Jørgensen, N., Levine, H., … & Chavarro, J. E. (2016). Intake of Fruits and Vegetables with Low-to-Moderate Pesticide Residues Is Positively Associated with Semen-Quality Parameters among Young Healthy Men–3. The Journal of nutrition, 146(5), 1084-1092.

60 Salas-Huetos, A., Babio, N., Carrell, D. T., Bulló, M., & Salas-Salvadó, J. (2019). Adherence to the Mediterranean diet is positively associated with sperm motility: A cross-sectional analysis. Scientific reports, 9(1), 3389.

61 Salas-Huetos, A., Bulló, M., & Salas-Salvadó, J. (2017). Dietary patterns, foods and nutrients in male fertility parameters and fecundability: a

systematic review of observational studies. Human reproduction update, 23(4), 371-389.

Nassan, F. L., Chavarro, J. E., & Tanrikut, C. (2018). Diet and men's fertility: does diet affect sperm quality?. Fertility and sterility, 110(4), 570-577.

62 Liu, C. Y., Chou, Y. C., Chao, J. C. J., Hsu, C. Y., Cha, T. L., & Tsao, C. W. (2015). The association between dietary patterns and semen quality in a general Asian population of 7282 males. PloS one, 10(7), e0134224.

63 Efrat, M., Stein, A., Pinkas, H., Unger, R., & Birk, R. (2022). Sugar Consumption Is Negatively Associated with Semen Quality. Reproductive Sciences, 29(10), 3000-3006.

Ghosh, I., Sharma, P. K., Rahman, M., & Lahkar, K. (2019). Sugar-sweetened beverage intake in relation to semen quality in infertile couples– a prospective observational study. Fertility Science and Research, 6(1), 40.

64 Hatch, E. E., Wesselink, A. K., Hahn, K. A., Michiel, J. J., Mikkelsen, E. M., Sorensen, H. T., ... & Wise, L. A. (2018). Intake of sugar-sweetened beverages and fecundability in a North American preconception cohort. Epidemiology (Cambridge, Mass.), 29(3), 369.

65 Salas-Huetos, A., Moraleda, R., Giardina, S., Anton, E., Blanco, J., Salas-Salvadó, J., & Bulló, M. (2018). Effect of nut consumption on semen quality and functionality in healthy men consuming a Western-style diet: a randomized controlled trial. The American journal of clinical nutrition, 108(5), 953-962.

66 Robbins, W. A., Xun, L., FitzGerald, L. Z., Esguerra, S., Henning, S. M., & Carpenter, C. L. (2012). Walnuts improve semen quality in men consuming a Western-style diet: randomized control dietary intervention trial. Biology of reproduction, 87(4), 101-1.

67 Gaur DS, Talekar MS, Pathak VP. Alcohol intake and cigarette smoking: Impact of two major lifestyle factors on male fertility. Indian J Pathol Microbiol. 2010;11:35–40.

Muthusami KR, Chinnaswamy P. Effect of chronic alcoholism on male fertility hormones and semen quality. Fertil Steril. 2005;11:919–924

68 Klonoff-Cohen H, Lam-Kruglick P, Gonzalez C. Effects of maternal and paternal alcohol consumption on the success rates of in vitro fertilization and gamete intrafallopian transfer. Fertil Steril. 2003;79:330–9.

69 Ricci, E., Al Beitawi, S., Cipriani, S., Candiani, M., Chiaffarino, F., Viganò, P., ... & Parazzini, F. (2017). Semen quality and alcohol intake: a systematic review and meta-analysis. Reproductive biomedicine online, 34(1), 38-47

Borges Jr, E., Braga, D. P. D. A. F., Provenza, R. R., Figueira, R. D. C. S., Iaconelli Jr, A., & Setti, A. S. (2018). Paternal lifestyle factors in relation to semen quality and in vitro reproductive outcomes. Andrologia, 50(9), e13090.

Braga DP, Halpern G, Figueira Rde C, Setti AS, Iaconelli A Jr, Borges E Jr. Food intake and social habits in male patients and its relationship to intracytoplasmic sperm injection outcomes. Fertil Steril. 2012 Jan;97(1):53-9.

70 Koch OR, Pani G, Borrello S et al. Oxidative stress and antioxidant defenses in ethanol-induced cell injury. Mol Aspects Med. 2004; 25: 191–8.

71 Zhang, S., Wang, L., Yang, T., Chen, L., Zhao, L., Wang, T., … & Qin, J. (2020). Parental alcohol consumption and the risk of congenital heart diseases in offspring: An updated systematic review and meta-analysis. European Journal of Preventive Cardiology, 27(4), 410-421.

72 Carter, T., Schoenaker, D., Adams, J., & Steel, A. (2023). Paternal preconception modifiable risk factors for adverse pregnancy and offspring outcomes: a review of contemporary evidence from observational studies. BMC Public Health, 23(1), 1-44.

73 Levine, H., Jørgensen, N., Martino-Andrade, A., Mendiola, J., Weksler-Derri, D., Jolles, M., … & Swan, S. H. (2023). Temporal trends in sperm count: A systematic review and meta-regression analysis of samples collected globally in the 20th and 21st centuries. Human reproduction update, 29(2), 157-176.

74 Levine, H., Jørgensen, N., Martino-Andrade, A., Mendiola, J., Weksler-Derri, D., Jolles, M., … & Swan, S. H. (2023). Temporal trends in sperm count: a systematic review and meta-regression analysis of samples collected globally in the 20th and 21st centuries. Human Reproduction Update, 29(2), 157-176.

75 Swan, S. H., Main, K. M., Liu, F., Stewart, S. L., Kruse, R. L., Calafat, A. M., … & Study for Future Families Research Team. (2005). Decrease in anogenital distance among male infants with prenatal phthalate exposure. Environmental health perspectives, 113(8), 1056-1061. Bustamante-Montes, L. P., Hernández-Valero, M. A., Flores-Pimentel, D., García-Fábila, M., Amaya-Chávez, A., Barr, D. B., & Borja-Aburto, V. H. (2013). Prenatal exposure to phthalates is associated with decreased anogenital distance and penile size in male newborns. Journal of developmental origins of health and disease, 4(4), 300-306.

76 Huang XF, Li Y, Gu YH, Liu M, Xu Y, Yuan Y, Sun F, Zhang HQ, Shi HJ. The effects of Di-(2-ethylhexyl)-phthalate exposure on fertilization and embryonic development in vitro and testicular genomic mutation in vivo. PLoS One. 2012;7(11):e50465;
Pant N, Pant A, Shukla M, Mathur N, Gupta Y, Saxena D. Environmental and experimental exposure of phthalate esters: the toxicological consequence on human sperm. Hum Exp Toxicol. 2011 Jun;30(6):507-14;
Duty S. M., Singh N. P., Silva M. J., Barr D. B., Brock J. W., Ryan L., Herrick R. F., Christiani D. C., Hauser R. 2003b. The relationship between environmental exposures to phthalates and DNA damage in human sperm using the neutral comet assay. Environ. Health Perspect.

111, 1164–1169. ("In conclusion, this study represents the first human data to demonstrate that urinary MEP, at environmental levels, is associated with increased DNA damage in sperm.")

77 Mendiola J, Meeker JD, Jørgensen N, Andersson AM, Liu F, Calafat AM, Redmon JB, Drobnis EZ, Sparks AE, Wang C, Hauser R, Swan SH. Urinary concentrations of di(2-ethylhexyl) phthalate metabolites and serum reproductive hormones: pooled analysis of fertile and infertile men. J Androl. 2012 May-Jun;33(3):488-98.
Meeker J. D., Calafat A.M., Hauser R. Urinary metabolites of di(2-ethylhexyl) phthalate are associated with decreased steroid hormone levels in adult men.. J Androl. 2009 May–Jun; 30(3): 287–297.

78 Ferguson KK, Loch-Caruso R, Meeker JD. Urinary phthalate metabolites in relation to biomarkers of inflammation and oxidative stress: NHANES 1999-2006. Environ Res. 2011 Jul;111(5):718-26.

79 Buck Louis G.M., Sundaram R., Sweeney A., Schisterman E.F., Kannan K. Bisphenol A, phthalates and couple fecundity, the life study. Fertil. Steril. 2013 Sep; 100(3): S1.

80 Rudel, R. A., Gray, J. M., Engel, C. L., Rawsthorne, T. W., Dodson, R. E., Ackerman, J. M., ... & Brody, J. G. (2011). Food packaging and bisphenol A and bis (2-ethyhexyl) phthalate exposure: findings from a dietary intervention. Environmental health perspectives, 119(7), 914-920.

81 Meeker JD, Ehrlich S, Toth TL, Wright DL, Calafat AM, Trisini AT, Ye X, Hauser R. Semen quality and sperm DNA damage in relation to urinary bisphenol A among men from an infertility clinic. Reprod Toxicol. 2010 Dec;30(4):532-9.

82 Knez J, Kranvogl R, Breznik BP, Vončina E, Vlaisavljević V. Are urinary bisphenol A levels in men related to semen quality and embryo development after medically assisted reproduction? Fertil Steril. 2014 Jan;101(1):215-221.e5Li DK, Zhou Z, Miao M, He Y, Wang J, Ferber J, Herrinton LJ, Gao E, Yuan W. Urine bisphenol-A (BPA) level in relation to semen quality. Fertil Steril. 2011 Feb;95(2):625-30.e1-4.

83 Sandhu RS, Wong TH, Kling CA, Chohan KR. In vitro effects of coital lubricants and synthetic and natural oils on sperm motility. Fertil Steril. 2014 Jan 23 [Epub ahead of print] ("Sandhu 2014");
Agarwal A, Deepinder F, Cocuzza M, Short RA, Evenson DP. Effect of vaginal lubricants on sperm motility and chromatin integrity: a prospective comparative study. Fertil Steril. 2008 Feb;89(2):375-9.

84 Mowat, A., Newton, C., Boothroyd, C., Demmers, K., & Fleming, S. (2014). The effects of vaginal lubricants on sperm function: an in vitro analysis. Journal of assisted reproduction and genetics, 31(3), 333-339.

85 Markram, J., Griessel, L., Girdler-Brown, B., & Outhoff, K. (2022). Sperm-friendly lubricant: Fact or fiction. International Journal of Gynecology & Obstetrics, 159(1), 111-115.

86 Rafaee, A., Kakavand, K., Sodeifi, N., Farrahi, F., & Sabbaghian, M. (2022). Effects of babydance lubricant on sperm parameters. Journal of Human Reproductive Sciences, 15(2), 133.

87 Sørensen, F., Melsen, L. M., Fedder, J., & Soltanizadeh, S. (2023). The Influence of Male Ejaculatory Abstinence Time on Pregnancy Rate, Live Birth Rate and DNA Fragmentation: A Systematic Review. Journal of Clinical Medicine, 12(6), 2219.

88 Setti, A. S., Braga, D. P. A. F., Iaconelli Junior, A., & Borges Junior, E. (2020). Increasing paternal age and ejaculatory abstinence length negatively influence the intracytoplasmic sperm injection outcomes from egg-sharing donation cycles. Andrology, 8(3), 594-601.

89 Setti, A. S., Braga, D. P. A. F., Iaconelli Junior, A., & Borges Junior, E. (2020). Increasing paternal age and ejaculatory abstinence length negatively influence the intracytoplasmic sperm injection outcomes from egg-sharing donation cycles. Andrology, 8(3), 594-601.

Sánchez-Martín, P., Sánchez-Martín, F., González-Martínez, M., & Gosálvez, J. (2013). Increased pregnancy after reduced male abstinence. Systems biology in reproductive medicine, 59(5), 256-260.

Barbagallo, F., Calogero, A. E., Condorelli, R. A., Farrag, A., Jannini, E. A., La Vignera, S., & Manna, C. (2021). Does a Very Short Length of Abstinence Improve Assisted Reproductive Technique Outcomes in Infertile Patients with Severe Oligo-Asthenozoospermia?. Journal of Clinical Medicine, 10(19), 4399.

Borges Jr, E., Braga, D. P. A. F., Zanetti, B. F., Iaconelli Jr, A., & Setti, A. S. (2019). Revisiting the impact of ejaculatory abstinence on semen quality and intracytoplasmic sperm injection outcomes. Andrology, 7(2), 213-219.

Gupta, S., Singh, V. J., Fauzdar, A., Prasad, K., Srivastava, A., & Sharma, K. (2021). Short ejaculatory abstinence in normozoospermic men is associated with higher clinical pregnancy rates in sub-fertile couples undergoing intra-cytoplasmic sperm injection in assisted reproductive technology: A retrospective analysis of 1691 cycles. Journal of Human Reproductive Sciences, 14(3), 273.

90 Gupta, S., Singh, V. J., Fauzdar, A., Prasad, K., Srivastava, A., & Sharma, K. (2021). Short ejaculatory abstinence in normozoospermic men is associated with higher clinical pregnancy rates in sub-fertile couples undergoing intra-cytoplasmic sperm injection in assisted reproductive technology: A retrospective analysis of 1691 cycles. Journal of Human Reproductive Sciences, 14(3), 273.

91 Dahan, M. H., Mills, G., Khoudja, R., Gagnon, A., Tan, G., & Tan, S. L. (2021). Three hour abstinence as a treatment for high sperm DNA fragmentation: a prospective cohort study. Journal of Assisted Reproduction and Genetics, 38, 227-233.

92 Carlsen E, Andersson AM, Petersen JH, Skakkebaek NE. History of febrile illness and variation in semen quality. Hum. Reprod. 2003; 18: 2089–92.

93 Jung A, Leonhardt F, Schill W, Schuppe H. Influence of the type of undertrousers and physical activity on scrotal temperature. Hum Reprod. 2005;11:1022–1027

94 Tiemessen CH, Evers JL, Bots RS. Tight-fitting underwear and sperm quality. Lancet. 1996;11:1844–1845.

95 Gebreegziabher, Y., Marcos, E., McKinon, W., & Rogers, G. (2004). Sperm characteristics of endurance trained cyclists. International journal of sports medicine, 25(04), 247-251.
Maleki, B. H., Tartibian, B., & Vaamonde, D. (2014). The effects of 16 weeks of intensive cycling training on seminal oxidants and antioxidants in male road cyclists. Clinical Journal of Sport Medicine, 24(4), 302-307.
Maleki, B. H., & Tartibian, B. (2015). Long-term low-to-intensive cycling training: impact on semen parameters and seminal cytokines. Clinical journal of sport medicine, 25(6), 535-540.

Chapter 14. Preparing for Embryo Transfer

1 Coates, A., Kung, A., Mounts, E., Hesla, J., Bankowski, B., Barbieri, E., ... & Munné, S. (2017). Optimal euploid embryo transfer strategy, fresh versus frozen, after preimplantation genetic screening with next generation sequencing: a randomized controlled trial. Fertility and sterility, 107(3), 723-730.
Shapiro, B. S., Daneshmand, S. T., Garner, F. C., Aguirre, M., Hudson, C., & Thomas, S. (2011). Evidence of impaired endometrial receptivity after ovarian stimulation for in vitro fertilization: a prospective randomized trial comparing fresh and frozen–thawed embryo transfer in normal responders. Fertility and sterility, 96(2), 344-348.
Roque, M., Lattes, K., Serra, S., Solà, I., Geber, S., Carreras, R., & Checa, M. A. (2013). Fresh embryo transfer versus frozen embryo transfer in in vitro fertilization cycles: a systematic review and meta-analysis. Fertility and sterility, 99(1), 156-162.
Roque, M., Valle, M., Guimarães, F., Sampaio, M., & Geber, S. (2015). Freeze-all policy: fresh vs. frozen-thawed embryo transfer. Fertility and sterility, 103(5), 1190-1193.
Wang, A., Santistevan, A., Cohn, K. H., Copperman, A., Nulsen, J., Miller, B. T., ... & Beim, P. Y. (2017). Freeze-only versus fresh embryo transfer in a multicenter matched cohort study: contribution of progesterone and maternal age to success rates. Fertility and sterility, 108(2), 254-261

2 Wang, A., Santistevan, A., Cohn, K. H., Copperman, A., Nulsen, J., Miller, B. T., ... & Beim, P. Y. (2017). Freeze-only versus fresh embryo transfer in a multicenter matched cohort study: contribution of

progesterone and maternal age to success rates. Fertility and sterility, 108(2), 254-261.

3   Wei, D., Liu, J. Y., Sun, Y., Shi, Y., Zhang, B., Liu, J. Q., ... & Chen, Z. J. (2019). Frozen versus fresh single blastocyst transfer in ovulatory women: a multicentre, randomised controlled trial. The lancet, 393(10178), 1310-1318.

4   Wong, K. M., Van Wely, M., Verhoeve, H. R., Kaaijk, E. M., Mol, F., Van der Veen, F., ... & Mastenbroek, S. (2021). Transfer of fresh or frozen embryos: a randomised controlled trial. Human reproduction, 36(4), 998-1006.
    Stormlund, S., Sopa, N., Zedeler, A., Bogstad, J., Prætorius, L., Nielsen, H. S., ... & Pinborg, A. (2020). Freeze-all versus fresh blastocyst transfer strategy during in vitro fertilisation in women with regular menstrual cycles: multicentre randomised controlled trial. Bmj, 370.

5   Zaat, T., Zagers, M., Mol, F., Goddijn, M., van Wely, M., & Mastenbroek, S. (2021). Fresh versus frozen embryo transfers in assisted reproduction. Cochrane Database of Systematic Reviews, (2).

6   Sadecki, E., Rust, L., Walker, D. L., Fredrickson, J. R., Krenik, A., Kim, T., ... & Zhao, Y. (2021). Comparison of live birth rates after IVF–embryo transfer with and without preimplantation genetic testing for aneuploidies. Reproductive BioMedicine Online, 43(6), 995-1001

7   Sadecki, E., Rust, L., Walker, D. L., Fredrickson, J. R., Krenik, A., Kim, T., ... & Zhao, Y. (2021). Comparison of live birth rates after IVF–embryo transfer with and without preimplantation genetic testing for aneuploidies. Reproductive BioMedicine Online, 43(6), 995-1001.

8   Ozgur, K., Berkkanoglu, M., Bulut, H., Yoruk, G. D. A., Candurmaz, N. N., & Coetzee, K. (2019). Single best euploid versus single best unknown-ploidy blastocyst frozen embryo transfers: a randomized controlled trial. Journal of Assisted Reproduction and Genetics, 36, 629-636.

9   Xiao, J. S., Healey, M., Talmor, A., & Vollenhoven, B. (2019). When only one embryo is available, is it better to transfer on Day 3 or to grow on?. Reproductive BioMedicine Online, 39(6), 916-923.

10 Greco, E., Minasi, M. G., & Fiorentino, F. (2015). Healthy babies after intrauterine transfer of mosaic aneuploid blastocysts. New England Journal of Medicine, 373(21), 2089-2090.

11 Barad, D. H., Albertini, D. F., Molinari, E., & Gleicher, N. (2022). IVF outcomes of embryos with abnormal PGT-A biopsy previously refused transfer: a prospective cohort study. Human Reproduction, 37(6), 1194-1206.
    Capalbo, A., Cimadomo, D., Rienzi, L., Garcìa-Velasco, J. A., Simòn, C., & Ubaldi, F. M. (2022). Avoid mixing apples and oranges: blastocysts diagnosed with uniform whole chromosome aneuploidies are reproductively incompetent and their transfer is harmful. Human Reproduction, 37(9), 2213-2214.

12 Yang, M., Rito, T., Naftaly, J., Hu, J., Albertini, D. F., Barad, D. H., ... & Gleicher, N. (2020). Self-correction of mosaicism in human self-organizing gastruloids as potential explanation for normal births after

transfer of chromosomal-abnormal embryos. Fertility and Sterility, 114(3), e14-e15.

13 Munné, S., Blazek, J., Large, M., Martinez-Ortiz, P. A., Nisson, H., Liu, E., ... & Fragouli, E. (2017). Detailed investigation into the cytogenetic constitution and pregnancy outcome of replacing mosaic blastocysts detected with the use of high-resolution next-generation sequencing. Fertility and sterility, 108(1), 62-71. Capalbo, A., Poli, M., Rienzi, L., Girardi, L., Patassini, C., Fabiani, M., ... & Simón, C. (2021). Mosaic human preimplantation embryos and their developmental potential in a prospective, non-selection clinical trial. The American Journal of Human Genetics, 108(12), 2238-2247.

Besser, A. G., Blakemore, J. K., Del Buono, E. J., McCaffrey, C., McCulloh, D. H., & Grifo, J. A. (2019). Four years of prospective mosaic embryo transfer: a single center's experience. Fertility and Sterility, 112(3), e230.

14 Viotti, M., Victor, A. R., Barnes, F. L., Zouves, C. G., Besser, A. G., Grifo, J. A., ... & Munné, S. (2021). Using outcome data from one thousand mosaic embryo transfers to formulate an embryo ranking system for clinical use. Fertility and Sterility, 115(5), 1212-1224.

15 Leigh, D., Cram, D. S., Rechitsky, S., Handyside, A., Wells, D., Munne, S., ... & Kuliev, A. (2022). PGDIS position statement on the transfer of mosaic embryos 2021. Reproductive BioMedicine Online, 45(1), 19-25. Kahraman, S., Cetinkaya, M., Yuksel, B., Yesil, M., & Pirkevi Cetinkaya, C. (2020). The birth of a baby with mosaicism resulting from a known mosaic embryo transfer: a case report. Human Reproduction, 35(3), 727-733.

16 Hashemi, Z., Sharifi, N., Khani, B., Aghadavod, E., & Asemi, Z. (2019). The effects of vitamin E supplementation on endometrial thickness, and gene expression of vascular endothelial growth factor and inflammatory cytokines among women with implantation failure. The Journal of Maternal-Fetal & Neonatal Medicine, 32(1), 95-102.

17 Takasaki, A., Tamura, H., Miwa, I., Taketani, T., Shimamura, K., & Sugino, N. (2010). Endometrial growth and uterine blood flow: a pilot study for improving endometrial thickness in the patients with a thin endometrium. Fertility and sterility, 93(6), 1851-1858.

18 El Refaeey, A., Selem, A., & Badawy, A. (2014). Combined coenzyme Q10 and clomiphene citrate for ovulation induction in clomiphene-citrate-resistant polycystic ovary syndrome. Reproductive biomedicine online, 29(1), 119-124.

19 Latifian, S., Hamdi, K., Totakneh, R., & Totakneh, R. (2015). Effect of addition of l-carnitine in polycystic ovary syndrome (PCOS) patients with clomiphene citrate and gonadotropin resistant. Int J Curr Res Acad Rev, 3(8), 469-476. Ismail, A. M., Hamed, A. H., Saso, S., & Thabet, H. H. (2014). Adding L-carnitine to clomiphene resistant PCOS women improves the quality of

ovulation and the pregnancy rate. A randomized clinical trial. European Journal of Obstetrics & Gynecology and Reproductive Biology, 180, 148-152.

Chaleshtori, M. H., Taheripanah, R., & Shakeri, A. (2022). Clomiphene citrate (CC) plus L-Carnitine improves clinical pregnancy rate along with glycemic status and lipid profile in clomiphene-resistant polycystic ovary syndrome patients: A triple-blind randomized controlled clinical trial. Obesity Medicine, 34, 100400.

20 Dirckx, K. A. A. T. J. E., Cabri, P., Merien, A., Galajdova, L., Gerris, J., Dhont, M., & De Sutter, P. (2009). Does low-dose aspirin improve pregnancy rate in IVF/ICSI? A randomized double-blind placebo controlled trial. Human reproduction, 24(4), 856-860.

Davar, R., Pourmasumi, S., Mohammadi, B., & Lahijani, M. M. (2020). The effect of low-dose aspirin on the pregnancy rate in frozen-thawed embryo transfer cycles: A randomized clinical trial. International journal of reproductive biomedicine, 18(9), 693.

Check, J. H., Dieterich, C., Lurie, D., Nazari, A., & Chuong, J. (1998). A matched study to determine whether low-dose aspirin without heparin improves pregnancy rates following frozen embryo transfer and/or affects endometrial sonographic parameters. Journal of assisted reproduction and genetics, 15, 579-582.

Gelbaya, T. A., Kyrgiou, M., Li, T. C., Stern, C., & Nardo, L. G. (2007). Low-dose aspirin for in vitro fertilization: a systematic review and meta-analysis. Human Reproduction Update, 13(4), 357-364.

21 Hasegawa, I., Yamanoto, Y., Suzuki, M., Murakawa, H., Kurabayashi, T., Takakuwa, K., & Tanaka, K. (1998). Prednisolone plus low-dose aspirin improves the implantation rate in women with autoimmune conditions who are undergoing in vitro fertilization. Fertility and sterility, 70(6), 1044-1048.

Wada, I., Hsu, C. C., Williams, G., Macnamee, M. C., & Brinsden, P. R. (1994). Pregnancy: the benefits of low-dose aspirin therapy in women with impaired uterine perfusion during assisted conception. Human Reproduction, 9(10), 1954-1957.

Weckstein, L. N., Jacobson, A., Galen, D., Hampton, K., & Hammel, J. (1997). Low-dose aspirin for oocyte donation recipients with a thin endometrium: prospective, randomized study. Fertility and sterility, 68(5), 927-930.

Hsieh, Y. Y., Tsai, H. D., Chang, C. C., Lo, H. Y., & Chen, C. L. (2000). Gynecology: low-dose aspirin for infertile women with thin endometrium receiving intraeuterine insemination: a prospective, randomized study. Journal of assisted reproduction and genetics, 17, 174-177.

22 Tao, Y., & Wang, N. (2020). Adjuvant vaginal use of sildenafil citrate in a hormone replacement cycle improved live birth rates among 10,069

women during first frozen embryo transfers. Drug Design, Development and Therapy, 5289-5297.

Eid, M. E. (2015). Sildenafil improves implantation rate in women with a thin endometrium secondary to improvement of uterine blood flow;"pilot study". Fertility and Sterility, 104(3), e342.

Mekled, A. K. H., Abd El-Rahim, A. M., & El-Sayed, A. (2017). Effect of Sildenafil Citrate on the Outcome of in vitro Fertilization after Multiple IVF Failures Attributed to Poor Endometrial Development: A Randomized Controlled Trial. Egyptian Journal of Hospital Medicine, 69(1).

23 de Castro Rocha, M. N., de Souza Florêncio, R., & Alves, R. R. F. (2020). The role played by granulocyte colony stimulating factor (G-CSF) on women submitted to in vitro fertilization associated with thin endometrium: systematic review. JBRA assisted reproduction, 24(3), 278.

Li, Y., Pan, P., Chen, X., Li, L., Li, Y., & Yang, D. (2014). Granulocyte colony-stimulating factor administration for infertile women with thin endometrium in frozen embryo transfer program. Reproductive Sciences, 21, 381-385.

24 Kunicki, M., Łukaszuk, K., Liss, J., Skowrońska, P., & Szczyptańska, J. (2017). Granulocyte colony stimulating factor treatment of resistant thin endometrium in women with frozen-thawed blastocyst transfer. Systems biology in reproductive medicine, 63(1), 49-57.

25 Samy, A., Abbas, A. M., Elmoursi, A., Elsayed, M., & Hussein, R. S. (2020). Effect of autologous platelet-rich plasma transfusion in the treatment of infertile women with thin endometrium and its implications in IVF cycles: a literature review. Middle East Fertility Society Journal, 25, 1-6.

26 Paulus, W. E., Zhang, M., Strehler, E., El-Danasouri, I., & Sterzik, K. (2002). Influence of acupuncture on the pregnancy rate in patients who undergo assisted reproduction therapy. Fertility and sterility, 77(4), 721-724.

27 Schwarze, J. E., Ceroni, J. P., Ortega-Hrepich, C., Villa, S., Crosby, J., & Pommer, R. (2018). Does acupuncture the day of embryo transfer affect the clinical pregnancy rate? Systematic review and meta-analysis. JBRA assisted reproduction, 22(4), 363.

Manheimer, E., van der Windt, D., Cheng, K., Stafford, K., Liu, J., Tierney, J., ... & Bouter, L. M. (2013). The effects of acupuncture on rates of clinical pregnancy among women undergoing in vitro fertilization: a systematic review and meta-analysis. Human reproduction update, 19(6), 696-713.

Shen, C., Wu, M., Shu, D., Zhao, X., & Gao, Y. (2015). The role of acupuncture in in vitro fertilization: a systematic review and meta-analysis. Gynecologic and obstetric investigation, 79(1), 1-12.

28 So, E. W. S., Ng, E. H. Y., Wong, Y. Y., Lau, E. Y. L., Yeung, W. S. B., & Ho, P. C. (2008). A randomized double blind comparison of real and placebo acupuncture in IVF treatment. Human Reproduction, 24(2), 341-348.

So, E. W. S., Ng, E. H. Y., Wong, Y. Y., Yeung, W. S. B., & Ho, P. C. (2010). Acupuncture for frozen–thawed embryo transfer cycles: a double-blind randomized controlled trial. Reproductive biomedicine online, 20(6), 814-821.

29 Domar, A. D., Meshay, I., Kelliher, J., Alper, M., & Powers, R. D. (2009). The impact of acupuncture on in vitro fertilization outcome. Fertility and sterility, 91(3), 723-726.

30 Craig, L. B., Rubin, L. E., Peck, J. D., Anderson, M., Marshall, L. A., & Soules, M. R. (2014). Acupuncture performed before and after embryo transfer: a randomized controlled trial. The Journal of reproductive medicine, 59(5-6), 313-320.

31 Rubin, L. E. H., Anderson, B. J., & Craig, L. B. (2018). Acupuncture and in vitro fertilisation research: current and future directions. Acupuncture in Medicine, acupmed-2016.
Magarelli, P. C., Cridennda, D. K., & Cohen, M. (2009). Changes in serum cortisol and prolactin associated with acupuncture during controlled ovarian hyperstimulation in women undergoing in vitro fertilization–embryo transfer treatment. Fertility and Sterility, 92(6), 1870-1879.
di Villahermosa, D. I. M., dos Santos, L. G., Nogueira, M. B., Vilarino, F. L., & Barbosa, C. P. (2013). Influence of acupuncture on the outcomes of in vitro fertilisation when embryo implantation has failed: a prospective randomised controlled clinical trial. Acupuncture in Medicine, 31(2), 157-161.

32 Magarelli, P. C., Cridennda, D. K., & Cohen, M. (2009). Changes in serum cortisol and prolactin associated with acupuncture during controlled ovarian hyperstimulation in women undergoing in vitro fertilization–embryo transfer treatment. Fertility and Sterility, 92(6), 1870-1879.

33 Cozzolino, M., Troiano, G., & Esencan, E. (2019). Bed rest after an embryo transfer: a systematic review and meta-analysis. Archives of Gynecology and Obstetrics, 300, 1121-1130.
Craciunas, L., & Tsampras, N. (2016). Bed rest following embryo transfer might negatively affect the outcome of IVF/ICSI: a systematic review and meta-analysis. Human Fertility, 19(1), 16-22.
Malhotra, N., & Sarkar, P. (2019). Pregnancy outcome after bed rest versus early ambulation following embryo transfer during IVF/ICSI cycles-a randomised controlled study. Fertility and Sterility, 112(3), e146.

34 Qasim, S. M., Callan, C., & Choe, J. K. (1996). The predictive value of an initial serum β human chorionic gonadotropin level for pregnancy outcome following in vitro fertilization. Journal of assisted reproduction and genetics, 13, 705-708.
Bjercke, S., Tanbo, T., Dale, P. O., Mørkrid, L., & Åbyholm, T. (1999). Human chorionic gonadotrophin concentrations in early pregnancy after in-vitro fertilization. Human reproduction, 14(6), 1642-1646.

Fridström, M., Garoff, L., Sjöblom, P., & Hillensjö, T. (1995). Human chorionic gonadotropin patterns in early pregnancy after assisted reproduction. Acta obstetricia et gynecologica Scandinavica, 74(7), 534-538.

Poikkeus, P., Hiilesmaa, V., & Tiitinen, A. (2002). Serum HCG 12 days after embryo transfer in predicting pregnancy outcome. Human Reproduction, 17(7), 1901-1905

35 Hughes, L. M., Schuler, A., Sharmuk, M., Schauer, J. M., Pavone, M. E., & Bernardi, L. A. (2022). Early β-hCG levels predict live birth after single embryo transfer. Journal of Assisted Reproduction and Genetics, 39(10), 2355-2364.

Chapter 15. Immune and Implantation Factors

1 Tessier, D. R., Yockell-Lelièvre, J., & Gruslin, A. (2015). Uterine spiral artery remodeling: the role of uterine natural killer cells and extravillous trophoblasts in normal and high-risk human pregnancies. American journal of reproductive immunology, 74(1), 1-11.

2 Moreno, I., Codoñer, F. M., Vilella, F., Valbuena, D., Martinez-Blanch, J. F., Jimenez-Almazán, J., ... & Simon, C. (2016). Evidence that the endometrial microbiota has an effect on implantation success or failure. American journal of obstetrics and gynecology, 215(6), 684-703.

Grewal, K., Lee, Y. S., Smith, A., Brosens, J. J., Bourne, T., Al-Memar, M., ... & Bennett, P. R. (2022). Chromosomally normal miscarriage is associated with vaginal dysbiosis and local inflammation. BMC medicine, 20(1), 1-15.

3 Chen, W., Wei, K., He, X., Wei, J., Yang, L., Li, L., ... & Tan, B. (2021). Identification of uterine microbiota in infertile women receiving in vitro fertilization with and without chronic endometritis. Frontiers in cell and developmental biology, 9, 693267.

Kitaya, K., Nagai, Y., Arai, W., Sakuraba, Y., & Ishikawa, T. (2019). Characterization of microbiota in endometrial fluid and vaginal secretions in infertile women with repeated implantation failure. Mediators of inflammation, 2019.

Cheah, F. C., Lai, C. H., Tan, G. C., Swaminathan, A., Wong, K. K., Wong, Y. P., & Tan, T. L. (2021). Intrauterine Gardnerella vaginalis infection results in fetal growth restriction and alveolar septal hypertrophy in a rabbit model. Frontiers in pediatrics, 8, 593802.

4 Liu, Y., Ko, E. Y. L., Wong, K. K. W., Chen, X., Cheung, W. C., Law, T. S. M., ... & Chim, S. S. C. (2019). Endometrial microbiota in infertile women with and without chronic endometritis as diagnosed using a quantitative and reference range-based method. Fertility and sterility, 112(4), 707-717.

5 Kitaya, K., Matsubayashi, H., Takaya, Y., Nishiyama, R., Yamaguchi, K., Takeuchi, T., & Ishikawa, T. (2017). Live birth rate following oral antibiotic treatment for chronic endometritis in infertile women with

repeated implantation failure. American Journal of Reproductive Immunology, 78(5), e12719.

6   Cheah, F. C., Lai, C. H., Tan, G. C., Swaminathan, A., Wong, K. K., Wong, Y. P., & Tan, T. L. (2021). Intrauterine Gardnerella vaginalis infection results in fetal growth restriction and alveolar septal hypertrophy in a rabbit model. Frontiers in pediatrics, 8, 593802.

7   Cicinelli, E.; Matteo, M.; Tinelli, R.; Lepera, A.; Alfonso, R.; Indraccolo, U.; Marrocchella, S.; Greco, P.; Resta, L. Prevalence of Chronic Endometritis in Repeated Unexplained Implantation Failure and the IVF Success Rate after Antibiotic Therapy. Hum. Reprod. 2015, 30, 323–330.
Cicinelli, E.; Matteo, M.; Trojano, G.; Mitola, P.C.; Tinelli, R.; Vitagliano, A.; Crupano, F.M.; Lepera, A.; Miragliotta, G.; Resta, L. Chronic Endometritis in Patients with Unexplained Infertility: Prevalence and Effects of Antibiotic Treatment on Spontaneous Conception. Am. J. Reprod. Immunol. 2018, 79, e12782.
Cheng, X., Huang, Z., Xiao, Z., & Bai, Y. (2022). Does antibiotic therapy for chronic endometritis improve clinical outcomes of patients with recurrent implantation failure in subsequent IVF cycles? A systematic review and meta-analysis. Journal of Assisted Reproduction and Genetics, 39(8), 1797-1813.
Bouet, P. E., El Hachem, H., Monceau, E., Gariépy, G., Kadoch, I. J., & Sylvestre, C. (2016). Chronic endometritis in women with recurrent pregnancy loss and recurrent implantation failure: prevalence and role of office hysteroscopy and immunohistochemistry in diagnosis. Fertility and sterility, 105(1), 106-110.
Kitaya, K., Matsubayashi, H., Takaya, Y., Nishiyama, R., Yamaguchi, K., Takeuchi, T., & Ishikawa, T. (2017). Live birth rate following oral antibiotic treatment for chronic endometritis in infertile women with repeated implantation failure. American Journal of Reproductive Immunology, 78(5), e12719.
Vitagliano, A.; Saccardi, C.; Noventa, M.; di Spiezio Sardo, A.; Saccone, G.; Cicinelli, E.; Pizzi, S.; Andrisani, A.; Litta, P.S. Effects of Chronic Endometritis Therapy on in Vitro Fertilization Outcome in Women with Repeated Implantation Failure: A Systematic Review and Meta-Analysis. Fertil. Steril. 2018, 110, 103–112.e1.
Yang, R., Du, X., Wang, Y., Song, X., Yang, Y., & Qiao, J. (2014). The hysteroscopy and histological diagnosis and treatment value of chronic endometritis in recurrent implantation failure patients. Archives of gynecology and obstetrics, 289, 1363-1369.

8   McQueen, D. B., Bernardi, L. A., & Stephenson, M. D. (2014). Chronic endometritis in women with recurrent early pregnancy loss and/or fetal demise. Fertility and sterility, 101(4), 1026-1030.

9   Sklyarova, V. O., Shatylovich, K. L., Filipyuk, A. L., Sklyarov, P. O., & Chajkivskyj, R. A. (2020). Platelet-Rich Plasma in the Management of

Chronic Endometritis Treatment in Women with Reproductive Health Disorders. European Journal of Medical and Health Sciences, 2(6).

Sfakianoudis, K., Simopoulou, M., Nitsos, N., Lazaros, L., Rapani, A., Pantou, A., ... & Pantos, K. (2019). Successful implantation and live birth following autologous platelet-rich plasma treatment for a patient with recurrent implantation failure and chronic endometritis. in vivo, 33(2), 515-521

Giulini, S., Grisendi, V., Sighinolfi, G., Di Vinci, P., Tagliasacchi, D., Botticelli, L., ... & Facchinetti, F. (2022). Chronic endometritis in recurrent implantation failure: Use of prednisone and IVF outcome. Journal of Reproductive Immunology, 153, 103673

10 Armstrong, E., Hemmerling, A., Miller, S., Burke, K. E., Newmann, S. J., Morris, S. R., ... & Kaul, R. (2022). Metronidazole treatment rapidly reduces genital inflammation through effects on bacterial vaginosis–associated bacteria rather than lactobacilli. The Journal of clinical investigation, 132(6).

11 Kadogami, D., Nakaoka, Y., & Morimoto, Y. (2020). Use of a vaginal probiotic suppository and antibiotics to influence the composition of the endometrial microbiota. Reproductive Biology, 20(3), 307-314.

Hashem, N. M., & Gonzalez-Bulnes, A. (2022). The use of probiotics for management and improvement of reproductive eubiosis and function. Nutrients, 14(4), 902.

12 Vujic, G., Knez, A. J., Stefanovic, V. D., & Vrbanovic, V. K. (2013). Efficacy of orally applied probiotic capsules for bacterial vaginosis and other vaginal infections: a double-blind, randomized, placebo-controlled study. European Journal of Obstetrics & Gynecology and Reproductive Biology, 168(1), 75-79.

Anukam, K. C., Osazuwa, E., Osemene, G. I., Ehigiagbe, F., Bruce, A. W., & Reid, G. (2006). Clinical study comparing probiotic Lactobacillus GR-1 and RC-14 with metronidazole vaginal gel to treat symptomatic bacterial vaginosis. Microbes and Infection, 8(12-13), 2772-2776.

Reid, G., Charbonneau, D., Erb, J., Kochanowski, B., Beuerman, D., Poehner, R., & Bruce, A. W. (2003). Oral use of Lactobacillus rhamnosus GR-1 and L. fermentum RC-14 significantly alters vaginal flora: randomized, placebo-controlled trial in 64 healthy women. FEMS Immunology & Medical Microbiology, 35(2), 131-134.

Saunders, S., Bocking, A., Challis, J., & Reid, G. (2007). Effect of Lactobacillus challenge on Gardnerella vaginalis biofilms. Colloids and Surfaces B: Biointerfaces, 55(2), 138-142.

Kamala, S., & Priya, S. (2009). Benefits of probiotic treatment in cases of bad obstetric history (BOH) and for prevention of post IVF pregnancy complications. J Obstet Gynecol India, 59(4), 336-339.

13 Kadogami, D., Nakaoka, Y., & Morimoto, Y. (2020). Use of a vaginal probiotic suppository and antibiotics to influence the composition of the endometrial microbiota. Reproductive Biology, 20(3), 307-314.

14 Likes, C. E., Cooper, L. J., Efird, J., Forstein, D. A., Miller, P. B., Savaris, R., & Lessey, B. A. (2019). Medical or surgical treatment before embryo transfer improves outcomes in women with abnormal endometrial BCL6 expression. Journal of Assisted Reproduction and Genetics, 36, 483-490.

15 Likes, C. E., Cooper, L. J., Efird, J., Forstein, D. A., Miller, P. B., Savaris, R., & Lessey, B. A. (2019). Medical or surgical treatment before embryo transfer improves outcomes in women with abnormal endometrial BCL6 expression. Journal of Assisted Reproduction and Genetics, 36, 483-490.

16 Evans, M. B., & Decherney, A. H. (2017). Fertility and endometriosis. Clinical obstetrics and gynecology, 60(3), 497-502.

17 Schwartz, A. S. K., Wölfler, M. M., Mitter, V., Rauchfuss, M., Haeberlin, F., Eberhard, M., ... & Leeners, B. (2017). Endometriosis, especially mild disease: a risk factor for miscarriages. Fertility and sterility, 108(5), 806-814. Santulli, P., Marcellin, L., Menard, S., Thubert, T., Khoshnood, B., Gayet, V., ... & Chapron, C. (2016). Increased rate of spontaneous miscarriages in endometriosis-affected women. Human Reproduction, 31(5), 1014-1023.

18 Almquist, L. D., Likes, C. E., Stone, B., Brown, K. R., Savaris, R., Forstein, D. A., ... & Lessey, B. A. (2017). Endometrial BCL6 testing for the prediction of in vitro fertilization outcomes: a cohort study. Fertility and sterility, 108(6), 1063-1069.

19 Evans-Hoeker, E., Lessey, B. A., Jeong, J. W., Savaris, R. F., Palomino, W. A., Yuan, L., ... & Young, S. L. (2016). Endometrial BCL6 overexpression in eutopic endometrium of women with endometriosis. Reproductive Sciences, 23(9), 1234-1241.

20 Id.

21 Dan, A. (2020). Outcomes in women with IVF failure who tested positive for BCL6 using ReceptivaDx™ testing: Effect of treatment on subsequent embryo transfer. Fertility and Sterility, 113(4), e13.

22 Dan, A. (2020). Outcomes in women with IVF failure who tested positive for BCL6 using ReceptivaDx™ testing: Effect of treatment on subsequent embryo transfer. Fertility and Sterility, 113(4), e13. Likes, C. E., Cooper, L. J., Efird, J., Forstein, D. A., Miller, P. B., Savaris, R., & Lessey, B. A. (2019). Medical or surgical treatment before embryo transfer improves outcomes in women with abnormal endometrial BCL6 expression. Journal of Assisted Reproduction and Genetics, 36, 483-490.

23 Mavrelos, D., & Saridogan, E. (2015). Treatment of endometriosis in women desiring fertility. The Journal of Obstetrics and Gynecology of India, 65, 11-16.

24 Id.

25 Lédée, N., Petitbarat, M., Chevrier, L., Vitoux, D., Vezmar, K., Rahmati, M., ... & Chaouat, G. (2016). The uterine immune profile may help

women with repeated unexplained embryo implantation failure after in vitro fertilization. American Journal of Reproductive Immunology, 75(3), 388-401.

Amjadi, F., Zandieh, Z., Mehdizadeh, M., Aghajanpour, S., Raoufi, E., Aghamajidi, A., & Aflatoonian, R. (2020). The uterine immunological changes may be responsible for repeated implantation failure. Journal of Reproductive Immunology, 138, 103080.

Wang, Q., Sun, Y., Fan, R., Wang, M., Ren, C., Jiang, A., & Yang, T. (2022). Role of inflammatory factors in the etiology and treatment of recurrent implantation failure. Reproductive Biology, 22(4), 100698.

Hill, J. A., Polgar, K., & Anderson, D. J. (1995). T-helper 1-type immunity to trophoblast in women with recurrent spontaneous abortion. Jama, 273(24), 1933-1936.

26 Birkenfeld, A., Mukaida, T., Minichiello, L., Jackson, M., Kase, N. G., & Yemini, M. (1994). Incidence of autoimmune antibodies in failed embryo transfer cycles. American Journal of Reproductive Immunology, 31(2-3), 65-68.

27 Deroux, A., Dumestre-Perard, C., Dunand-Faure, C., Bouillet, L., & Hoffmann, P. (2017). Female infertility and serum auto-antibodies: a systematic review. Clinical reviews in allergy & immunology, 53, 78-86.

28 Practice Committee of the American Society for Reproductive Medicine. (2012). Evaluation and treatment of recurrent pregnancy loss: a committee opinion. Fertility and sterility, 98(5), 1103-1111.

29 Bobircă, A., Dumitrache, A., Alexandru, C., Florescu, A., Ciobotaru, G., Bobircă, F., ... & Ancuța, I. (2022). Pathophysiology of Placenta in Antiphospholipid Syndrome. Physiologia, 2(3), 66-79.

30 Practice Committee of the American Society for Reproductive Medicine. (2012). Evaluation and treatment of recurrent pregnancy loss: a committee opinion. Fertility and sterility, 98(5), 1103-1111.

31 Stern, C., Chamley, L., Hale, L., Kloss, M., Speirs, A., & Baker, H. G. (1998). Antibodies to β2 glycoprotein I are associated with in vitro fertilization implantation failure as well as recurrent miscarriage: results of a prevalence study. Fertility and sterility, 70(5), 938-944.

Jarne-Borràs, M., Miró-Mur, F., Anunciación-Llunell, A., & Alijotas-Reig, J. (2022). Antiphospholipid antibodies in women with recurrent embryo implantation failure: A systematic review and meta-analysis. Autoimmunity Reviews, 21(6), 103101.

Papadimitriou, E., Boutzios, G., Mathioudakis, A. G., Vlahos, N. F., Vlachoyiannopoulos, P., & Mastorakos, G. (2022). Presence of antiphospholipid antibodies is associated with increased implantation failure following in vitro fertilization technique and embryo transfer: A systematic review and meta-analysis. Plos one, 17(7), e0260759.

32 Hamulyák, E. N., Scheres, L. J., Marijnen, M. C., Goddijn, M., & Middeldorp, S. (2020). Aspirin or heparin or both for improving pregnancy outcomes in women with persistent antiphospholipid

antibodies and recurrent pregnancy loss. Cochrane Database of Systematic Reviews, (5).

Wu, L., Fang, X., Lu, F., Zhang, Y., Wang, Y., & Kwak-Kim, J. (2022). Anticardiolipin and/or anti-β2-glycoprotein-I antibodies are associated with adverse IVF outcomes. Frontiers in Immunology, 13, 6671.

Geva, E., et al., (2000). Prednisone and aspirin improve pregnancy rate in patients with reproductive failure and autoimmune antibodies: a prospective study. American Journal of Reproductive Immunology, 43(1), 36-40.

Hamulyák, E. N., Scheres, L. J., Marijnen, M. C., Goddijn, M., & Middeldorp, S. (2020). Aspirin or heparin or both for improving pregnancy outcomes in women with persistent antiphospholipid antibodies and recurrent pregnancy loss. Cochrane Database of Systematic Reviews, (5).

Bramham, K., Thomas, M., Nelson-Piercy, C., Khamashta, M., & Hunt, B. J. (2011). First-trimester low-dose prednisolone in refractory antiphospholipid antibody–related pregnancy loss. Blood, The Journal of the American Society of Hematology, 117(25), 6948-6951.

Yang, Z., Shen, X., Zhou, C., Wang, M., Liu, Y., & Zhou, L. (2021). Prevention of recurrent miscarriage in women with antiphospholipid syndrome: A systematic review and network meta-analysis. Lupus, 30(1), 70-79.

33 Wu, L., Fang, X., Lu, F., Zhang, Y., Wang, Y., & Kwak-Kim, J. (2022). Anticardiolipin and/or anti-β2-glycoprotein-I antibodies are associated with adverse IVF outcomes. Frontiers in Immunology, 13, 6671.

34 Geva, E., et al., (2000). Prednisone and aspirin improve pregnancy rate in patients with reproductive failure and autoimmune antibodies: a prospective study. American Journal of Reproductive Immunology, 43(1), 36-40.

35 La Villa G, Pantaleo P, Tarquini R, Cirami L, Perfetto F, Man- cuso F, Laffi G. Multiple immune disorders in unrecognized celiac disease: a case report. World J Gastroenterol, 2003;9(6): 1377-1380. ("La Villa 2003").

36 La Villa 2003.

37 Łukaszuk, K., Kunicki, M., Kulwikowska, P., Liss, J., Pastuszek, E., Jaszczołt, M., ... & Skowroński, K. (2015). The impact of the presence of antithyroid antibodies on pregnancy outcome following intracytoplasmatic sperm injection-ICSI and embryo transfer in women with normal thyreotropine levels. Journal of endocrinological investigation, 38, 1335-1343.

Monteleone, P., Parrini, D., Faviana, P., Carletti, E., Casarosa, E., Uccelli, A., ... & Artini, P. G. (2011). Female infertility related to thyroid autoimmunity: the ovarian follicle hypothesis. American journal of reproductive immunology, 66(2), 108-114.

Bellver, J., Soares, S. R., Alvarez, C., Munoz, E., Ramírez, A., Rubio, C., ... & Pellicer, A. (2008). The role of thrombophilia and thyroid autoimmunity in unexplained infertility, implantation failure and recurrent spontaneous abortion. Human reproduction, 23(2), 278-284.

Chen CW, Huang YL, Tzeng CR, Huang RL, Chen CH 2017 Idiopathic low ovarian reserve is associated with more frequent positive thyroid peroxidase antibodies. Thyroid 27:1194–1200.

38 Monteleone, P., Parrini, D., Faviana, P., Carletti, E., Casarosa, E., Uccelli, A., ... & Artini, P. G. (2011). Female infertility related to thyroid autoimmunity: the ovarian follicle hypothesis. American journal of reproductive immunology, 66(2), 108-114.

Zhong, Y. P., Ying, Y., Wu, H. T., Zhou, C. Q., Xu, Y. W., Wang, Q., ... & Li, J. (2012). Relationship between antithyroid antibody and pregnancy outcome following in vitro fertilization and embryo transfer. International journal of medical sciences, 9(2), 121-125.

39 Rahnama, R., Mahmoudi, A. R., Kazemnejad, S., Salehi, M., Ghahiri, A., Soltanghoraee, H., ... & Zarnani, A. H. (2021). Thyroid peroxidase in human endometrium and placenta: a potential target for anti-TPO antibodies. Clinical and Experimental Medicine, 21, 79-88.

Spinillo, A., De Maggio, I., Ruspini, B., Bellingeri, C., Cavagnoli, C., Giannico, S., ... & Beneventi, F. (2021). Placental pathologic features in thyroid autoimmunity. Placenta, 112, 66-72

40 Jha, V., & Goswami, D. (2016). Premature ovarian failure: an association with autoimmune diseases. Journal of Clinical and Diagnostic Research: JCDR, 10(10), QC10.

Hsieh, Y. T., & Ho, J. Y. (2021). Thyroid autoimmunity is associated with higher risk of premature ovarian insufficiency—a nationwide health insurance research database study. Human Reproduction, 36(6), 1621-1629.

Monteleone, P., Parrini, D., Faviana, P., Carletti, E., Casarosa, E., Uccelli, A., ... & Artini, P. G. (2011). Female infertility related to thyroid autoimmunity: the ovarian follicle hypothesis. American journal of reproductive immunology, 66(2), 108-114.

Zhong, Y. P., Ying, Y., Wu, H. T., Zhou, C. Q., Xu, Y. W., Wang, Q., ... & Li, J. (2012). Relationship between antithyroid antibody and pregnancy outcome following in vitro fertilization and embryo transfer. International journal of medical sciences, 9(2), 121-125

Saglam, F., Onal, E. D., Ersoy, R., Koca, C., Ergin, M., Erel, O., & Cakir, B. (2015). Anti-Müllerian hormone as a marker of premature ovarian aging in autoimmune thyroid disease. Gynecological Endocrinology, 31(2), 165-168

Pogačnik, R. K., Vrtovec, H. M., Vizjak, A., Levičnik, A. U., Slabe, N., & Ihan, A. (2014). Possible role of autoimmunity in patients with premature ovarian insufficiency. International journal of fertility & sterility, 7(4), 281

41 Kim, N. Y., Cho, H. J., Kim, H. Y., Yang, K. M., Ahn, H. K., Thornton, S., ... & Kwak-Kim, J. (2011). Thyroid autoimmunity and its association

with cellular and humoral immunity in women with reproductive failures. American Journal of Reproductive Immunology, 65(1), 78-87.

Miko, E., Meggyes, M., Doba, K., Farkas, N., Bogar, B., Barakonyi, A., ... & Mezosi, E. (2017). Characteristics of peripheral blood NK and NKT-like cells in euthyroid and subclinical hypothyroid women with thyroid autoimmunity experiencing reproductive failure. Journal of reproductive immunology, 124, 62-70.

42 Zhou, G., Zhou, M., Duan, X., & Li, W. (2021). Glucocorticoid supplementation improves reproductive outcomes in infertile women with antithyroid autoimmunity undergoing ART: a meta-analysis. Medicine, 100(16).

Pearce, E. N. (2015). Prednisolone Treatment May Improve In Vitro Fertilization Outcomes in Women with Antithyroid Antibodies. Clinical Thyroidology, 27(1), 17-19.

Turi, A., Giannubilo, S. R., Zanconi, S., Mascetti, A., & Tranquilli, A. L. (2010). Preconception steroid treatment in infertile women with antithyroid autoimmunity undergoing ovarian stimulation and intrauterine insemination: a double-blind, randomized, prospective cohort study. Clinical therapeutics, 32(14), 2415-2421

43 Revelli, A., Casano, S., Piane, L. D., Grassi, G., Gennarelli, G., Guidetti, D., & Massobrio, M. (2009). A retrospective study on IVF outcome in euthyroid patients with anti-thyroid antibodies: effects of levothyroxine, acetyl-salicylic acid and prednisolone adjuvant treatments. Reproductive biology and endocrinology, 7(1), 1-6

Turi, A., Giannubilo, S. R., Zanconi, S., Mascetti, A., & Tranquilli, A. L. (2010). Preconception steroid treatment in infertile women with antithyroid autoimmunity undergoing ovarian stimulation and intrauterine insemination: a double-blind, randomized, prospective cohort study. Clinical therapeutics, 32(14), 2415-2421

44 Zhou, P., Yao, Q., Zhao, Q., Yang, L., Yu, Y., Xie, J., ... & Jin, M. (2022). IVF/ICSI outcomes of euthyroid infertile women with thyroid autoimmunity: does treatment with aspirin plus prednisone matter?. BMC Pregnancy and Childbirth, 22(1), 263.

45 Zhou, P., Yao, Q., Zhao, Q., Yang, L., Yu, Y., Xie, J., ... & Jin, M. (2022). IVF/ICSI outcomes of euthyroid infertile women with thyroid autoimmunity: does treatment with aspirin plus prednisone matter?. BMC Pregnancy and Childbirth, 22(1), 263.

Litwicka, K., Arrivi, C., Varricchio, M. T., Mencacci, C., & Greco, E. (2015). In women with thyroid autoimmunity, does low-dose prednisolone administration, compared with no adjuvant therapy, improve in vitro fertilization clinical results?. Journal of Obstetrics and Gynaecology Research, 41(5), 722-728.

46 Liu, H., Shan, Z., Li, C., Mao, J., Xie, X., Wang, W., ... & Teng, W. (2014). Maternal subclinical hypothyroidism, thyroid autoimmunity, and the

risk of miscarriage: a prospective cohort study. Thyroid, 24(11), 1642-1649.

47 Kacharava, T., Giorgadze, E., Janjgava, S., Lomtadze, N., & Taboridze, I. (2023). Correlation between Vitamin B12 Deficiency and Autoimmune Thyroid Diseases. Endocrine, Metabolic & Immune Disorders-Drug Targets (Formerly Current Drug Targets-Immune, Endocrine & Metabolic Disorders), 23(1), 86-94.

Zhang, J., Chen, Y., Li, H., & Li, H. (2021). Effects of vitamin D on thyroid autoimmunity markers in Hashimoto's thyroiditis: systematic review and meta-analysis. Journal of International Medical Research, 49(12), 03000605211060675.

Aktaş, H. Ş. (2020). Vitamin B12 and vitamin D levels in patients with autoimmune hypothyroidism and their correlation with anti-thyroid peroxidase antibodies. Medical Principles and Practice, 29(4), 364-370.

48 Hu, Y., Feng, W., Chen, H., Shi, H., Jiang, L., Zheng, X., ... & Cui, D. (2021). Effect of selenium on thyroid autoimmunity and regulatory T cells in patients with Hashimoto's thyroiditis: A prospective randomized-controlled trial. Clinical and Translational Science, 14(4), 1390-1402.

49 Krysiak, R., Szkróbka, W., & Okopień, B. (2019). The effect of gluten-free diet on thyroid autoimmunity in drug-naïve women with Hashimoto's thyroiditis: a pilot study. Experimental and Clinical Endocrinology & Diabetes, 127(07), 417-422.

50 Hollywood, J. B., Hutchinson, D., Feehery-Alpuerto, N., Whitfield, M., Davis, K., & Johnson, L. M. (2022). The Effects of the Paleo Diet on Autoimmune Thyroid Disease: A Mixed Methods Review. Journal of the American Nutrition Association, 1-10.

51 Ostrowska, L., Gier, D., & Zyśk, B. (2021). The influence of reducing diets on changes in thyroid parameters in women suffering from obesity and hashimoto's disease. Nutrients, 13(3), 862.

52 Ostrowska, L., Gier, D., & Zyśk, B. (2021). The influence of reducing diets on changes in thyroid parameters in women suffering from obesity and hashimoto's disease. Nutrients, 13(3), 862.

53 Whitfield, M., Hollywood, J., & Keister, A. (2021). Nutritional Management of Hashimoto's Thyroiditis: A Case Report. Available at SSRN 3990138.

54 Stern, C., Chamley, L., Hale, L., Kloss, M., Speirs, A., & Baker, H. G. (1998). Antibodies to β2 glycoprotein I are associated with in vitro fertilization implantation failure as well as recurrent miscarriage: results of a prevalence study. Fertility and sterility, 70(5), 938-944

Ticconi, C., Inversetti, A., Logruosso, E., Ghio, M., Casadei, L., Selmi, C., & Di Simone, N. (2023). Antinuclear antibodies positivity in women in reproductive age: from infertility to adverse obstetrical outcomes–A meta-analysis. Journal of Reproductive Immunology, 103794.

Cavalcante, M. B., Cavalcante, C. T. D. M. B., Sarno, M., da Silva, A. C. B., & Barini, R. (2020). Antinuclear antibodies and recurrent miscarriage: systematic review and meta-analysis. American Journal of Reproductive Immunology, 83(3), e13215

55 Yoshihara, H., Sugiura-Ogasawara, M., Kitaori, T., & Goto, S. (2021, July). Association between antinuclear antibodies and pregnancy prognosis in recurrent pregnancy loss patients. In HUMAN REPRODUCTION (Vol. 36, pp. 307-308).
Sun S, Li C, Kou X, Chen C, Guo F, Zhao A. Association of Prednisone and Antinuclear Antibodies With Pregnancy Outcomes in Women With Unexplained Recurrent Pregnancy Loss. Int J Gynaecol Obstet (2021) 154:492–99. doi: 10.1002/ijgo.13556

56 Fan, J., Zhong, Y., & Chen, C. (2016). Combined treatment of prednisone and aspirin, starting before ovulation induction, may improve reproductive outcomes in ANA-positive patients. American Journal of Reproductive Immunology, 76(5), 391-395.
Zhu, Q., Wu, L., Xu, B., Hu, M. H., Tong, X. H., Ji, J. J., & Liu, Y. S. (2013). A retrospective study on IVF/ICSI outcome in patients with anti-nuclear antibodies: the effects of prednisone plus low-dose aspirin adjuvant treatment. Reproductive Biology and Endocrinology, 11(1), 1-9.

57 Fan, J., Zhong, Y., & Chen, C. (2016). Combined treatment of prednisone and aspirin, starting before ovulation induction, may improve reproductive outcomes in ANA-positive patients. American Journal of Reproductive Immunology, 76(5), 391-395.
Zhu, Q., Wu, L., Xu, B., Hu, M. H., Tong, X. H., Ji, J. J., & Liu, Y. S. (2013). A retrospective study on IVF/ICSI outcome in patients with anti-nuclear antibodies: the effects of prednisone plus low-dose aspirin adjuvant treatment. Reproductive Biology and Endocrinology, 11(1), 1-9.

58 Gao, R., Deng, W., Meng, C., Cheng, K., Zeng, X., & Qin, L. (2021). Combined treatment of prednisone and hydroxychloroquine may improve outcomes of frozen embryo transfer in antinuclear antibody-positive patients undergoing IVF/ICSI treatment. Lupus, 30(14), 2213-2220.

59 Sun, S., Li, C., Kou, X., Chen, C., Guo, F., & Zhao, A. (2021). Association of prednisone and antinuclear antibodies with pregnancy outcomes in women with unexplained recurrent pregnancy loss. International Journal of Gynecology & Obstetrics, 154(3), 492-499.

60 D'Ippolito, S., Ticconi, C., Tersigni, C., Garofalo, S., Martino, C., Lanzone, A., ... & Di Simone, N. (2020). The pathogenic role of autoantibodies in recurrent pregnancy loss. American Journal of Reproductive Immunology, 83(1), e13200.

61 Vomstein, K., Aulitzky, A., Strobel, L., Bohlmann, M., Feil, K., Rudnik-Schöneborn, S., ... & Toth, B. (2021). Recurrent spontaneous miscarriage: a comparison of international guidelines. Geburtshilfe und Frauenheilkunde, 81(07), 769-779.

62 Kim, N. Y., Cho, H. J., Kim, H. Y., Yang, K. M., Ahn, H. K., Thornton, S., ... & Kwak-Kim, J. (2011). Thyroid autoimmunity and its association with cellular and humoral immunity in women with reproductive failures. American Journal of Reproductive Immunology, 65(1), 78-87.
Miko, E., Meggyes, M., Doba, K., Farkas, N., Bogar, B., Barakonyi, A., ... & Mezosi, E. (2017). Characteristics of peripheral blood NK and NKT-like cells in euthyroid and subclinical hypothyroid women with thyroid autoimmunity experiencing reproductive failure. Journal of reproductive immunology, 124, 62-70.
Wu, L., Fang, X., Lu, F., Zhang, Y., Wang, Y., & Kwak-Kim, J. (2022). Anticardiolipin and/or anti-β2-glycoprotein-I antibodies are associated with adverse IVF outcomes. Frontiers in Immunology, 13, 6671

63 Fukui, A., Fujii, S., Yamaguchi, E., Kimura, H., Sato, S., & Saito, Y. (1999). Natural killer cell subpopulations and cytotoxicity for infertile patients undergoing in vitro fertilization. American journal of reproductive immunology, 41(6), 413-422.
Coulam, C. B., & Roussev, R. G. (2003). Correlation of NK cell activation and inhibition markers with NK cytoxicity among women experiencing immunologic implantation failure after in vitro fertilization and embryo transfer. Journal of assisted reproduction and genetics, 20, 58-62.
Lee, S. K., Na, B. J., Kim, J. Y., Hur, S. E., Lee, M., Gilman-Sachs, A., & Kwak-Kim, J. (2013). Determination of clinical cellular immune markers in women with recurrent pregnancy loss. American journal of reproductive immunology, 70(5), 398-411.

64 Lee SK, Kim JY, Hur SE, Kim CJ, Na BJ, Lee M, et al. An imbalance in interleukin-17-producing T and Foxp3(+) regulatory T cells in women with idiopathic recurrent pregnancy loss. Hum Reprod. (2011) 26:2964–71.
Sereshki, N., Gharagozloo, M., Ostadi, V., Ghahiri, A., Roghaei, M. A., Mehrabian, F., ... & Rezaei, A. (2014). Variations in T-helper 17 and regulatory T cells during the menstrual cycle in peripheral blood of women with recurrent spontaneous abortion. International journal of fertility & sterility, 8(1), 59.
Wang, W., Sung, N., Gilman-Sachs, A., & Kwak-Kim, J. (2020). T helper (Th) cell profiles in pregnancy and recurrent pregnancy losses: Th1/Th2/Th9/Th17/Th22/Tfh cells. Frontiers in immunology, 11, 2025.
Kuroda, K., Nakagawa, K., Horikawa, T., Moriyama, A., Ojiro, Y., Takamizawa, S., ... & Sugiyama, R. (2021). Increasing number of implantation failures and pregnancy losses associated with elevated Th1/Th2 cell ratio. American Journal of Reproductive Immunology, 86(3), e13429.

65 Singh, N., Davis, A. A., Kumar, S., & Kriplani, A. (2019). The effect of administration of intravenous intralipid on pregnancy outcomes in women with implantation failure after IVF/ICSI with non-donor

oocytes: a randomised controlled trial. European Journal of Obstetrics & Gynecology and Reproductive Biology, 240, 45-51.

Dakhly DMR, Bayoumi YA, Sharkawy M, et al. Intralipid supplementation in women with recurrent spontaneous abortion and elevated levels of natural killer cells. Int J Gynaecol Obstet. 2016;135(3):324-327.

El-Khayat, W., & El Sadek, M. (2015). Intralipid for repeated implantation failure (RIF): a randomized controlled trial. Fertility and Sterility, 104(3), e26.

66 Sung, N., Khan, S. A., Yiu, M. E., Jubiz, G., Salazar, M. D., Skariah, A., ... & Kwak-Kim, J. (2021). Reproductive outcomes of women with recurrent pregnancy losses and repeated implantation failures are significantly improved with immunomodulatory treatment. Journal of Reproductive Immunology, 148, 103369.

67 Mekinian, A., Cohen, J., Alijotas-Reig, J., Carbillon, L., Nicaise-Roland, P., Kayem, G., ... & Bornes, M. (2016). Unexplained recurrent miscarriage and recurrent implantation failure: is there a place for immunomodulation?. American Journal of Reproductive Immunology, 76(1), 8-28.

68 Turocy, J., & Williams, Z. (2021). Novel therapeutic options for treatment of recurrent implantation failure. Fertility and Sterility, 116(6), 1449-1454.

Busnelli, A., Somigliana, E., Cirillo, F., Baggiani, A., & Levi-Setti, P. E. (2021). Efficacy of therapies and interventions for repeated embryo implantation failure: a systematic review and meta-analysis. Scientific Reports, 11(1), 1747

69 Nazari, L., Salehpour, S., Hosseini, S., Sheibani, S., & Hosseinirad, H. (2022). The effects of autologous platelet-rich plasma on pregnancy outcomes in repeated implantation failure patients undergoing frozen embryo transfer: a randomized controlled trial. Reproductive Sciences, 1-8. Turocy, J., & Williams, Z. (2021). Novel therapeutic options for treatment of recurrent implantation failure. Fertility and Sterility, 116(6), 1449-1454

70 Scarpellini, F., Klinger, F. G., Rossi, G., & Sbracia, M. (2019). Immunohistochemical study on the expression of G-CSF, G-CSFR, VEGF, VEGFR-1, Foxp3 in first trimester trophoblast of recurrent pregnancy loss in pregnancies treated with G-CSF and controls. International journal of molecular sciences, 21(1), 285.

Busnelli, A., Somigliana, E., Cirillo, F., Baggiani, A., & Levi-Setti, P. E. (2021). Efficacy of therapies and interventions for repeated embryo implantation failure: a systematic review and meta-analysis. Scientific Reports, 11(1), 1747

71 Ji, J., Zhai, H., Zhou, H., Song, S., Mor, G., & Liao, A. (2019). The role and mechanism of vitamin D-mediated regulation of Treg/Th17

balance in recurrent pregnancy loss. American journal of reproductive immunology, 81(6), e13112.

Kwak-Kim, J., Skariah, A., Wu, L., Salazar, D., Sung, N., & Ota, K. (2016). Humoral and cellular autoimmunity in women with recurrent pregnancy losses and repeated implantation failures: a possible role of vitamin D. Autoimmunity reviews, 15(10), 943-947.

72 Ota, K., Dambaeva, S., Han, A. R., Beaman, K., Gilman-Sachs, A., & Kwak-Kim, J. (2014). Vitamin D deficiency may be a risk factor for recurrent pregnancy losses by increasing cellular immunity and autoimmunity. Human reproduction, 29(2), 208-219.

73 Ota, K., Han, A., Gilman-Sachs, A., Kenneth, B., & Kwak-Kim, J. (2012). Vitamin D deficiency (VDd) and immune parameters in recurrent pregnancy losses. Fertility and Sterility, 98(3), S27.

74 Yang, T., Yang, Y., Zhang, Q., Liu, D., Liu, N., Li, Y., ... & Li, Y. (2022). Homeostatic model assessment for insulin resistance is associated with late miscarriage in non-dyslipidemic women undergoing fresh IVF/ICSI embryo transfer. Frontiers in Endocrinology, 1124.

Edugbe, A. E., James, B., Akunaeziri, U. A., Egbodo, C. O., Imoh, C. L., Ajen, A. S., ... & Samaila, M. (2020). Beta-cell dysfunction and abnormal glucose metabolism among non-diabetic women with recurrent miscarriages. Archives of Gynecology and Obstetrics, 301, 559-564.

Ispasoiu, C. A., Chicea, R., Stamatian, F. V., & Ispasoiu, F. (2013). High fasting insulin levels and insulin resistance may be linked to idiopathic recurrent pregnancy loss: a case-control study. International Journal of Endocrinology, 2013.

Craig LB , Ke RW, Kutteh WH. (2002). Increased prevalence of insulin resistance in women with a history of recurrent pregnancy loss. Fertil Steril, 2002;78:487–490.

75 Columbia University (2019), Study reports that high insulin levels are toxic to placenta cells, potentially causing miscarriages. https://www. obgyn.columbia.edu/news/study-reports-high-insulin-levels-are-toxic-placenta-cells-potentially-causing-miscarriages

76 Vega, M., Mauro, M., & Williams, Z. (2019). Direct toxicity of insulin on the human placenta and protection by metformin. Fertility and Sterility, 111(3), 489-496.

77 Fruzzetti, F., Perini, D., Russo, M., Bucci, F., & Gadducci, A. (2017). Comparison of two insulin sensitizers, metformin and myo-inositol, in women with polycystic ovary syndrome (PCOS). Gynecological Endocrinology, 33(1), 39-42.

Formoso, G., Baldassarre, M. P., Ginestra, F., Carlucci, M. A., Bucci, I., & Consoli, A. (2019). Inositol and antioxidant supplementation: Safety and efficacy in pregnancy. Diabetes/metabolism research and reviews, 35(5), e3154.

78   Practice Committee of the American Society for Reproductive Medicine. (2012). Evaluation and treatment of recurrent pregnancy loss: a committee opinion. Fertility and sterility, 98(5), 1103-1111.

79   Pritchard, A. M., Hendrix, P. W., & Paidas, M. J. (2016). Hereditary thrombophilia and recurrent pregnancy loss. Clinical obstetrics and gynecology, 59(3), 487-497.

80   Zarfeshan Fard, Y., Kooshkaki, O., Kordi Tammandani, D., & Anani Sarab, G. (2019). Investigation of the association between C677T polymorphism of the MTHFR gene and plasma homocysteine level in recurrent fetal miscarriage. Journal of Obstetrics and Gynaecology Research, 45(8), 1442-1447.
Govindaiah, V., Naushad, S. M., Prabhakara, K., Krishna, P. C., & Devi, A. R. R. (2009). Association of parental hyperhomocysteinemia and C677T Methylene tetrahydrofolate reductase (MTHFR) polymorphism with recurrent pregnancy loss. Clinical biochemistry, 42(4-5), 380-386.
Sah, A. K., Shrestha, N., Joshi, P., Lakha, R., Shrestha, S., Sharma, L., ... & Rijal, B. (2018). Association of parental methylenetetrahydrofolate reductase (MTHFR) C677T gene polymorphism in couples with unexplained recurrent pregnancy loss. BMC research notes, 11(1), 1-5.

81   Gris, J. C., Quéré, I., Monpeyrou, F., Mercier, E., Ripart-Neveu, S., Tailland, M. L., ... & Marès, P. (1999). Case-control study of the frequency of thrombophilic disorders in couples with late foetal loss and no thrombotic antecedent. Thrombosis and haemostasis, 81(06), 891-899.

82   Clément, A., Amar, E., Brami, C., Clément, P., Alvarez, S., Jacquesson-Fournols, L., ... & Menezo, Y. (2022). MTHFR SNPs (Methyl Tetrahydrofolate Reductase, Single Nucleotide Polymorphisms) C677T and A1298C Prevalence and Serum Homocysteine Levels in> 2100 Hypofertile Caucasian Male Patients. Biomolecules, 12(8), 1086.
Govindaiah, V., Naushad, S. M., Prabhakara, K., Krishna, P. C., & Devi, A. R. R. (2009). Association of parental hyperhomocysteinemia and C677T Methylene tetrahydrofolate reductase (MTHFR) polymorphism with recurrent pregnancy loss. Clinical biochemistry, 42(4-5), 380-386.

83   Practice Committee of the American Society for Reproductive Medicine. (2012). Evaluation and treatment of recurrent pregnancy loss: a committee opinion. Fertility and sterility, 98(5), 1103-1111.

84   Hirahara F, Andoh N, Sawai K, Hirabuki T, Uemura T, Minaguchi H. Hyperprolactinemic recurrent miscarriage and results of randomized bromocriptine treatment trials. Fertil Steril 1998;70:246–52.

85   Lin, X., Wei, M., Li, T. C., Huang, Q., Huang, D., Zhou, F., & Zhang, S. (2013). A comparison of intrauterine balloon, intrauterine contraceptive device and hyaluronic acid gel in the prevention of adhesion reformation following hysteroscopic surgery for Asherman syndrome: a cohort study. European Journal of Obstetrics & Gynecology and Reproductive Biology, 170(2), 512-516.

Guo, E. J., Chung, J. P. W., Poon, L. C. Y., & Li, T. C. (2019). Reproductive outcomes after surgical treatment of asherman syndrome: A systematic review. Best practice & research Clinical obstetrics & gynaecology, 59, 98-114.

86 Khan, Z., & Goldberg, J. M. (2018). Hysteroscopic management of Asherman's syndrome. Journal of minimally invasive gynecology, 25(2), 218-228.

87 Baradwan, S., Baradwan, A., & Al-Jaroudi, D. (2018). The association between menstrual cycle pattern and hysteroscopic march classification with endometrial thickness among infertile women with Asherman syndrome. Medicine, 97(27).

88 Willis, O. (April 21, 2023.) Asherman's syndrome can affect fertility. But many women say they struggled to get diagnosed. ABC News Australia. https://www.abc.net.au/news/health/2023-04-22/ashermans-syndrome-fertility-dilation-curettage-scarring-uterus/102243858

89 Gharibeh, N., Aghebati-Maleki, L., Madani, J., Pourakbari, R., Yousefi, M., & Ahmadian Heris, J. (2022). Cell-based therapy in thin endometrium and Asherman syndrome. Stem Cell Research & Therapy, 13(1), 33.

Puente Gonzalo, E., Alonso Pacheco, L., Vega Jiménez, A., Vitale, S. G., Raffone, A., & Laganà, A. S. (2021). Intrauterine infusion of platelet-rich plasma for severe Asherman syndrome: a cutting-edge approach. Updates in Surgery, 73, 2355-2362.

Aghajanova, L., Sundaram, V., Kao, C. N., Letourneau, J. M., Manvelyan, E., Cedars, M. I., & Huddleston, H. G. (2021). Autologous platelet-rich plasma treatment for moderate-severe Asherman syndrome: the first experience. Journal of Assisted Reproduction and Genetics, 38, 2955-2963.

Gleicher, N., Vidali, A., & Barad, D. H. (2011). Successful treatment of unresponsive thin endometrium. Fertility and sterility, 95(6), 2123-e13.

90 Arian, S. E., Hessami, K., Khatibi, A., To, A. K., Shamshirsaz, A. A., & Gibbons, W. (2022). Endometrial receptivity array before frozen embryo transfer cycles: a systematic review and meta-analysis. Fertility and Sterility.

Riestenberg, C., Kroener, L., Quinn, M., Ching, K., & Ambartsumyan, G. (2021). Routine endometrial receptivity array in first embryo transfer cycles does not improve live birth rate. Fertility and Sterility, 115(4), 1001-1006.

Doyle, N., Combs, J. C., Jahandideh, S., Wilkinson, V., Devine, K., & O'Brien, J. E. (2022). Live birth after transfer of a single euploid vitrified-warmed blastocyst according to standard timing vs. timing as recommended by endometrial receptivity analysis. Fertility and Sterility, 118(2), 314-321.

91 Stern, C., Pertile, M., Norris, H., Hale, L., & Baker, H. W. G. (1999). Chromosome translocations in couples with in-vitro fertilization implantation failure. Human Reproduction, 14(8), 2097-2101.
Shaulov, T., Sierra, S., & Sylvestre, C. (2020). Recurrent implantation failure in ivf: A canadian fertility and andrology society clinical practice guideline. Reproductive biomedicine online, 41(5), 819-833.

92 Meuleman, T., Lashley, L. E., Dekkers, O. M., van Lith, J. M., Claas, F. H., & Bloemenkamp, K. W. (2015). HLA associations and HLA sharing in recurrent miscarriage: a systematic review and meta-analysis. Human immunology, 76(5), 362-373.

93 Balasch, J., Coll, O., Martorell, J., Jove, I. C., Gaya, A., & Vanrell, J. A. (1989). Further data against HLA sharing in couples with recurrent spontaneous abortion. Gynecological Endocrinology, 3(1), 63-69.
Aruna, M., Sudheer, P. S., Andal, S., Tarakeswari, S., Reddy, A. G., Thangaraj, K., ... & Reddy, B. M. (2010). HLA-G polymorphism patterns show lack of detectable association with recurrent spontaneous abortion. Tissue Antigens, 76(3), 216-222.
Dizon,, Nelson, L., Scott, J. R., Branch, D. W., & Ward, K. (1995). Human leukocyte antigen DQ α sharing is not increased in couples with recurrent miscarriage. American Journal of Reproductive Immunology, 34(4), 209-212.

94 Meuleman, T., Lashley, L. E., Dekkers, O. M., van Lith, J. M., Claas, F. H., & Bloemenkamp, K. W. (2015). HLA associations and HLA sharing in recurrent miscarriage: a systematic review and meta-analysis. Human immunology, 76(5), 362-373.

95 Cavalcante, M. B., Sarno, M., Araujo Júnior, E., Da Silva Costa, F., & Barini, R. (2017). Lymphocyte immunotherapy in the treatment of recurrent miscarriage: systematic review and meta-analysis. Archives of gynecology and obstetrics, 295, 511-518.
Wong, L. F., Porter, T. F., & Scott, J. R. (2014). Immunotherapy for recurrent miscarriage. Cochrane Database of Systematic Reviews, (10).

Chapter 16. Troubleshooting Low Ovarian Reserve

1   Lliberos, C., Liew, S. H., Mansell, A., & Hutt, K. J. (2021). The inflammasome contributes to depletion of the ovarian reserve during aging in mice. Frontiers in Cell and Developmental Biology, 8, 628473.
Navarro-Pando, J. M., Alcocer-Gómez, E., Castejón-Vega, B., Navarro-Villarán, E., Condés-Hervás, M., Mundi-Roldan, M., ... & Cordero, M. D. (2021). Inhibition of the NLRP3 inflammasome prevents ovarian aging. Science advances, 7(1), eabc7409.

2   Favero, G., Franceschetti, L., Bonomini, F., Rodella, L. F., & Rezzani, R. (2017). Melatonin as an anti-inflammatory agent modulating inflammasome activation. International journal of endocrinology, 2017.

3   Li, G., Jiao, J., Xiang, S., Dong, S., Fu, L., Zuo, N., ... & Wang, X. (2022). Effect of various types of gut microbiota in patients on the diminished ovarian reserve.
Wu, J., Zhuo, Y., Liu, Y., Chen, Y., Ning, Y., & Yao, J. (2021). Association between premature ovarian insufficiency and gut microbiota. BMC Pregnancy and Childbirth, 21(1), 418.

4   O'Keefe, J. H., Gheewala, N. M., & O'Keefe, J. O. (2008). Dietary strategies for improving post-prandial glucose, lipids, inflammation, and cardiovascular health. Journal of the American College of Cardiology, 51(3), 249-255.

5   Kim, E. R., Kim, S. R., Cho, W., Lee, S. G., Kim, S. H., Kim, J. H., ... & Lee, Y. H. (2022). Short term isocaloric ketogenic diet modulates NLRP3 inflammasome via B-hydroxybutyrate and fibroblast growth factor 21. Frontiers in Immunology, 13, 843520.

6   Palafox-Gómez, C., Ortiz, G., Madrazo, I., & López-Bayghen, E. (2023). Adding a ketogenic dietary intervention to IVF treatment in patients with polycystic ovary syndrome improves implantation and pregnancy. Reproductive Toxicology, 108420.

7   Kiltz, R. (2020). The Fertile Feast, Waterside Productions.

8   Id.

9   Li, C., Zhang, H., Wu, H., Li, R., Wen, D., Tang, Y., ... & Ma, B. (2023). Intermittent fasting reverses the declining quality of aged oocytes. Free Radical Biology and Medicine, 195, 74-88.

10 Kalam, F., Akasheh, R. T., Cienfuegos, S., Ankireddy, A., Gabel, K., Ezpeleta, M., ... & Varady, K. A. (2023). Effect of time-restricted eating on sex hormone levels in premenopausal and postmenopausal females. Obesity, 31, 57-62.

11 Lie, M. R., van der Giessen, J., Fuhler, G. M., de Lima, A., Peppelenbosch, M. P., van der Ent, C., & van der Woude, C. J. (2018). Low dose Naltrexone for induction of remission in inflammatory bowel disease patients. Journal of Translational Medicine, 16, 1-11.

12 https://www.ldnscience.org/resources/interviews/interview-phil-boyle

13 Hsu CC, Hsu L, Hsu I, Chiu YJ, Dorjee S. Live birth in woman with premature ovarian insufficiency receiving ovarian administration of platelet-rich plasma (PRP) in combination with gonadotropin: a case report. Front Endocrinol (Lausanne). 2020;11:50

14 Pantos K, Simopoulou M, Pantou A, Rapani A, Tsioulou P, Nitsos N, Syrkos S, Pappas A, Koutsilieris M, Sfakianoudis K. A case series on natural conceptions resulting in ongoing pregnancies in menopausal and prematurely menopausal women following platelet-rich plasma treatment. Cell Transplant. 2019;28(9–10):1333–40.

15 Cakiroglu, Y., Saltik, A., Yuceturk, A., Karaosmanoglu, O., Tayyar, A. T., Scott, R. T., ... & Seli, E. (2019). Effects of intraovarian injection of autologous platelet rich plasma on ovarian reserve and IVF outcomes

in women with premature ovarian insufficiency. Fertility and Sterility, 112(3), e72.

Cakiroglu, Y., Saltik, A., Yuceturk, A., Karaosmanoglu, O., Kopuk, S. Y., Scott Jr, R. T., ... & Seli, E. (2020). Effects of intraovarian injection of autologous platelet rich plasma on ovarian reserve and IVF outcome parameters in women with primary ovarian insufficiency. Aging (Albany NY), 12(11), 10211.

16 Garavelas, A., Mallis, P., Michalopoulos, E., & Nikitos, E. (2023). Clinical benefit of autologous platelet-rich plasma infusion in ovarian function rejuvenation: evidence from a before-after prospective pilot study. Medicines, 10(3), 19.

Panda, S. R., Sachan, S., & Hota, S. (2020). A systematic review evaluating the efficacy of intra-ovarian infusion of autologous platelet-rich plasma in patients with poor ovarian reserve or ovarian insufficiency. Cureus, 12(12).

Tremellen, K., & Pacella-Ince, L. (2022). An audit of clinical outcomes following ovarian administration of platelet-rich plasma (PRP) in women with severe diminished ovarian reserve. Australian and New Zealand Journal of Obstetrics and Gynaecology, 62(5), 767-772.

17 Seckin, S., Ramadan, H., Mouanness, M., Kohansieh, M., & Merhi, Z. (2022). Ovarian response to intraovarian platelet-rich plasma (PRP) administration: hypotheses and potential mechanisms of action. Journal of Assisted Reproduction and Genetics, 39(1), 37-61.

Melo, P., Navarro, C., Jones, C., Coward, K., & Coleman, L. (2020). The use of autologous platelet-rich plasma (PRP) versus no intervention in women with low ovarian reserve undergoing fertility treatment: a non-randomized interventional study. Journal of assisted reproduction and genetics, 37, 855-863.

Cakiroglu, Y., Yuceturk, A., Karaosmanoglu, O., Kopuk, S. Y., Korun, Z. E. U., Herlihy, N., ... & Seli, E. (2022). Ovarian reserve parameters and IVF outcomes in 510 women with poor ovarian response (POR) treated with intraovarian injection of autologous platelet rich plasma (PRP). Aging (Albany NY), 14(6), 2513.

Stojkovska, S., Dimitrov, G., Stamenkovska, N., Hadzi-Lega, M., & Petanovski, Z. (2019). Live birth rates in poor responders' group after previous treatment with autologous platelet-rich plasma and low dose ovarian stimulation compared with poor responders used only low dose ovarian stimulation before in vitro fertilization. Open access Macedonian journal of medical sciences, 7(19), 3184.

Garavelas, A., Mallis, P., Michalopoulos, E., & Nikitos, E. (2023). Clinical benefit of autologous platelet-rich plasma infusion in ovarian function rejuvenation: evidence from a before-after prospective pilot study. Medicines, 10(3), 19.

Tremellen, K., & Pacella-Ince, L. (2022). An audit of clinical outcomes following ovarian administration of platelet-rich plasma (PRP) in women with severe diminished ovarian reserve. Australian and New Zealand Journal of Obstetrics and Gynaecology, 62(5), 767-772.

18 Sills ES, Rickers NS, Wood SH. Intraovarian insertion of autologous platelet growth factors as cell-free concentrate: fertility recovery and first unassisted conception with term delivery at age over 40. Int J Reprod Biomed. 2020;18(12):1081–6

19 Merhi, Z., Seckin, S., & Mouanness, M. (2022). Intraovarian platelet-rich plasma administration could improve blastocyst euploidy rates in women undergoing in vitro fertilization. Clinical and Experimental Reproductive Medicine, 49(3), 210-214.

20 Cakiroglu, Y., Saltik, A., Yuceturk, A., Karaosmanoglu, O., Kopuk, S. Y., Scott Jr, R. T., ... & Seli, E. (2020). Effects of intraovarian injection of autologous platelet rich plasma on ovarian reserve and IVF outcome parameters in women with primary ovarian insufficiency. Aging (Albany NY), 12(11), 10211.

21 Seckin, S., Ramadan, H., Mouanness, M., Kohansieh, M., & Merhi, Z. (2022). Ovarian response to intraovarian platelet-rich plasma (PRP) administration: hypotheses and potential mechanisms of action. Journal of Assisted Reproduction and Genetics, 39(1), 37-61.

22 Hamblin, M. R. (2017). Mechanisms and applications of the anti-inflammatory effects of photobiomodulation. AIMS biophysics, 4(3), 337.

23 Ash, C., Dubec, M., Donne, K., & Bashford, T. (2017). Effect of wavelength and beam width on penetration in light-tissue interaction using computational methods. Lasers in medical science, 32, 1909-1918.

24 Oubiña, G., Pascuali, N., Scotti, L., Di Pietro, M., La Spina, F. A., Buffone, M. G., ... & Parborell, F. (2019). Low level laser therapy (LLLT) modulates ovarian function in mature female mice. Progress in biophysics and molecular biology, 145, 10-18.

25 Ohshiro, T. (2012). Personal overview of the application of LLLT in severely infertile Japanese females. Laser Therapy, 21(2), 97-103.
Ohshiro, T. (2012). The proximal priority theory: an updated technique in low level laser therapy with an 830 nm GaAlAs laser. Laser Therapy, 21(4), 275-285.
Iwahata, H., Endoh, S., & Hirai, Y. (2006). Treatment of female infertility incorporating low-reactive laser therapy (LLLT): An initial report. Laser Therapy, 15(1), 37-41.

26 Grinsted (2019), PhotoBioModulation (Low Level Laser) for Infertility, EC GYNAECOLOGY. 8.9: 875-879.

27 Mourad, A., Jamal, W., Hemmings, R., Tadevosyan, A., Phillips, S., & Kadoch, I. J. (2022). GROWTH HORMONE IS USELESS IN IVF: THE LARGEST RANDOMIZED CONTROLLED TRIAL. Fertility and Sterility, 118(4), e3.

28   He, F., Wang, F., Yang, Y., Yuan, Z., Sun, C., Zou, H., ... & Han, T. L. (2023). The effect of growth hormone on the metabolome of follicular fluid in patients with diminished ovarian reserve. Reproductive Biology and Endocrinology, 21(1), 1-11.
Cai, M. H., Gao, L. Z., Liang, X. Y., Fang, C., Wu, Y. Q., & Yang, X. (2019). The effect of growth hormone on the clinical outcomes of poor ovarian reserve patients undergoing in vitro fertilization/ intracytoplasmic sperm injection treatment: A retrospective study based on POSEIDON criteria. Frontiers in Endocrinology, 10, 775.
Yang, X., & Cai, M. H. (2020). THE EFFECT OF GROWTH HORMONE ON CLINICAL OUTCOMES OF POOR OVARIAN RESPONDER UNDERGOING IN VITRO FERTILIZATION/INTRACYTOPLASMIC SPERM INJECTION TREATMENT: A RETROSPECTIVE STUDY BASED ON POSEIDON CRITERIA. Fertility and Sterility, 114(3), e335.
Cozzolino, M., Cecchino, G. N., Troiano, G., & Romanelli, C. (2020). Growth hormone cotreatment for poor responders undergoing in vitro fertilization cycles: a systematic review and meta-analysis. Fertility and sterility, 114(1), 97-109.

29   Yovich, J. L., Regan, S. L., Zaidi, S., & Keane, K. N. (2019). The concept of growth hormone deficiency affecting clinical prognosis in IVF. Frontiers in Endocrinology, 10, 650.

30   Id.

31   Regan, S. L., Knight, P. G., Yovich, J. L., Arfuso, F., & Dharmarajan, A. (2018). Growth hormone during in vitro fertilization in older women modulates the density of receptors in granulosa cells, with improved pregnancy outcomes. Fertility and Sterility, 110(7), 1298-1310.

32   Silva, J. R. V., Figueiredo, J. R., & Van den Hurk, R. (2009). Involvement of growth hormone (GH) and insulin-like growth factor (IGF) system in ovarian folliculogenesis. Theriogenology, 71(8), 1193-1208.

33   Pekarovics, S., Romans, J., Beres, A., Kelly, C., Heaton, A., & Greenway, F. (2019). SUN-439 improvement in insulin-like growth factor-1 and clinical symptoms: Results of an open-label, single-arm study of a human growth hormone-enhancing amino acid supplement. Journal of the Endocrine Society, 3(Supplement_1), SUN-439.

34   Pekarovics, S., Romans, J., Beres, A., Kelly, C., Heaton, A., & Greenway, F. (2019). SUN-439 improvement in insulin-like growth factor-1 and clinical symptoms: Results of an open-label, single-arm study of a human growth hormone-enhancing amino acid supplement. Journal of the Endocrine Society, 3(Supplement_1), SUN-439.
Tam, C. S., Johnson, W. D., Rood, J., Heaton, A. L., & Greenway, F. L. (2020). Increased human growth hormone following oral consumption of an amino acid supplement: results of a randomized, placebo-controlled, double-blind, crossover study in healthy subjects. American journal of therapeutics, 27(4), e333.

35 So, S., Yamaguchi, W., Murabayashi, N., Miyano, N., Tawara, F., & Kanayama, N. (2020). Beneficial effect of l-arginine in women using assisted reproductive technologies: a small-scale randomized controlled trial. Nutrition Research, 82, 67-73.

36 Hwang, P. S., Machek, S. B., Cardaci, T. D., Wilburn, D. T., Kim, C. S., Suezaki, E. S., & Willoughby, D. S. (2020). Effects of pyrroloquinoline quinone (PQQ) supplementation on aerobic exercise performance and indices of mitochondrial biogenesis in untrained men. Journal of the American College of Nutrition, 39(6), 547-556.

37 Nakano, M., Murayama, Y., Hu, L., Ikemoto, K., Uetake, T., & Sakatani, K. (2016). Effects of antioxidant supplements (BioPQQ™) on cerebral blood flow and oxygen metabolism in the prefrontal cortex. In Oxygen Transport to Tissue XXXVIII (pp. 215-222). Springer International Publishing.
Harris, C. B., Chowanadisai, W., Mishchuk, D. O., Satre, M. A., Slupsky, C. M., & Rucker, R. B. (2013). Dietary pyrroloquinoline quinone (PQQ) alters indicators of inflammation and mitochondrial-related metabolism in human subjects. The Journal of nutritional biochemistry, 24(12), 2076-2084.

38 Dai, X., Yi, X., Wang, Y., Xia, W., Tao, J., Wu, J., ... & Chen, L. (2022). PQQ dietary supplementation prevents alkylating agent-induced ovarian dysfunction in mice. Frontiers in Endocrinology, 13, 781404.

39 Lane, S. L., Parks, J. C., Khan, S. A., Yuan, Y., Schoolcraft, W. B., & Katz-Jaffe, M. G. (2021). Restoring ovarian antioxidant balance to combat female reproductive aging. Fertility and Sterility, 116(3), e40.

40 Katz-Jaffe, M. G., Parks, J. C., McCallie, B. R., Lane, S. L., Makloski, R., & Schoolcraft, W. B. (2020). THERAPEUTIC STRATEGY TO IMPROVE THE QUALITY OF AGED OOCYTES. Fertility and Sterility, 114(3), e218-e219.

41 Katz-Jaffe, M. G., Lane, S. L., Parks, J. C., McCallie, B. R., Makloski, R., & Schoolcraft, W. B. (2020). Antioxidant intervention attenuates aging-related changes in the murine ovary and oocyte. Life, 10(11), 250.

42 Ochiai, A., Kuroda, K., Ikemoto, Y., Ozaki, R., Nakagawa, K., Nojiri, S., ... & Sugiyama, R. (2019). Influence of resveratrol supplementation on IVF–embryo transfer cycle outcomes. Reproductive BioMedicine Online, 39(2), 205-210.

43 Ochiai, A., Kuroda, K., Ikemoto, Y., Ozaki, R., Nakagawa, K., Nojiri, S., ... & Sugiyama, R. (2019). Influence of resveratrol supplementation on IVF–embryo transfer cycle outcomes. Reproductive BioMedicine Online, 39(2), 205-210.

44 Yang, Q., Cong, L., Wang, Y., Luo, X., Li, H., Wang, H., ... & Sun, Y. (2020). Increasing ovarian NAD+ levels improve mitochondrial functions and reverse ovarian aging. Free Radical Biology and Medicine, 156, 1-10.

45 Miao, Y., Cui, Z., Gao, Q., Rui, R., & Xiong, B. (2020). Nicotinamide mononucleotide supplementation reverses the declining quality of maternally aged oocytes. Cell reports, 32(5), 107987.
    Bertoldo, M. J., Listijono, D. R., Ho, W. H. J., Riepsamen, A. H., Goss, D. M., Richani, D., ... & Wu, L. E. (2020). NAD+ repletion rescues female fertility during reproductive aging. Cell reports, 30(6), 1670-1681.
46 Bertoldo, M. J., Listijono, D. R., Ho, W. H. J., Riepsamen, A. H., Goss, D. M., Richani, D., ... & Wu, L. E. (2020). NAD+ repletion rescues female fertility during reproductive aging. Cell reports, 30(6), 1670-1681.
47 Shen, H. (2019). Cancer Research Points to Key Unknowns about Popular 'Antiaging' Supplements. Scientific American. Scientific American, May, 30.
48 Maric, T., Bazhin, A., Khodakivskyi, P., Mikhaylov, G., Solodnikova, E., Yevtodiyenko, A., ... & Goun, E. (2023). A bioluminescent-based probe for in vivo non-invasive monitoring of nicotinamide riboside uptake reveals a link between metastasis and NAD+ metabolism. Biosensors and Bioelectronics, 220, 114826.
49 Ratajczak, J., Joffraud, M., Trammell, S. A., Ras, R., Canela, N., Boutant, M., ... & Cantó, C. (2016). NRK1 controls nicotinamide mononucleotide and nicotinamide riboside metabolism in mammalian cells. Nature communications, 7(1), 13103.
50 Liu, L., Su, X., Quinn, W. J., Hui, S., Krukenberg, K., Frederick, D. W., ... & Rabinowitz, J. D. (2018). Quantitative analysis of NAD synthesis-breakdown fluxes. Cell metabolism, 27(5), 1067-1080.
    Chellappa, K., McReynolds, M. R., Lu, W., Zeng, X., Makarov, M., Hayat, F., ... & Baur, J. A. (2022). NAD precursors cycle between host tissues and the gut microbiome. Cell Metabolism, 34(12), 1947-1959.
    Sauve, A. A. (2022). Metabolic Disease, NAD Metabolism, Nicotinamide Riboside, and the Gut Microbiome: Connecting the Dots from the Gut to Physiology. Msystems, 7(1), e01223-21.
51 Petrack, B., Greengard, P., & Kalinsky, H. (1966). On the relative efficacy of nicotinamide and nicotinic acid as precursors of nicotinamide adenine dinucleotide. Journal of Biological Chemistry, 241(10), 2367-2372.
    Micheli V, Simmonds HA, Sestini S, Ricci C. Importance of nicotinamide as an NAD precursor in the human erythrocyte. Arch Biochem Biophys. 1990; 283(1): 40- 45.
52 Min, H., Lee, M., Cho, K. S., Lim, H. J., & Shim, Y. H. (2021). Nicotinamide supplementation improves oocyte quality and offspring development by modulating mitochondrial function in an aged Caenorhabditis elegans model. Antioxidants, 10(4), 519.
    Lee AR, Kishigami S, Amano T, Matsumoto K, Wakayama T, Hosoi Y. Nicotinamide: a class III HDACi delays in vitro aging of mouse oocytes. J Reprod Dev 2013; 59: 238–244.
53 Nikas, I. P., Paschou, S. A., & Ryu, H. S. (2020). The role of nicotinamide in cancer chemoprevention and therapy. Biomolecules, 10(3), 477.

Damian, D. L. (2017). Nicotinamide for skin cancer chemoprevention. Australasian journal of dermatology, 58(3), 174-180.

Galbraith, A. R., Seabloom, D. E., Wuertz, B. R., Antonides, J. D., Steele, V. E., Wattenberg, L. W., & Ondrey, F. G. (2019). Chemoprevention of Lung Carcinogenesis by Dietary Nicotinamide and Inhaled BudesonideNicotinamide and Budesonide for Lung Cancer Prevention. Cancer Prevention Research, 12(2), 69-78.

54 Allen, N. C., Martin, A. J., Snaidr, V. A., Eggins, R., Chong, A. H., Fernandéz-Peñas, P., ... & Damian, D. L. (2023). Nicotinamide for Skin-Cancer Chemoprevention in Transplant Recipients. New England Journal of Medicine, 388(9), 804-812.

55 Pollard, C. L., Gibb, Z., Swegen, A., & Grupen, C. G. (2022). NAD+, Sirtuins and PARPs: enhancing oocyte developmental competence. Journal of Reproduction and Development, 68(6), 345-354.

56 El Sheikh M, Mesalam AA, Idrees M, Sidrat T, Mesalam A, Lee KL, Kong IK. Nicotinamide supplementation during the in vitro maturation of oocytes improves the developmental competence of preimplantation embryos: potential link to SIRT1/AKT signaling. Cells 2020; 9: E1550.

Index

I

ICSI (intracytoplasmic sperm injection), and sperm quality, 208

IGF-1 (insulin-like growth factor 1), growth hormone and, 301

IL(s) (interleukins), 268–269

Immature eggs, myo-inositol for, 18, 19, 129–132

Immature follicles, AMH and, 72

Immune activity, vitamin D and, 63

Immune issues, 20–21
  gluten and, 185, 191–192
  implantation dysfunction due to, 258–269

Immune-mediated miscarriage, diet for, 192

Immune-signaling molecules, 268–269

Immune system, and placental development, 248

Immunology, vitamin D and, 271

Immunology testing, 258–269
  for autoimmune antibodies, 259–266
  cellular immune testing in, 266–269

Immunology treatments, 269–271

Immunotherapy, lymphocyte, 282

Implantation, 12, 26
  late, 242–243
  progesterone and, 78
  resveratrol and, 154–155

Implantation dysfunction, 226, 247–284
  action plan for, 283–284
  defined, 248–249
  due to endometriosis, 254–258
  due to hidden infections and chronic endometritis, 250–253
  due to hormone and clotting issues, 272–275
  due to immune factors, 258–271

due to parental genetic issues, 278–282

testing for, 249–269

due to uterine issues and Asherman's syndrome, 276–278

Implantation factors, 20–21

Inchauspé, Jessie, 184

Infections
  hidden, 250–253
  and implantation dysfunction, 250–253
  silent, 21
  and sperm quality, 203–204, 206
  uterine lining and, 226, 238
  vitamin D and, 62, 63, 213

Infertility
  age-related. See Age-related infertility
  male, 199–224
  secondary, 204
  unexplained. See Unexplained infertility

Inflammasome, 288

Inflammation, 20
  alpha-lipoic acid and, 121
  due to antiphospholipid antibodies, 261
  diet and, 191
  and diminished ovarian reserve, 288–295
  due to endometriosis, 255
  gluten and dairy and, 185
  gut microbiome and, 290
  ketogenic diet for, 292
  low-dose naltrexone for, 294–295
  Mediterranean diet and, 186
  and miscarriage, 189–190
  omega-3 fats and, 188
  red light therapy for, 299
  systemic, 290

Inflammatory bacteria, and sperm quality, 203–204, 206

Inhibin B, 74